Selenium in Food and Health

Selenium in Food and Health

Second Edition

Conor Reilly
B.Sc., Lic. Phil., H.Dip.Ed., PhD, FAIFST
Emeritus Professor of Public Health
Queensland University of Technology, Brisbane, Australia

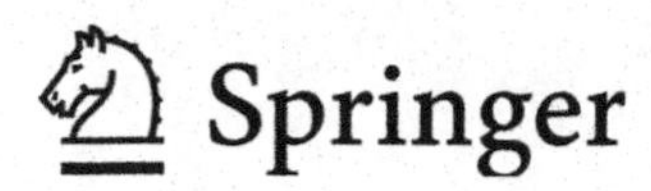

ISBN 978-1-4419-4117-6 e-ISBN 0-387-33244-8
e-ISBN 978-0-387-33244-4

Printed in the United States of America. (SPI/MVY)

9 8 7 6 5 4 3 2 1

springer.com

To the memory of Ann Reilly (1933–2005)

Preface

Selenium is a contradictory nutrient. It has been called *the essential poison*—too much of it in the diet can be toxic; too little can result in chronic, and sometimes fatal, deficiency. Even health authorities have at times been confused. Although today in the USA, as in most other countries, selenium appears among the trace elements for which recommended dietary allowances (RDAs) have been established, it was at one time declared by the Food and Drug Administration (FDA) to be a carcinogen and banned as an additive in food.

Selenium is considered by some to be a serious hazard to the environment and to animal health. Selenium-contaminated water has brought deformity and death to wildlife in nature reserves in western USA. There is even concern that because of selenium contamination of soil, crops supplied to the great cities of California could become unfit for human consumption. In large areas of China, endemic selenium toxicity is a hazard for locals who depend on crops grown on selenium-rich soil. Yet, in the UK, and in other parts of Europe, fears are expressed that soil selenium levels are inadequate. There are demands that the example of Finland should be followed and soil selenium levels increased by the addition of selenium to fertilizers.

There may be controversy among the experts and health authorities about selenium, but this has not deterred the general public from deciding that the element has an important role to play in health. In New Zealand, when the use of selenium was first permitted to prevent deficiency in farm animals, but was still not approved as a supplement for humans, people took the matter into their own hands. Veterinary preparations containing selenium were used by those who believed that what was good for animals must also be good for humans.

Undeterred by reports of their possible toxic effects, today millions of people worldwide consume selenium supplements. They are encouraged to do so, not only by articles in the popular media but also by the results of investigations by reputable scientists which indicate that selenium has a vital role to play in human health, not least in the prevention of cancer. Their findings indicate that selenium is a key player in cellular metabolism, is an essential component of enzymes that protect the body against oxidative damage, and has important roles in thyroid metabolism, human fertility, and many other vital functions.

But not all the experts are convinced by such findings. They point out that there is still a great deal we do not know about selenium and its relation to body function and human health. They argue that not all the evidence supports the claims, for instance, of selenium's anticancer role. It must not be forgotten, they point out, that selenium is both a toxic and an essential element and that the difference between the two is measured in minute amounts.

Thus, though selenium is probably the most widely investigated of all the trace element nutrients, it continues to be highly controversial. Indeed, it has been so all through the nearly 200 years since it was first identified by the Swedish scientist, Jöns Jakob Berzelius. He named his new discovery selenium after the moon goddess, Selēnē—an appropriate name, since, like the moon, the element has two faces—dark and light, good and bad. It is because of the interactions of those opposing faces that selenium remains a controversial topic to the present day.

It has been estimated that more than 100,000 scientific papers, not to mention popular articles and books, about selenium have been published over the past 50 years. These publications continue to appear without showing any sign of diminution today. This mass of writing makes it very difficult for anyone who is not a dedicated and specialized scientist to get a clear picture of what is now known about the element and its role in human health. Not only for the general reader who wants to make an informed judgment about the competing claims for and against its value as a nutritional supplement, but even for some professionals who want to keep abreast of the latest findings about its potential role in the management of human health, this is a serious deterrent to their quest for knowledge.

The first edition of this book was written with the intention of providing reliable and up-to-date information to readers who wanted to learn more about selenium, but who were deterred by either a lack of time or, they believed, by their inadequate scientific background, from wading through the extensive literature then available. Its aim was to present, in a readable and user-friendly manner, a review, based on a wide range of scientific and other literature. It would, it was hoped, provide all that was essential for readers who wanted to know more about selenium, as a component of food and diet, its biological significance, and its role in health and disease.

Ten years later, this new edition of *Selenium in Food and Health* is written with the same aim, to provide readers with a clear and reliable account of the extraordinary story of selenium and its role in human health. It is based on the author's more than 3 decades of teaching undergraduate and graduate students about trace elements and his active participation in selenium research, as well as on extensive reading of the pertinent literature and information gathering at workshops and conferences in many different countries.

This new edition takes into account the considerable amount of fresh information that has been published over the past decade, by investigators from a wide range of specialisms, not all of which might at first glance appear to have much to do with human health. For readers who have the background to do so, and are willing to search further, many references to original and up-to-date reports and reviews in the scientific literature are provided. The book will not tell the final story—much is still to be discovered. Even as I write, new findings are being reported and new discoveries about selenium are being made, especially as modern bioinformatics and genetic techniques are brought to bear. It is hoped that what has been produced will help to make the picture clear and help readers to form their own, informed, opinion about the importance of selenium in human food and health, and that the text is readable and comprehensible, bringing clarity without distortion or oversimplification. It is intended for a wide audience, including dietitians, nutritionists, and other health professionals, food scientists, medical practitioners, and, not least, general readers who want to learn about the element that is so often in the news.

This book is dedicated to the memory of my late wife, Ann, who not only encouraged me to write but also took part in some of the research on which it is based, and also in the days when literature searches required more than sitting at a computer keyboard, spent long hours reference checking in the library stacks. The book owes much to the generous help of the library staff of the Queensland University of Technology, especially to the wonders of the Internet that allowed me to access journals and other publications in the library's databases, even when I was more than 12,000 miles away from the antipodes. I also thank the staff of the Bodleian Library of Oxford University, where I had the special pleasure of being able to read, in the original, the earliest of the publications on selenium, including the key paper in which Berzelius announced, in 1818, his discovery of the element.

Gratitude is due also to others who contributed to the writing of the book. I thank several of my academic colleagues and friends in many countries, in particular Dr. Fiona Cumming and Dr. Ujang Tinggi, Professor John Arthur, Professor Jim Oldfield, Dr. Margaret Rayman, and several others who prefer to be nameless. They helped in different ways, by taking part in my research activities, supplying copies of their publications, discussing my ideas, and in some cases reading and commenting on sections of the text. The views expressed in this book, however, are solely mine and do not necessarily reflect their opinions.

Conor Reilly
Enstone, Oxfordshire, UK
January 31, 2006

Contents

Preface vii

1. Introduction **1**
1.1 The element selenium 1
1.2 The discovery of selenium: the Swedish connection 1
1.2.1 Predecessors of Berzelius 2
1.3 Selenium chemistry 3
1.3.1 Allotropic forms of selenium 3
1.3.2 Physical properties of selenium 4
1.3.3 Inorganic compounds of selenium 4
1.3.4 Organo-selenium compounds 5
1.3.5 Isotopes of selenium 6
1.4 Distribution of selenium in the lithosphere 7
1.4.1 Selenium in soil 7
1.4.2 Selenium in water 7
1.5 Sources and production of selenium 8
1.6 Industrial and other applications of selenium 8
1.7 Selenium analysis 10
1.7.1 Sample preparation 10
1.7.1.1 Dry ashing 10
1.7.1.2 Wet ashing 11
1.7.2 End-determination methods for selenium analysis 12
1.7.2.1 Spectrofluorimetry 12
1.7.2.2 Atomic absorption spectrophotometry 12
1.7.2.3 Inductively coupled plasma atomic emission spectrophotometry 13
1.7.2.4 Inductively coupled plasma mass spectrometry 13
1.7.3 Speciation analysis 14
1.7.4 Analytical quality control 15

2. The biology of selenium **20**
2.1 A belated recognition 20
2.2 The biological role of selenium in prokaryotes 20
2.3 Selenium in plants 21
2.3.1 Selenium in higher plants 21
2.3.1.1 Selenium accumulators and nonaccumulators 22
2.3.2 Selenium metabolism in plants 22
2.3.2.1 Selenium uptake and transport in plants 23
2.3.2.2 Selenium assimilation and modification within plant tissues 23
2.3.2.3 Selenium toxicity and tolerance in plants 24
2.3.2.4 Volatilization of selenium by plants 25
2.3.3 Selenium in food plants 25
2.3.3.1 Crops grown on low-selenium soils 25
2.3.3.2 Crops grown on adequate-selenium soils 26
2.3.3.3 Crops grown on high-selenium soils 26
2.3.3.4 The risk of selenosis in humans from eating selenium-rich crops 27
2.4 Selenium in animal tissues 28
2.4.1 Absorption, transport, and excretion of selenium 28
2.4.2 Enteric absorption of selenium 29
2.4.3 Transport of selenium in the body 29
2.4.4 Selenium distribution and retention in the human body 30
2.4.5 Selenium levels in blood 31
2.4.5.1 Selenium in whole blood 31
2.4.5.2 Selenium in serum and plasma 31
2.4.5.3 Selenium levels in other blood fractions 33
2.4.6 Selenium retention and excretion from the body 34
2.4.6.1 Urinary excretion of selenium 34
2.4.6.2 Fecal excretion of selenium 35
2.4.6.3 Pulmonary excretion of selenium 36
2.4.6.4 Losses of selenium in hair and nails 36
2.4.7 Selenium pools and stores in the body 36

3. Selenium metabolism **43**
3.1 The metabolic roles of selenium 43
3.1.1 Selenoproteins 43
3.1.1.1 The glutathione peroxidases 44
3.1.1.2 The iodothyronine deiodinases 46
3.1.1.3 Thioredoxin reductases 47
3.1.1.4 Selenophosphate synthetase 48
3.1.1.5 Selenoprotein P 48
3.1.1.6 Other selenoproteins 49
3.2 Selenoprotein synthesis 50
3.2.1 Selenocysteine: the 21st amino acid 50

3.2.1.1 Dual functions of the UGA codon 51
3.2.2 Selenoprotein synthesis in prokaryotes 51
3.2.3 Selenoprotein synthesis in eukaryotes 53
3.3 Regulation of selenoprotein expression 53
3.3.1 Complexities of regulation of selenoprotein synthesis 55
3.3.1.1 A regulatory role for $tRNA^{[Ser]Sec}$ in selenoprotein synthesis 56
3.3.1.2 Single nucleotide polymorphisms and regulation of selenoprotein synthesis 56
3.4 Selenium status 57
3.4.1 Assessment of selenium status 57
3.4.1.1 Use of blood selenium levels to assess selenium status 58
3.4.1.2 Hair, nail, and urinary selenium 58
3.4.1.3 Use of functional indicators of selenium status 59
3.4.1.4 Other potential markers of selenium functional status 60

4. Selenium in health and disease I: The agricultural connection 67
4.1 Selenium and agriculture 67
4.2 Selenium toxicity in farm animals 67
4.2.1 Alkali disease and blind staggers 68
4.2.2 Selenosis in farm animals outside the USA 70
4.2.2.1 Selenosis in Irish farms 70
4.3 The other face of selenium—an essential nutrient 72
4.3.1 Selenium as an essential nutritional factor 72
4.4 Selenium-responsive conditions in farm animals 74
4.4.1 White muscle disease 74
4.4.2 Exudative diathesis 75
4.4.3 Hepatosis dietetica 76
4.4.4 Pancreatic degeneration 76
4.4.5 Ill thrift 76
4.4.6 Impaired reproduction 77
4.4.7 Impaired immune response 77
4.5 Subclinical selenium deficiencies 79
4.6 Selenium supplementation of livestock 79

5. Selenium in health and disease II: Endemic selenium-related conditions in humans 85
5.1 Selenium toxicity 85
5.1.1 Selenium toxicity in humans in seleniferous regions of North America 85
5.1.2 Human selenosis in Latin America 86
5.1.3 Endemic selenosis in China 87
5.1.4 Other consequences of large-scale selenium intake 88

5.1.4.1 Dental caries 89
5.1.4.2 Amyotrophic lateral sclerosis (motor neuron disease) 89
5.1.4.3 Defective reproduction 90
5.2 Endemic diseases related to selenium deficiency in humans 90
5.2.1 Keshan disease 91
5.2.1.1 Regional studies of Keshan disease in China 92
5.2.1.2 Features of Keshan disease 93
5.2.1.3 Etiology of Keshan disease 93
5.2.2 Selenium status of residents of Keshan disease areas 95
5.2.3 Interventions in the management of Keshan disease 96
5.2.4 Keshan disease in Russia 98
5.3 Kashin–Beck disease 98
5.3.1 The etiology of Kashin–Beck disease 99
5.4 Combined endemic selenium and iodine deficiencies 100
5.4.1 Selenium, Kashin–Beck disease, and goiter 100
5.4.2 The role of selenium deficiency in endemic goiter 101
5.4.3 Thyroid biochemistry and selenium 104
5.4.3.1 Selenium supplementation and iodine deficiency: a caution 104

6. Selenium in health and disease III: Nonendemic selenium-responsive conditions, cancer, and coronary vascular disease 111
6.1 Nonendemic selenium deficiency 111
6.1.1 TPN-induced selenium deficiency 111
6.1.1.1 TPN-related KD-like cardiomyopathies 112
6.1.1.2 Other causes of selenium deficiency-associated cardiomyopathies 112
6.1.1.3 Low selenium intake and muscular problems in New Zealand 113
6.2 Other iatrogenic selenium deficiencies 113
6.3 Selenium and cancer 114
6.3.1 Epidemiological studies of the relation between selenium and cancer 115
6.3.2 Case-control studies of selenium and cancer associations 115
6.3.3 "Nested" case-control studies 116
6.3.4 Intervention trials 117
6.3.4.1 The Linxian intervention trials 117
6.3.4.2 Qidong intervention trial 118
6.3.4.3 The nutritional prevention of cancer with selenium trial 118
6.3.4.4 The PRECISE intervention trial 120
6.3.4.5 The SELECT intervention trial 120

6.3.4.6 The SU.VI.MAX trial 121
6.3.5 Evidence for an association between cancer-prevention and selenium 121
6.3.5.1 Baseline selenium levels and dose size in cancer prevention Trials 122
6.4 The carcinostatic properties of selenium compounds 122
6.4.1 How selenium compounds may prevent cancer 123
6.4.1.1 Hypotheses of cancer prevention by dietary selenium 123
6.5 Selenium and cardiovascular disease 125
6.5.1 Epidemiological studies of CVD incidence 126
6.5.2 Prospective epidemiological studies of selenium and CVD associations 126

7. Selenium in health and disease IV: The immune response and other selenium-related conditions 134
7.1 The immune system 134
7.1.1 Components of the immune system 134
7.1.2 The role of selenium in the immune response 137
7.1.2.1 Selenium and the immune response to infection 139
7.1.2.2 Selenium and inflammatory diseases in humans 140
7.2 Selenium and viral infections 141
7.2.1 Selenium, human immunodeficiency virus, and acquired immunodeficiency syndrome 142
7.3 Selenium and human fertility 143
7.4 Selenium and preeclampsia 144

8. Selenium in health and disease V: Selenium deficiency in search of a disease? 149
8.1 Selenium and other health conditions 149
8.2 Selenium and ageing 149
8.3 Selenium and age-related degenerative disorders of the eye 150
8.3.1 Age-related macular degeneration 150
8.3.2 Cataract 151
8.4 Sudden infant death syndrome 151
8.5 Selenium and brain function 152
8.6 Other possible selenium-related conditions 153
8.7 Other health conditions and selenium 155

9. Selenium in foods 158
9.1 Selenium in food 158
9.1.1 Selenium in foods: national and international databases 158
9.1.2 Selenium in food composition databases 159
9.1.2.1 Selenium in total diet studies 160
9.1.3 Variations in levels of selenium in foods 160

9.1.4 Selenium levels in individual foodstuffs 161
9.1.4.1 Selenium levels in cow's milk 161
9.1.4.2 Selenium levels in human milk 161
9.1.4.3 Selenium in infant formula 162
9.1.4.4 Selenium in bread and flour 163
9.1.4.5 Selenium levels in other cereals 164
9.1.4.6 Selenium in meat and meat products 165
9.1.4.7 Selenium in fish and other seafoods 165
9.1.4.8 The relation between selenium and mercury in seafoods 166
9.1.4.9 Selenium in vegetables and fruits 167
9.1.4.10 Selenium in Brazil and other nuts 168
9.2 Selenium in drinking water 168

10. Selenium in diets 173
10.1 Selenium status and dietary intakes 173
10.2 Dietary intakes of selenium in different countries 174
10.3 Variations in dietary intakes between countries and population groups 175
10.3.1 Selenium intake by vegans and other vegetarians 176
10.3.2 Selenium intake by young Swedish vegans 176
10.3.3 Selenium intake by Sikh vegetarians 177
10.3.4 Selenium intake in fish-eating populations 177
10.4 Changes in dietary intakes of selenium 178
10.4.1 Changes in selenium intake in Finland 178
10.4.2 The changing selenium status of the UK population 180
10.4.3 Effect of changes in wheat imports on selenium intakes 181
10.4.4 Changing selenium status in New Zealand 181
10.5 Use of dietary supplements to change selenium intake 182
10.5.1 Selenium-enriched yeast 183
10.5.2 Selenomethionine in selenium yeast 184
10.5.3 Variations in levels of selenium in supplements 185
10.6 Enhancing selenium content of foods 185
10.6.1 Selenium in functional foods 187
10.6.2 Chemical forms of selenium used to fortify foods 187
10.6.2.1 Use of selenomethione as a food fortificant 187
10.7 Dietary reference values for selenium 188
10.8 The future—is supplementation the way forward? 190

Index 199

1
Introduction

1.1 The Element Selenium

Selenium is one of the rarest elements. It is about 70th in abundance among the 88 elements that naturally occur in the earth's crust (Shriver and Atkins, 1999). Yet, in spite of its scarcity, selenium plays a key role in all animal life. It is an essential component of the human diet, though only in minute amounts. If this intake is exceeded by relatively little, disastrous consequences can follow. Selenium is a two-faced element. Like the moon, after which it is named, it has both a dark and a bright side. This duality has, right from the time the element was first isolated, presented science with a dilemma: how to reconcile its apparently contradictory properties and roles? Now, nearly 200 years later, in spite of thousands of hours of research and the publication of great numbers of scientific studies, the dilemma has not yet been fully resolved. Nevertheless, the gaps in our understanding of selenium are rapidly being filled by the efforts of an extraordinary array of investigators, working in a range of disciplines, aided by powerful new research tools and techniques. The purpose of this book is to look at the findings of those investigators and to show how selenium, once known only for its toxicity, has come to be recognized as one of the important key players in human health.

1.2 The Discovery of Selenium: The Swedish Connection

Selenium began its formal scientific life in controversy, in a laboratory in Uppsala, during an era when Swedish scientists were world leaders in the rapidly developing field of chemistry. Preeminent among them was Jöns Jakob Berzelius, an outstanding theorist and skilled experimenter. The electrochemical theory and the use of chemical symbols to represent the elements are among the valuable contributions he made to science. His laboratory skills, under conditions that may be hard for modern researchers to visualize, enabled him to determine atomic and molecular weights with such accuracy that many of his calculations are very close to those in use today. He also discovered, or isolated for the first time, several new elements, including silicon, cerium, thorium, vanadium, zirconium, and, in 1817, selenium (Hurd and Kipling, 1964).

A few years earlier, a German chemist, M.H. Klaproth, who had come to work in Sweden with Berzelius had examined a reddish material found in the residue after copper pyrites had been roasted in a lead chamber during the manufacture of sulfuric acid. The residue had an unpleasant smell, described as rotten radishes, and blistered the skin of those who handled it. Klaproth, who had already made a name for himself as the discoverer of several new elements, including titanium, uranium, and zirconium, concluded that the deposit contained tellurium, another of his discoveries. This had also been found as a residue of copper ore roasting and, like the new material, had an unpleasant smell. But his friend Berzelius disagreed. In collaboration with another Swedish chemist, J.G. Gahn, who had discovered manganese, Berzelius reexamined the residue. As he explained in a letter to the French chemist Claude-Louis Berthollet, he found no evidence of the presence of tellurium, but rather of "an unknown substance with properties very like those of tellurium. For this reason I gave it the name *selenium* from the Greek word Σεληνη (Selēnē), which signifies the moon, while *tellus* is the name of our own planet" (Berzelius, 1818). The letter, which was published in the French scientific journal, *Annales de Chimie et de Physique* in 1818, was the first of more than 100,000 papers on selenium to appear in the scientific press over the following 2 centuries.

1.2.1 Predecessors of Berzelius

While Berzelius was the first to isolate and chemically characterize selenium, he was probably not its original discoverer. That achievement should, perhaps, be attributed to the 13th-century Italian scholar, Arnold of Villanova, who, in his book *Rosarium Philosophorum,* described a "red sulfur" sometimes found on the walls of chambers in which native yellow sulfur was heated to make "flowers of sulfur." This "red sulfur," it has been argued by Hoefer (1842), could have been the same type of deposit investigated by Berzelius 500 years later. However, even of it were, Villanova was in no position to isolate and study the element (Crombie, 1959).

Another 13th-century Italian, the Venetian traveler Marco Polo, may also have stumbled across selenium, or at least evidence of its less desirable qualities, at about the same time as Villanova. On one of his journeys through Cathay, as China was then known to Europeans, Polo came, according to the journal he produced after his return home, to "Succuir in the province of Tanguth. . . . a country where there are few inhabitants, and little of any kind worthy of remark" (Polo, 1967). Added to the problems of travel in such a wild area was another hazard, well known to merchants who had to pass through the district: "when they take the road they cannot venture among the mountains with any beasts of burden, on account of a poisonous plant growing there, which, if eaten by them, has the effect of causing hoofs of the animals to drop off."

The plant mentioned by Polo was probably what is known today as a *selenium accumulator*, able to take up the element from soil and concentrate it to toxic levels in its leaves (Trelase, 1942). Lameness and sloughing of hooves are typical symptoms of selenium poisoning in animals. In parts of the Midwest, and in a few other parts of the world where the soil contains high levels of available selenium, certain plants such as the vetch *Astragalus* have been shown to be selenium accumulators. Farm animals that graze on them suffer from selenium poisoning, a condition known to US farmers as *blind staggers* and to Australians as *change hoof disease* (Knott and McCray, 1959).

We cannot know for certain which particular plant Polo was referring to, or where exactly was "Succuir in the province of Tanguth." The place may have been what is known today as So-cheu, in the province of Shaanxi or possibly Gansu (Mizutani et al., 1992). Whatever be the correct interpretation of the location, or of the plant species, what is certain is that in the 20th century areas of endemic selenium intoxication of both animals and humans, where some crops and other plants accumulate high levels of selenium, were found by Chinese investigators in both Shaaxi and Gansu provinces. These modern investigators graciously acknowledged that Polo had predated their discovery by more than 700 years (Yang et al., 1983).

1.3 Selenium Chemistry

Selenium has an atomic weight of 78.96 and its atomic number is 34. It occurs along with oxygen, sulfur, tellurium, and polonium in Group 16/VIA, and between arsenic and bromine in Period 4 of the Periodic Table of the elements. This location accounts for many of its biological interactions with sulfur, as well as with arsenic and its neighbor phosphorus, and, as was noted by an eminent biochemist more than 3 decades ago (Frost, 1972), places selenium in "a frontier that will challenge advances in biochemistry." Subsequent research has confirmed the accuracy of that prediction.

The outer electronic configuration of the element is $3d^{10}4s^{2}4p^{4}$, with three completely filled inner shells. Its chemical properties are intermediate between those of sulfur and tellurium, and its compounds resemble the corresponding sulfur and tellurium compounds in behavior. Its electronic configuration and position in the Periodic Table place selenium in the important group of half metals, or metalloids, elements that are neither fully metals nor nonmetals, but share chemical and physical properties of both.

1.3.1 Allotropic Forms of Selenium

Selenium, like sulfur, has several allotropes. They include monoclinic or red selenium, an amorphous powder that exists in two forms, one of which is comparable to crystalline "flowers of sulfur." There is also a black amorphous form. A vitreous form that changes to gray selenium on heating also occurs. Gray, also known as metallic selenium is stable at ordinary temperatures and is the most common allotrope.

1.3.2 Physical Properties of Selenium

Selenium has unique electrical properties. Its conductivity, which is low in the dark, is increased several 100-fold on exposure to light which also generates a small electrical current in the element. It is, in addition, a semiconductor, possessing what is known as asymmetrical conductivity, able to conduct more easily in one direction than in the other. These properties account for the element's exceptional usefulness to the electrical and electronic industries.

Elemental selenium boils at the relatively low temperature of 684°C. As a consequence, atmospheric pollution can be caused by industrial processes that involve heating the element or its compounds (Crystal, 1973). However, elemental selenium itself is very stable and highly insoluble. These properties are important from an environmental point of view since, under reducing conditions, selenates and other soluble compounds of selenium that occur in certain soils can be converted into elemental selenium and thus become unavailable for absorption by plants. The process can also remove selenium from active recycling and thus reduce the possibility of environmental pollution (World Health Organization, 1987).

1.3.3 Inorganic Compounds of Selenium

The chemical properties of selenium are similar to, though not identical with, those of sulfur (Greenwood and Earnshaw, 1984). Compared with the sulfur atom, with a radius of 0.37Å, the selenium atom is slightly larger, with a radius of 0.5Å.

Like sulfur, selenium reacts with metals and nonmetals, gaining electrons to form ionic compounds containing the selenide ion, Se^{2-}, for example, FeSe, Al_3Se_2, and Na_2Se. Several of these compounds are notorious among chemists for their foul odor and toxicity. Selenium also forms covalent compounds with most of the other substances. Naturally occurring oxidation states of selenium in elemental and combined forms are −2 (e.g., Na_2Se, sodium selenide), 0 (Se, elemental selenium), +4 (e.g., Na_2SeO_3, sodium selenite), and +6 (e.g., Na_2SeO_4, sodium selenate).

Binary compounds of selenium are formed with heavy and other metals, as well as with other elements. Metallic selenides occur widely in nature and are the most common mineral form of the element. Sodium selenide can be formed by (very vigorous) direct action between sodium and selenium. Selenides of the alkali and alkaline earth metals are water-soluble and many are readily decomposed by water and dilute acids, producing hydrogen selenide. This property can be of significance for the use of such compounds in agriculture and medicine. H_2Se is a colorless, inflammable gas with a foul odor. It has strong reducing properties and is a relatively strong acid with a pK_a of 3.73. It is also highly toxic. Exposure to H_2Se can cause olfactory fatigue so that those who inhale it may become unaware of its presence, in spite of its strong odor, with possibly fatal results (Howard, 1971).

Selenides of heavy metals are naturally present in many minerals. Iron selenide, which is found in some soils, is highly insoluble and can account in certain circumstances for the element's unavailability for absorption by plant roots.

Selenium forms halides by direct combination with fluorine, chlorine, and bromine, but not with iodine. It also forms oxyhalides. One of these, selenium oxychloride ($SeOCl_2$), is a powerful chlorinating agent and oxidant, capable of reacting with other substances explosively. It is a universal solvent.

The oxides and oxyacids of selenium correspond to those of sulfur. Selenium dioxide (SeO_2) is formed when the element is burned in air. It is a white, crystalline, and stable substance and is a strong oxidizing agent. It is used by analysts to catalyze oxidation of nitrogen compounds in Kjeldahl digestions. The dioxide must be handled with care since it can cause acute dermatitis. It sublimes at a temperature of 317°C and, since it may be formed during incineration of selenium-containing waste, can cause environmental pollution.

Selenium dioxide dissolves readily in water to form selenous acid (H_2SeO_3) and gives rise to two series of compounds, selenites, e.g., sodium selenite (Na_2SeO_3) and hydrogen selenites, e.g., potassium hydrogenselenite ($NaHSeO_3$). The selenites tend to oxidize slowly to the +6 state when exposed to air under acidic or neutral conditions. They are readily reduced to elemental selenium by ascorbate, sulfur dioxide, and other reducing agents. Selenites bind tightly to iron and aluminum oxides, a reaction that accounts for the element's unavailability in some soils and low concentration in natural waters. They also react readily with certain organic compounds such as *o*-diamines. This reaction is the basis for the spectrofluorimetric analytical procedure in which selenium in biological samples is first reduced to the +4 state by hydrogen peroxide and then complexed with 2,3-diaminonaphthalene (DAN).

Selenium trioxide (SeO_3) is produced by the action of sulfur trioxide on potassium selenate. It is a white, crystalline, hygroscopic compound that dissolves in water to form selenic acid (H_2SeO_4). The acid is a strong oxidant and can react with many organic and inorganic substances to form two series of compounds, the selenates, e.g., sodium selenate (Na_2SeO_4), and the hydrogen selenates, e.g., potassium hydrogen selenate ($KHSeO_4$). Selenium in the +6 state is stable under both acidic and alkaline conditions. This is of significance with regard to the availability for absorption by plant roots in alkaline soils in which selenates naturally occur. Selenates are also the most common form of the element in alkaline waters.

1.3.4 Organo-Selenium Compounds

The organic compounds of selenium are of considerable chemical and biochemical interest. They are similar in chemical and physical properties to, but not identical with, the corresponding organo-sulfur compounds. Since an increase in atomic number results in a decrease in bond stability, selenium compounds are less stable on exposure to light or heat and are more easily oxidized than their sulfur analogs. Selenols and selenide anions are more potent nucleophiles, with a greater facility for carbon bonding than their corresponding S-anions (Monahan et al., 1987). Selenols, moreover, are much stronger acids than thiols (the pK_a for the selenohydryl group of selenocysteine is 5.5 compared to 8.3 for the sulfydryl group of cysteine, the corresponding S-acid). In addition, selenols are readily ionized at physiological pH, whereas the corresponding thiols are mostly protonated, with implications for catalytic function (Ursini and Bindoli, 1987).

Of less scientific, but possibly of more practical interest, is the fact that many organo-selenium compounds are blessed with extremely unpleasant and pervasive odors. To some extent this was one of the reasons that discouraged chemists from undertaking studies of these compounds in the past, understandably so, if we are to judge by a story related by Frost (1972). This tells of the unfortunate experience of an organic chemist who worked on selenium at the University of Cambridge in the UK some time in the early 20th century. His efforts at synthesis led to such a stench that he was obliged to move his apparatus out of his laboratory and on to the roof of the building. "There, however, the horrible odor permeated all of Cambridge and even disrupted a ceremony at the university in memory of Darwin." As a result, the chemist and his smelly synthesis were banished to the open fens, well away from the university.

In spite of the odor problem, there is today a remarkable level of interest, among chemists and biochemists, in organoselenium compounds, as a scan of the current literature will show. This has been increasing particularly with the growing recognition of their key roles in biological processes, not least their potential as possible anticarcinogens.

A considerable number of selenium analogs of organosulfur compounds are known. Many have been isolated from biological materials and their properties investigated. Although some aspects of the metabolism of organosulfur compounds resemble those of their sulfur analogs, their metabolic pathways diverge considerably (Levander, 1976). Many have also been synthesized and their possible uses, industrially and medicinally, have been investigated (Klayman and Gunther, 1973). Of particular interest from the nutrition point of view are the selenoaminocarboxylic acids, selenium-containing peptides, and selenium derivatives of nucleic acids that occur naturally in body cells and tissues.

1.3.5 Isotopes of Selenium

Selenium has six naturally occurring stable isotopes, ^{74}Se, ^{76}Se, ^{77}Se, ^{78}Se, ^{80}Se, and ^{82}Se. The two most abundant are ^{80}Se (49.82%) and ^{78}Se (23.52%). Availability of these isotopes has enabled significant advances to be made in recent years in our understanding of the biological roles of selenium. They have been particularly useful in the investigation of selenium bioavailability (Fairweather-Tait, 1997). An increasing use is in the study of selenium metabolism and status as well as in the assessment of body-pool compartments. The ability to label specific chemical forms of selenium with stable isotopes is also helping our understanding of the role these different species play in the complex biochemistry of the element (Crews, 2001).

A number of artificial radioactive isotopes of selenium have been prepared by neutron activation. The gamma-emitting ^{75}Se, with a half-life of 120.4 days, is used as a diagnostic tool in biological investigations, for example, as an in vivo label for proteins.

1.4 Distribution of Selenium in the Lithosphere

Selenium is widely, though unevenly, distributed over the surface of the earth. It is about 70th in order of abundance of the minerals, the average in crustal rocks being 0.05 mg/kg. It occurs in igneous rocks, normally as selenide. In volcanic sulfur deposits it occurs in sulfides where it is isomorphous with sulfur. It is present in small concentrations, though in total in large amounts, in sulfide and porphyry copper deposits. In certain sedimentary rocks, such as sandstones and carbonaceous siltstones, selenium is syngenetic, that is, it was introduced during deposition, probably by absorption on precipitated ferric hydroxide (Elkin, 1980). Coal can contain up to 12 mg/kg. Selenium can also be present in crude oil, but usually at less than 0.5 mg/kg (Bapu, 1975).

1.4.1 Selenium in Soil

In soils, the concentration of selenium is generally low at about 50 to 200 μg/kg. In some discrete areas, however, it can be present in considerably higher concentrations, depending on geological and other factors. Significant amounts often occur in soils derived from the pyrite and marcasite of sedimentary formations. It is concentrated in soils of drier regions, such as the North American great plains from Mexico north into Canada, especially in Wyoming and South Dakota. Similar seleniferous soils occur in China, the Amazon basin, Columbia and Venezuela in South America, and less extensively in Australia, Russia, and other countries (Oldfield, 1999). Some of the most seleniferous soils in the world, with concentrations up to 1,250 mg/kg have been found in Ireland (Fleming, 1962).

Selenium occurs in well-drained alkaline soils chiefly as selenates, which are highly available for absorption by plant roots. In contrast, in acid, poorly drained soils it is present mainly as unavailable selenides and sometimes as elemental selenium (National Research Council, 1971). An insoluble ferric iron–selenite complex can also form under these conditions. Elemental selenium is generally stable in soil and, apart from slight oxidation by microbial action, is not converted into soluble forms (Watkinson and Davies, 1967).

1.4.2 Selenium in Water

Selenium levels in natural waters are normally low, usually less than 1 μg/l in potable fresh water. In seawater, levels are about ten times lower. Concentrations can be higher in well waters in seleniferous areas and especially in some rivers where irrigation drainage from seleniferous soils occurs (Elkin, 1980).

1.5 Sources and Production of Selenium

Selenium forms natural compounds with several other elements and is a constituent of more than 60 mineral species, chiefly sulfides. However, selenium minerals, the most common of which is clausthalite (PbSe), are finely disseminated and do not form economically exploitable deposits. Primary commercial sources are sulfide deposits of copper and other base metals with which small amounts of selenium are associated. The element is recovered as a by-product from slimes produced during electrolytic refining, particularly of copper ores, along with a variety of precious metals, including silver, gold, platinum, and germanium. In some ores in which it is present as the double selenide CuAgSe, selenium may make up more than 50% of the total metal content of the slime (Oldfield, 1990). Other lesser sources are sludges and dusts produced during the manufacture of sulfuric acid. This was the source from which selenium was first isolated by Berzelius. Treatment of such slimes and dusts requires that the selenium be converted into a water-soluble form, followed by reduction to the elemental state. This can be achieved by a number of different processes such as heating with soda ash or sulfuric acid as well as by direct oxidation.

A growing, but still relatively small amount of selenium is recovered by recycling from discarded electronic equipment and other scrap machinery. It can be recovered mechanically by milling, sandblasting, by use of high-pressure water jets, or by solution in aqueous sodium sulfite, fused caustic soda, or other such solvents.

Most of the world's selenium is produced in the USA, Japan, and Canada, with smaller amounts coming from China, Russia, Belgium, Finland, Australia, Peru, Zambia, and other countries with a copper refining industry. Production has been increasing in recent years as new uses for the element, especially in the electronic and related industries, have been found. World production in the late 20th century was estimated to be about 2,300 tonnes per year, up from the approximate half tonne produced in 1910. Although ultra-pure selenium of, it is claimed, 99.9999% purity is available, most marketed refined grades contain >99.5% selenium with, as impurities, up to 0.2% tellurium and lesser amounts of iron, lead, and copper. Several compounds of selenium are commercially available, including ferro- and nickel-selenide, selenium dioxide, cadmium sulfoselenide, and selenium diethyldithiocarbamate, as well as sodium selenite and selenate (Selenium Tellurium Development Association, 1993).

1.6 Industrial and Other Applications of Selenium

As long ago as 1873 it was discovered by two British engineers, W. Smith and J. May, that on exposure to light the electrical resistance of selenium was decreased (van der Krogt, 2004). A selenium photovoltaic cell was constructed in 1883 and the application of the element in rectifiers described in 1909. Industrial exploitation of the element's photoelectric and semiconducting properties began in the 1920s when the first commercially available selenium rectifier was produced. Today, the electrical and electronic industries are major users of selenium, taking about a third of the world's production. Until recently, large amounts of selenium were also used on photoreceptor drums of plain paper copiers, in the process known as "xerography" or dry photocopying (Zingaro and Cooper, 1974). However, this use has decreased, mainly for health and economic reasons, as selenium is replaced by more environment-friendly photosensitive materials.

Selenium is also used in laser printers, solar photovoltaic cells, and X-ray machines. Significant amounts are used by the glass industry, both to decolorize and to color glass. Selenium ruby glass is one of the most brilliant reds known and is used in airfield and other warning lights and in decorative stained glass. Selenium compounds added to the glass mix can also produce other colors as well as the bronze and smoky plate glass used in curtain walls of many modern buildings to block solar heat transmission.

Selenium compounds, such as cadmium sulfide-selenide, are used in a range of pigments in ceramics, paints, and plastics. These pigments are highly valued because of their long life, brilliancy and their stability to heat, sunlight, and chemical action. Finely ground metallic selenium as well as certain selenium compounds are used in the vulcanization of both natural and synthetic rubber. Lubricating oils and greases, especially those used at high temperatures, may also contain selenium. In metallurgy, small amounts of selenium are added to improve the machinability of wrought iron and steel castings. It is also used to harden the grids of lead storage batteries. Other industrial uses are as oxidizing agents in a variety of reactions, including synthesis of organic chemical and pharmaceutical compounds.

Selenium has a number of important agricultural and horticultural applications. These include the use of sodium selenite and selenate as additives and dietary supplements in animal feeds. Soil deficiencies are corrected by adding selenium compounds to fertilizers and top dressings. Potassium ammonium sulfoselenide has considerable pesticidal properties and was one of the first systemic insecticides to be marketed in the 1930s. It was recommended for use on a variety of glasshouse and other crops. It is still in use, but is restricted to nonfood crops because of its toxicity. Sodium selenate has also been used for a similar purpose in commercial greenhouses growing flowers for cutting. The selenate is added to irrigation water and is taken up through the roots of the plants. It is converted in the leaves into volatile selenide, which is released by the plant to repel red spiders, aphids, and similar pests.

Considerable amounts of selenium are employed in the pharmaceutical industry for the manufacture of prescribed as well as over-the-counter (OTC) dietary supplements. A number of different compounds are used in this way, including sodium selenite and selenate, selenomethionine, and selenium-enriched yeast. A surprisingly large amount of selenium is used for the treatment of seborrheic dermatitis and tinea versicolor. A buffered solution of selenide sulfide is marketed as an antidandruff shampoo (Selenium Tellurium Development Association, 1993).

1.7 Selenium Analysis

A major problem that contributed to the apparent lack of interest in selenium displayed by many biological scientists until well into the 20th century was the difficulty they experienced in trying to analyze the element in the materials they studied. Even as recently as the 1980s accurate determination of concentrations in biological tissues was a challenge beyond the ability of not a few analysts (Versieck and Cornelis, 1989). This was largely because, in addition to the normally low levels of selenium found in biological materials, it is very volatile and is easily lost during sample preparation. Modern analytical equipment, allied with improved laboratory procedure and careful quality control and the availability of appropriate certified reference materials (CRMs), has largely overcome these difficulties. Today methods for determining total selenium levels are well established (Crews, 1997). However, while analytical techniques have been considerably improved, unless they have been applied critically and results presented with sufficient background information, including analytical reliability and data treatment, published data may, even today, be of little use or misleading (Alfthan and Nève, 1996).

1.7.1 Sample Preparation

Although a few methods of analysis for selenium can be performed without destroying the sample, in most procedures, apart from neutron activation analysis (NAA) and X-ray fluorescence (XRF) analysis, the sample must be subjected to certain preliminary steps to remove organic matter and bring the element into the mineralized state in solution (Alt and Messerschmidt, 1988). This destructive preparation usually involves some form of oxidation. This can be either a dry procedure, in which the sample is incinerated at high temperature in a furnace or in some other type of heating apparatus in the presence of air or oxygen, or wet digestion, in which it is heated with various acids or mixtures of them.

1.7.1.1 Dry Ashing

Although open, dry ashing is not normally recommended, because of the risk of loss of the selenium through volatilization, it is still considered a convenient and versatile method, for example, for preparing food samples for instrumental analysis, provided care is taken to control the incineration temperature (Tinggi et al., 1992). A particular advantage of the method is that it allows use of relatively large sample sizes. It also reduces the possibility of contamination of the sample by reagents, since normally only dilute acids are used to dissolve the ash. Steps that can be taken to improve reliability and effectiveness of dry ashing, such as the use of ashing aids, have been reported (Connolly et al., 2004). Use of a programmable electric oven in which samples are incinerated in a series of mineralization stages for different times and temperatures has been found to prevent volatilization losses and to give excellent recoveries (Amaro et al., 1998).

1.7.1.2 Wet Ashing

A "wet" digestion, in which samples are prepared by heating with acid, is the method of choice in most analytical laboratories. The procedure, which is applicable to most sample matrices, is rapid, and generally has a high recovery rate compared to dry ashing. It has, however, the disadvantage that only small sample sizes can normally be used and relatively large volumes of digestion fluids are required, with the resulting possibility of high blanks and sample contamination.

The composition of the digestion fluid used will depend on the nature of the sample to be analyzed. Nitric acid, or a nitric–sulfuric acid mixture, is frequently used. Since selenium tends to form stable organic compounds in biological tissues, nitric acid on its own may not always achieve complete digestion. The addition of sulfuric acid, which has a boiling point of 330°C, greatly improves the oxidizing process (Hansson et al., 1987). However, even a nitric–sulfuric acid mixture may not be fully effective in releasing selenium from certain tissues (Tinggi et al., 1992a). The addition of perchloric acid to the mixture has been found to overcome this difficulty, though there can be problems because of the explosive nature of perchloric acid. Moreover, under certain conditions its presence may result in the loss of selenium through volatilization (Jones et al., 1975).

Digestion can be carried out in open vessels, for example, on a temperature-controlled heating block or plate heater, using an appropriate exhaust system to remove fumes. In recent years closed digestion systems have been widely adopted, with resulting reduction in time required for digestion and of the likelihood of contamination from external sources. Various digestion apparatus can be used, such as an oxygen bomb or microwave-heated sealed polytetrafluoroethylene (PTFE) tubes (Oles and Graham, 1991).

The use of microwave heating for sample digestion has been an important development in mineral analysis (Lachica, 1990). Initially ovens developed for domestic purposes were adapted for use in the laboratory (Abu-Samara et al., 1975) but these have largely been replaced by purpose-built systems, with appropriate fume extraction and other attachments. They have many advantages over traditional equipment, especially in reducing heating times. The systems are also adaptable, relatively easily to automation. Since samples in microwave ovens are usually contained in closed vessels such as low- or high-pressure tubes fitted with pressure-release valves, losses due to volatilization are minimized and the likelihood of external contamination is considerably reduced (Neas and Collins, 1985). The method has been shown to be particularly effective for the preparation of food samples for analysis of volatile elements such as selenium (Tinggi and Craven, 1996) and is used routinely in many large scale commercial and government analytical laboratories, such as the UK's Central Science Laboratory (Ysart et al., 1999).

1.7.2 End-Determination Methods for Selenium Analysis

As even a brief scan of the large number of papers on selenium in the current scientific literature will show, many different instrumental techniques can be used for its determination in biological materials. Some of these are listed in Table 1.1. The choice of method will depend largely on the laboratory facilities and the technical expertise available to the investigators, as well as on the particular object of their study. Details of the different techniques can be found by readers who wish to do so in the original publications. Here we will concentrate on some of the most widely used and generally more practical end-determinations currently available.

1.7.2.1 Spectrofluorimetry

A widely used method for the determination of selenium in foods and other biological materials, especially in small-scale studies, is spectrofluorimetry. It is based on the reaction of selenites with diamines to produce a piazoselenol that is fluorescent. The most commonly used diamine for the reaction is DAN. It is a highly sensitive method and can measure selenium concentrations down to nanogram quantities in many different biological matrices. It also has the advantage of requiring only small sample sizes. However, the method is somewhat cumbersome and requires careful supervision and has to a great extent been replaced by techniques such as hydride generation atomic absorption spectrophotometry (HGAAS) (Tinggi et al., 1992b).

1.7.2.2 Atomic Absorption Spectrophotometry

Atomic absorption spectrophotometry (AAS) in one of its various modes is the most commonly used technique for the determination of a wide range of trace

TABLE 1.1 Analytical techniques for trace elements

Neutron activation analysis (NAA)
X-ray fluorescence (XRF) spectrometry
Atomic absorption spectrophotometry-flame/graphite furnace/hydride generation/cold vapor (FAAS/GFAAS/HGAAS/CVAAS)
Atomic/optical emission spectrometry (AES/OES) with or without inductively coupled plasma (ICP)
Atomic fluorescence spectrometry (AFS)
Mass spectrometry (MS)
Voltammetry:
Differential pulse anodic/cathodic stripping voltammetry (DPASV/DPCSV)
Potentiometric stripping analysis (PSA)
Square wave anodic stripping voltammetry (SWASV)
Fluorimetry

After Schramel, P., 2000, New sensitive methods in the determination of trace elements, in: Roussel, A.M., Anderson, R.A., and Favier, A.E. (eds), *Trace Elements in Man and Animals—TEMA10*, pp. 1091–1097, Kluwer/Plenum, New York.

elements, including selenium, in biological materials. It has replaced the formerly, almost universally, used flame atomic emission spectrophotometry (FAES), except for the determination of alkali metals. Its popularity has largely been due to the relatively low cost of the instrumentation required and, possibly more, to the fact that it is easily learned by investigators who have not been formally trained as analysts. Graphite furnace or electrothermal AAS (GFAAS/ETAAS) is a rapid and efficient method and allows determination of selenium levels in biological materials down to the microgram per gram range with ease (Tinggi et al., 1992a). Problems can be experienced because of matrix interferences, particularly from the presence of phosphates, as well as from excessive volatilization. Procedures for overcoming these difficulties have been reported (Kumpulainen et al., 1983). The use of HGAAS can also avoid such problems (Tinggi et al., 1992a). An efficient form of background correction, such as Zeeman mode, is essential, especially with GFAAS, for overcoming spectral interference (Tinggi et al., 1992b).

1.7.2.3 Inductively Coupled Plasma Atomic Emission Spectrophotometry

A significant enhancement of analytical capabilities was achieved in the late 1980s with the replacement of the acetylene or other gas flame by a plasma discharge for atomization–excitation in FAES and related instruments. The plasma consists of ions, electrons, and neutral particles formed from argon gas and operates at far higher temperatures than does the gas flame of FAES. Inductively coupled plasma atomic/optical emission spectrophotometry (ICP-AES/OES) allows simultaneous multi element analysis with accuracy in many cases similar to that of ETAAS. It is the method of choice for laboratories with a high sample load and a need to determine multiple elements per sample. Early versions of ICP-AES lacked sufficient sensitivity to determine concentrations at the very low levels found in some biological samples (Kumpulainen, 1990).

1.7.2.4 Inductively Coupled Plasma Mass Spectrometry

The problem of relatively low sensitivity has been overcome by the coupling of ICP with the techniques of mass spectrometry (MS) in inductively coupled plasma mass spectrometry (ICP-MS). This is a very powerful tool for trace and ultra-trace element analysis, capable, for example, of determining selenium down to levels of 10 pg/g, compared to microgram per gram achieved using FAAS. Unfortunately, the equipment is expensive and requires for its operation a level of technical expertise often unavailable in many research laboratories. However, spare capacity makes it possible for large commercial and other laboratories that do possess ICP-MS to undertake analyses, usually for a fee, to meet the needs of less well-endowed establishments.

In ICP-MS the ions produced by the plasma are passed through a series of apertures (cones) into a high-vacuum mass analyzer. The isotopes of the elements are identified by their mass/charge ratio and the intensity of a specific peak in the mass spectrum is proportional to the amount of the element in the original sample. Several different methods of analysis can be employed, depending on the particular model of the instrument. The quadripole mass analyser (PQ) is capable of handling high-volume samples and is suitable for the majority of applications, while a high-resolution mass analyzer (HRMA) provides higher sensitivities and higher mass resolutions, but with a smaller throughput than PQ (University of Missouri Research Reactor Center, 2004). A problem encountered in the determination of selenium using earlier versions of quadripole instruments was that the dimer from the ICP's argon plasma, $^{40}Ar_2$, has the same mass as the most abundant selenium isotope, ^{80}Se, thus precluding measurement of this isotope (Crews et al., 1996).

Several different plasma sources have been developed to meet different analytical requirements. These include microwave-induced plasma (MIP), glow-discharge (GD) and electrospray ionization (ESI). Technical aspects and advantages of these different techniques, especially for speciation analysis, are, however, more the concern of analytical experts than of most nutritionists and biological research scientists. Those who wish to do so should consult the appropriate technical literature for further information (Ray et al., 2004).

Several other well-tried instrumental methods of analysis for selenium are available and have been described in the literature. They include instrumental neutron activation analysis (INAA), which has the advantage of requiring only minimal sample preparation. It is a powerful analytical technique, which has been shown to be especially useful for determining low levels of selenium, for example, in human breast milk (Cumming et al., 1992). However, it requires access to sophisticated equipment, including a nuclear reactor. Nevertheless, when these are available, even on a commercial basis, INAA is recommended as a valuable quality control reference method against which routine laboratory methods can be evaluated (World Health Organization, 1987).

Other instrumental techniques, normally available only in well-endowed laboratories, include isotope dilution mass spectrometry (IDMS) and XRF. Hybrid systems, in which two or more analytical techniques are interfaced to enhance analytical capabilities, are also in use. In several of these, high-performance liquid chromatography (HPLC) is joined to AAS, ICP, MS, and other procedures, for example, HPLC-fluorimetry, and the triple hybrid HPLC-ICP-MS. These are powerful analytical tools, especially useful in the determination of different chemical species of elements (Crews et al., 1997).

1.7.3 Speciation Analysis

Food composition databases normally include only information on levels of total selenium. Until relatively recently, research reports and other studies appearing in the scientific literature followed the same practice and rarely presented data on the different selenium species present in the biological materials under investigation. Similarly, official dietary reference values published in different countries present intake recommendations and safe levels for selenium, as for other trace elements, normally in terms of total amounts, not of different chemical species. It is now recognized that this practice needs to be at least modified, if not abandoned. As has been commented by Crews (1998), information about total amounts of an element in a particular food may tell little, for example, about how well that element is absorbed and utilized by the body. This, however, is the sort of information that is required to allow consumers informed choice and to provide authorities with the basis for good advice and legislation. It may be, as Crews noted elsewhere, "that one day essential trace element species will be listed on food composition labels or that legislation for potentially toxic elements will be based on the chemical species rather than the total concentration" (Crews, 1997). Unfortunately, that day may be long in coming. Compared to the determination of total amounts of elements, the quantitative determination of elemental species is both costly and complicated. Routine analytical procedures for total element determinations, often automated with multi element capabilities, already set up in government and other laboratories, are unlikely to be abandoned, to be replaced by as yet cumbersome, costly and not yet fully validated speciation analysis procedures for many years to come (Berg and Larsen, 1999).

Although progress in the development of methods that will allow routine speciation analysis of trace elements is slow, advances have been made. Several methods currently available in specialist laboratories could be adopted for this purpose. Among them are hybrid systems in which a separation process is coupled with a well-established analytical procedure, such as ICP-MS. Among separation techniques found to be effective for selenium are ion exchange (IX), size-exclusion chromatography (SEC), HPLC, and capillary electrophoresis (CE); detectors used include MS, NAA, and atomic fluorescence spectrometry (AFS) (Slejkovec et al., 2000). Other techniques are also in use, but are mainly confined to well-equipped specialist laboratories (Lobinski et al., 2000). A complex procedure used to determine selenium species in yeast has been described. It includes high-resolution fractionation of water extracts using size-exclusion chromatography and characterization by combined matrix-assisted laser desorption ionization (MADDI)-time-of-flight mass spectrometry (TOF MS) and electrospray quadrupole-TOF tandem MS (Encinar et al., 2003). It is to be hoped that less complex techniques will eventually become available for use by a wider range of investigators than at present are able to perform these operations. Otherwise the study of elemental speciation in foods, as well as in clinical and environmental samples, will remain largely the preserve of the specialist, and multidisciplinary studies, so important for advances in human physiology and nutrition, will be seriously impeded.

1.7.4 Analytical Quality Control

No matter how technically advanced or how modern the equipment and procedures used to determine levels of selenium, or any other element, in biological samples may be, the quality of the data generated must always be checked by a robust quality assurance programme. Knowledge of the accuracy of its data is the foundation of a laboratory's quality control (Alvarez, 1984).

TABLE 1.2 Reference materials for total selenium

Material	Selenium concentration	Reference code
Skim-milk powder		
(Spiked)	(127 μg/kg)[a]	BCR-150
Bovine muscle	183 ± 12 μg/kg	BCR-184
Bovine liver	1680 ± 140 μg/kg	BCR-185R
Pig kidney	10300 ± 500 μg/kg	BCR-186
Cod muscle	1.63 ± 0.07 mg/kg	BCR-422

Source: Data from IRMM: Certified Reference Materials 2005. http://www.irmm.jrc.be.
[a] Values in brackets are not certified.

In addition to the standard techniques to ensure the quality of laboratory work and to keep to a minimum the potential for accidental loss or contamination, it is essential that analytical procedures be validated and results checked against appropriate CRMs. They are powerful tools for instrument calibration, validation of analytical procedures and achieving reliability, and they play a key role in quality control and/or quality assurance (QC/QA). The importance of having appropriate reference standards has been underlined in a report presented to BERM, the international symposium on biological and environmental reference materials (Roelandts, 1998).

Until recently, reference materials for selenium, of appropriate concentration ranges and in different matrices, were not readily available. That situation no longer exists, at least for total concentrations, though not for individual chemical species of the element. CRMs can be obtained from a number of international reference centers and agencies, such as the Institute for Reference Materials and Measurements (IRMM) of the European Community, formerly known as the Bureau Communautaire des Références (BCR), the National Institute of Standards and Technology (NIST) in the USA, and the International Atomic Energy Agency (IAEA) in Vienna. Table 1.2 lists a number of standards, certified for total selenium content, available from IRRM.

References

Abu-Samara, A., Morris, J.S., and Koirtyohann, S.R., 1975, Wet ashing of some biological samples in a microwave oven, *Anal. Chem.* **47**, 1475–1477.

Alfthan, G. and Nève, J., 1996, Reference values for serum selenium in various areas—evaluated according to the TRACY protocol, *J. Trace Elem. Med. Biol.* **10**, 77–87.

Alt, F. and Messerschmidt, J., 1988, Selenium, in: McKenzie, H.A. and Smythe, L.E. (eds), *Quantitative Trace Analysis of Biological Materials*, Elsevier, Amsterdam, p. 487.

Alvarez, R., 1984, NBS Standard Reference Materials for food analysis, in: Steward, K.K. and Whitaker, J.R. (eds), *Modern Methods of Food Analysis*, Avi, Westport, CT, pp. 35–40.

Amaro, M.A., Moreno, R., and Zurera, C., 1998, Nutritional estimation of changes in mineral content during storage of white asparagus, *J. Food Qual.* **21**, 445–458.

Bapu, S.P., 1975, Trace elements in fuel, in: *Advances in Chemistry,* Series 141, American Chemical Society, Washington, DC, pp. 121–147.

Berg, T. and Larsen, E.H., 1999, Speciation and legislation—where we are today and what do we need for tomorrow? *Fresenius J. Anal. Chem.* **363**, 431–434.

Berzelius, J.J., 1818, Lettre de M. Berzelius à M. Berthollet sur deux métaux nouveaux, *Annales de Chimie et de Physique, Série 2,* **7**, 199–202.

Connolly, C.D., Power, R.F., and Hynes, M.J., 2004, Validation of method for total selenium determination in yeast by flame atomic absorption spectrometry, *Biol. Trace Elem. Res.* **100**, 87–93.

Crews, H.M., 1997, The analyst's viewpoint with special reference to selenium, *Nutr. Food Sci.* **6**, 221–228.

Crews, H.M., 1998, Speciation of trace elements in foods, with special reference to selenium: is it necessary? *Spectrochim. Acta,* Part B, **53**, 213–219.

Crews, H.M., 2001, Use of stable isotopes of selenium to investigate selenium status, in: Lowe, N. and Jackson, M. (eds), *Advances in Isotope Methods for the Analysis of Trace Elements in Man*, CRC Press, Boca Raton, FL, pp. 130–150.

Crews, H.M., Luten, J.B., and McGaw, B.A., 1996, Inductively coupled plasma-mass spectrometry, in: Mellon, F.A. and Sandström, B. (eds), *Stable Isotopes in Human Nutrition: Inorganic Nutrient Metabolism,* Academic Press, London, pp. 37–52.

Crews, H.M., Baxter, M.J., Lewis, D.J., et al., 1997, Multi-element and isotope ratio determination in foods and clinical samples using inductively coupled plasma-mass spectrometry, in: Fischer, P.W.P., L'Abbé, M.R., Cockell, K.A., and Gibson, R.S. (eds), *Trace Elements in Man and Animals 9*, NRC Research Press, Ottawa, Canada, pp. 88–93.

Crombie, A.C., 1959, *Medieval and Early Modern Science*, Vol. 1, Doubleday, New York, pp. 137 and 230.

Crystal, R.G., 1973, Elemental selenium: structure and properties, in: Klayman, D.L. and Gunther, W.H.H. (eds), *Organic Selenium Compounds: their Chemistry and Biology*, Wiley, New York, pp. 107–167.

Cumming, F.J., Fardy, J.J., and Florence, T.M., 1992, Selenium and human lactation in Australia: milk and blood levels in lactating women, and selenium intakes of their breast-fed infants, *Acta Paediatr.* **81**, 292–295.

Elkin, E.M., 1980, Selenium and selenium compounds, in: *Kirk-Othmer Encyclopedia of Chemical Technology*, 3rd edn., Wiley, New York, pp. 575–601.

Encinar, J.R., Śliwka-Kaszyńska, M.M., Polatajko, M.M., et al., 2003, Methodological advances for selenium analysis in yeast, *Anal. Chim. Acta* **500**, 171–183.

Fairweather-Tait, S.J., 1997, Bioavailability of selenium, *Eur. J. Clin. Nutr.* **51**, S20–S23.

Fleming, G.A., 1962, Selenium in Irish soils and plants, *Soil Sci.* **94**, 28–35.

Frost, D.V., 1972, Two faces of selenium—can selenophobia be cured? in: Hemphill, D. (ed), *CRC Critical Reviews in Toxicology*, CRC Press, Boca Raton, FL, pp. 467–514.

Greenwood, N.N. and Earnshaw, A., 1984, *Chemistry of the Elements,* Pergamon Press, Oxford, pp. 882–899.

Hansson, L., Pettersson, J., and Olin, A, 1987, A comparison of two digestion procedures for the determination of selenium in biological materials, *Talanta* **34**, 829–833.

Hoefer, F., 1842, *Histoire de la Chimie*, Vol. 1, p. 389, cited in, Mellor, J.W., 1934, *A Comprehensive Treatise on Inorganic and Theoretical Chemistry*, Vol. x, Longmans Green, London, pp. 693–696.

Howard, J.H., 1971, Control of geochemical behavior of selenium in natural waters by adsorption on hydrous ferric oxides, in: Hemphill, D.D. (ed), *Trace Substances in Environmental Health,* University of Missouri Press, Columbia, MO, p. 485.

Hurd, D.L. and Kipling, J.J., 1964, *Origins and Growth of Physical Science,* Part 2, Penguin Books, Harmondsworth.

Jones, G.B., Buckley, R.A., and Chandler, C.S., 1975, The volatility of chromium from brewer's yeast during assay, *Anal. Chim. Acta* **80**, 389–392.

Klayman, D.L. and Gunther, W.H.H. (eds), 1973, *Organic Selenium Compounds: their Chemistry and Biology,* Wiley, New York.

Knott, S.G. and McCray, C.W.R., 1959, Two naturally occurring outbreaks of selenosis in Queensland, *Aust. Vet. J.* **35**, 161–165.

Kumpulainen, J., 1990, Summary of new analytical techniques and general discussion, in: Tomita, H. (ed), *Trace Elements in Clinical Medicine*, Springer, Tokyo, pp. 541–546.

Kumpulainen, J., Raittila, A., Lehto, J., and Koivistoinen, P., 1983, Electrothermal atomic absorption spectrometric determination of selenium in foods and diets, *JAOAC.* **66**, 1129–1135.

Lachica, M., 1990, Use of microwave oven for the determination of mineral elements in biological materials, *Analusis* **18**, 331–333.

Levander, O.A., 1976, Selective aspects of the comparative metabolism and biochemistry of selenium and sulfur, in: Prasad, A.S. (ed.), *Trace Elements in Human Health and Disease*, Vol. 2, Academic Press, New York, pp. 135–163.

Lobinski, R., Edmonds, J.S., Suzuki, K.T., and Uden, P.C., 2000, Species-selective determination of selenium compounds in biological materials, *Pure Appl. Chem.* **72**, 447–461.

Mizutani, T., Kishimoto, M., and Yamada, K., 1992, Selenium levels in Chinese plants relating to the travels of Marco Polo, in: *Fifth Int Symp. Se Biol. Med, Abstracts.* July 20–23 1992, Vanderbilt University, Nashville, TN, p. 143.

National Research Council, 1971, *Selenium in Nutrition,* National Academy Press, Washington, DC.

Neas, E.D. and Collins, M.J., 1985, Microwave heating: theoretical concepts and equipment design, in: Kingston, H.M. and Jassie, L.B. (eds), *Introduction to Microwave Sample Preparation: Theory and Practice*, ACS Professional Book, American Chemical Society, Washington, DC, pp. 23–40.

Oldfield, J.M., 1990, *Selenium: its Uses in Agriculture, Nutrition and Health and the Environment,* Selenium-Tellurium Development Association, Grimbergen, Belgium.

Oldfield, J.E., 1999, *Selenium World Atlas,* Selenium-Tellurium Development Association, Grimbergen, Belgium.

Oles, P.J. and Graham, W.M., 1991, Microwave acid digestion of various food matrices for nutrient determination by atomic absorption spectrophotometry, *JAOAC* **74**, 812–814.

Polo, M., 1967, *The Travels of Marco Polo*, translated by Marsden, E.W., revised by Wright, T., Everyman's Library, Dent, London, pp. 110–111.

Ray, S.J., Andrade, F., Gamez, G., et al., 2004, Plasma-source mass spectrometry for speciation analysis: state of the art, *J. Chromatogr.* **1050**, 3–23.

Roelandts, I., 1998, Seventh International Symposium on Biological and Environmental Reference Materials (BERM-7), Antwerp, Belgium, 21–25 April 1997, *Spectrochim. Acta, Part B,* **53**, 1365–1368.

Selenium Tellurium Development Association, 1993, *Information on the Handling and Storage of Selenium,* Selenium Tellurium Development Association, Grimbergen, Belgium.

Shriver, D.F. and Atkins, P.W. 1999, *Inorganic Chemistry,* 3rd edn., Oxford University Press, Oxford.

Slejkovec, Z., Van Elteren, J.T., Woroniecka, U.D., et al., 2000, Preliminary study of the determination of selenium compounds in some selenium-accumulating mushrooms, *Biol. Trace Elem. Res.* **75**, 139–155.

Tinggi, U. and Craven, G., 1996, Determination of total mercury in biological materials by cold vapor atomic absorption spectrometry after microwave digestion, *Microchem. J.* **54**, 168–173.

Tinggi, U., Reilly, C., Hahn, S., and Capra, M., 1992a, Comparison of wet digestion procedures for the determination of cadmium and lead in marine biological tissues by Zeeman graphite furnace atomic absorption spectrophotometry, *Sci. Total Environ.* **125**, 15–23.

Tinggi, U., Reilly, C., and Patterson, C.M., 1992b, Determination of selenium in foodstuffs using spectrofluorimetry and hydride generation atomic absorption spectrometry, *J. Food Comp. Anal.* **5**, 269–280.

Trelase, S.F., 1942, Bad earth, *Sci. Monthly* **54**, 12–28.

University of Missouri Research Reactor Center, 2004, *Inductively Coupled Mass Spectrometry,* http://www.missouri.edu/~murrwww/pages/ac_icpms1.shtml.

Ursini, R. and Bindoli, A., 1987, The role of selenium peroxidases in the protection against oxidative damage of membranes, *Chem. Phys. Lipids* **44**, 255–276.

van der Krogt, P., 2004, *Elementology and Elements Multidictionary,* http://vanderkrogt.net/elements/elem/se.html.

Versieck, J. and Cornelis, R., 1989, *Trace Elements in Human Plasma or Serum,* CRC Press, Boca Raton, FL, p. 76.

Watkinson, J.H. and Davies, E.B., 1967, Uptake of native and applied selenium by pasture plants III. Uptake of selenium from various carriers. *NZ J. Agric. Res.* **10**, 116–121.

World Health Organization, 1987, *Environmental Health Criteria 58*: *Selenium,* WHO, Geneva.

Yang, G., Wang, S., Zhou, R., and Sun, S., 1983, Endemic selenium toxicity of humans in China, *Am. J. Clin. Nutr.* **37**, 872–881.

Ysart, G., Miller, P., Crews, H., et al., 1999, Dietary exposure estimates of 30 elements from the UK Total Diet Study, *Food Add. Contam.* **16**, 391–403.

Zingaro, R.A. and Cooper, R., 1974, *Selenium*, Van Nostrand Reinhold, New York, pp. 788–807.

2
The Biology of Selenium

2.1 A Belated Recognition

The first clear indication that selenium plays a vital role in the metabolism of animals was obtained in the late 1950s when the element was shown by Schwartz and Foltz (1957) to be a key component of the so-called Factor 3, an active principle found in brewer's yeast able to replace vitamin E in preventing liver necrosis in rats and chickens. The discovery was a milestone in our understanding of the biological significance of selenium. Until then, it had been known only as a toxin, but was now shown to have a positive and presumably essential role in health. In quick succession, researchers were able to demonstrate that a variety of enzootic myopathies in cattle and sheep, as well as exudative diathesis in chickens (Patterson et al., 1957), that had been found to respond to vitamin E, could be controlled even more effectively by selenium (Andrews et al., 1968).

Another major step was taken in the early 1970s, when selenium was shown to be an essential component of glutathione peroxidase (GPX), an enzyme that provides antioxidant protection by reducing levels of hydroperoxides in cells (Rotruck et al., 1972). About the same time, it was reported that GPX was a tetramer containing about 4 g atoms of selenium per mole (Flohé et al., 1973). As well as demonstrating for the first time the central position of selenium in the structure of a functional protein, this finding appeared to offer an explanation for the "sparing" of vitamin E by selenium which also protected cells against oxidative damage (Combs, 2001). It seemed that now all that was needed to be known about the biological role of selenium had been discovered. How wrong this belief was has been shown by results of the vast amount of research on selenium that was to be carried out over the following 3 decades.

2.2 The Biological Role of Selenium in Prokaryotes

About the same time that mammalian GPX was demonstrated to be a selenoenzyme, selenium-dependent enzymes were also identified in certain microorganisms. One of these was the anaerobic bacterium *Clostridium sticklandii*, which requires selenium for the synthesis of a key protein in its glycine reductase enzyme complex (Turner and Stadman, 1973). Of even more significance, in the light of subsequent findings, was the identification by Stadman's group of selenocysteine as the selenium moiety in the polypeptide of the glycine reductase. This was the first demonstration of the role of selenoamino acid as an essential residue in a selenoenzyme (Cone et al., 1976).

Selenoenzymes have subsequently been identified and isolated from other microorganisms. One of these, formate dehydrogenase in *Eschericia coli*, has been studied extensively, with results that have contributed considerably to our understanding of the biological role of selenium. Of particular significance was the discovery, again by Stadman's group, that genes for formate dehydrogenase contain an in-frame UGA codon that directs the cotranslational insertion of selenocysteine into protein (Zinoni et al., 1986).

2.3 Selenium in Plants

Certain lower plants, such as plankton algae, require selenium for growth (Lindström, 1948). One of these organisms, the obligate selenium-dependent dinoflagellate *Peridinium gatuense* has been used in ecological studies in Sweden as a bioassay of selenium bioavailability in freshwater (Lindström and Johansson, 1995). Selenium does not appear to be required for growth of *Saccharomyces cerevisiae*, although the yeast can take up large amounts from the medium in which it is cultured. The selenium is assimilated in competition with sulfur and is metabolized into a number of different organic compounds, the major product being selemomethionine (Demirici, 1999). Fungi, including those used as human food, can also accumulate and metabolize selenium, though apparently not requiring it for growth (Piepponen et al., 1983). Levels of about 10 μg/g (dry weight) are commonly recorded in mushrooms cultivated in normal compost, while those in compost enriched with sodium selenite more than 1,000 μg/g (dry weight) can be accumulated (László and Csába, 2004), Much of the selenium in mushrooms appears to be in the form of selenomethionine, with some in other organic forms (Werner and Beelman, 2001).

2.3.1 Selenium in Higher Plants

Selenium is apparently not required for growth by majority of higher plants, though there is still some doubt about this (Novoselov et al., 2002). It is, in fact, toxic to many plants, which cannot grow on seleniferous soils. However, a small number of species actually thrive on high-selenium soils and these do appear to require the element (Trelase and Trelase, 1939). These unusual plants are sometimes called *primary indicator plants* because their presence indicates that selenium is a component of the soil in potentially large amounts. Some of them are *hyperaccumulators* (Baker and Brookes, 1989), able to accumulate extraordinarily high levels of selenium, even, in some cases, from soil that contains relatively little of the element (Brown and Shrift, 1982). Certain species of the vetch *Astragalus*, for example, have been found to contain more than 3,000 mg/kg (dry weight) in their leaves (Broyer et al., 1972). Ingestion of these so-called *locoweeds* by grazing animals can cause acute poisoning (Rosenfeld and Beath, 1961).

2.3.1.1 Selenium Accumulators and Nonaccumulators

Another group of plants can also grow on selenium-rich soils, but do not require it for growth. These can accumulate the element in their tissues, in some cases to relatively high levels. It is a somewhat ill-defined group, to which the names *secondary converter plants* and *facultative* or *secondary selenium absorbers* have been given. Among them are a number of grasses and other forage plants, such as alfalfa and clover, and plants used as human foods, such as garlic, onions, Swiss chard, broccoli, and other *brassicae*, as well as cereals, including barley, wheat, and rice. Since they are capable of accumulating potentially toxic levels of selenium, such plants can, in some seleniferous soil areas, pose a health problem to farm animals and humans (Ullrey, 1981).

Under normal field conditions, in the absence of high-selenium soil, forage and other crop plants will accumulate selenium, even though it is not required for their growth. Levels of uptake will depend on soil concentrations, as well as on certain other factors such as the chemical form of selenium present, as well as soil pH and moisture content. Crop plants grown on nonseleniferous soils normally contain between 0.01 and 1.0 mg/kg (dry weight) of selenium (Marschner, 1995). Even on soils with somewhat higher than normal levels of selenium, concentrations rarely exceed an upper limit of 1.0 mg/kg (Burau et al., 1988). In certain regions where selenium levels are low, such as in Finland and New Zealand, farmers add selenium to fertilizers used on their fields. This is not to promote plant growth, which the selenium will not do, but to increase levels in crops to meet the nutritional needs of consumers, both farm animals and humans (Oldfield, 1992).

2.3.2 Selenium Metabolism in Plants

In recent years, a considerable amount of research has been carried out on the uptake and metabolism of selenium by plants. The trigger for much of this work was the recognition, not only by scientists, but also by administrators, politicians, and, not least, the general public, especially in the USA, of the importance of selenium as an environmental contaminant. It followed the wide publicity given to the finding of extensive selenium pollution of water and plants, with disastrous consequences for birds and fish, in the wildlife refuge at Kesterton Reserve in California. The contamination resulted from high selenium levels in agricultural drainage water, runoff from neighboring farms that had been allowed to flow into the reservoir (Saiki and Lowe, 1987). There was considerable concern that vegetables and other crops produced in quantity on intensively irrigated farms in the San Joaquin Valley, one of the most productive agricultural areas in the country

(Oldfield, 1999), and other areas in central California might also be contaminated and be a health hazard for consumers. This concern triggered a significant escalation in interest among environmental scientists, encouraged by generous financial assistance from government and private sources. An informative review of the resulting research, especially as it relates to selenium metabolism in accumulator and nonaccumulator plants, by Terry and colleagues has been used to provide the basis of the following brief outline (Terry et al., 2000). The full paper, which cites some 175 original studies, is recommended to readers who wish to follow up aspects of the subject that are only briefly covered here.

2.3.2.1 Selenium Uptake and Transport in Plants

Selenate is taken up by plant roots from the soil by a process of active transport (Brown and Shrift, 1982). It competes with sulfur for uptake, both anions using a sulfate transporter in the root plasma membrane (Arvy, 1993). Organic forms of selenium, such as selenomethionine, are also taken up actively by plant roots. In contrast, transport of selenite does not appear to require the use of a sulfur transporter (Abrams et al., 1990).

Subsequent translocation of selenium within the plant is related to the form in which the element is supplied to the root. Selenate is more easily transported from the roots and much more is accumulated in the leaves than either selenite or organic selenium. Much of the selenite is retained in the roots where it is rapidly converted into organic forms, particularly selenomethionine (Zayed et al., 1998).

Distribution of selenium in various tissues differs between accumulator and nonaccumulator plants. In the former, the selenium is accumulated especially in young leaves, but later appears at higher levels in seeds than in other tissues, while, in nonaccumulators, such as cereals, levels in seeds and roots are usually the same (Beath, 1937).

2.3.2.2 Selenium Assimilation and Modification Within Plant Tissues

Although there is no strong evidence that selenium is an essential requirement for plant growth, it is nevertheless metabolized in a variety of ways once it is taken up into the plant tissues. These include, for example, nonspecific incorporation into selenoaminoacids and proteins, as well as synthesis of certain volatile selenium compounds, which can be released into the atmosphere from the plant's external surfaces (Zayed et al., 1999).

Selenium is translocated from the roots to the leaves via the xylem without undergoing any chemical transformation (De Souza et al., 1998). It is then reduced to selenide in the leaf chloroplasts, in a series of both enzymatic and nonenzymatic reactions, via glutathione (GSH) and the intermediate compound selenodiglutathione (GS-Se-SG). The selenide can then be converted into the selenoamino acid selenocysteine by coupling with *o*-acetylserine and then non specifically incorporated into protein (Ng and Anderson, 1979). Selenocysteine is also believed to be metabolized into selenomethionine, which likewise can be incorporated into proteins, in place of methionine. The nonspecific replacement of cysteine and methionine in proteins by selenocysteine and selenomethione has been shown to occur readily in non accumulator plants treated with selenium (Eustice et al., 1981).

The volatile compound dimethylselenide (DMSe) is produced by methylation of selenomethionine in an enzymatic reaction that apparently occurs in the cytosol. Since roots volatilize selenium at a much faster rate than other tissues, DMSe precursors, which are synthesized in chloroplasts, must be transported downwards from the leaves for this to occur (Zayed and Terry, 1994).

While the initial steps in selenium uptake and conversion to selenocysteine are believed to be the same in both selenium accumulators and non accumulators, subsequent metabolic pathways differ. Unlike nonaccumulators, accumulators metabolize selenocysteine primarily into different nonprotein selenoamino acids (Brown and Shrift, 1982). Among these are selenomethylselenocysteine (Se-methylSeCys), selenocystathione, and the dipeptide, γ-glutamyl-seleno-methyl-selenocysteine (Terry et al., 2000).

2.3.2.3 Selenium Toxicity and Tolerance in Plants

Concentration of selenium in the tissues of plants at which they begin to show symptoms of toxicity, such as stunting, chlorosis, and withering of leaves, range from 2 mg/kg in nonaccumulators, such as rice, and 330 mg/kg in white clover (Mikkelson et al., 1989), to several thousand mg/kg in the accumulator *Astragalus bisulcatus* (Shrift, 1969).

In addition to selenium concentrations, other factors, such as the stage of growth, levels of sulphate in the soil, and the chemical form of selenium accumulated, determine the susceptibility of a particular plant to toxicity. Both selenite and selenate are the major forms that are toxic to nonaccumulators because they are readily absorbed and assimilated by the plants (Wu et al., 1998). The major mechanism of selenium toxicity is believed to be the incorporation of selenoamino acids, selenocysteine, and selenomethionine, into proteins in place of cysteine and methionine. Alterations in tertiary structure, resulting from differences in size and ionization properties between the sulfur and selenium atoms, probably have a negative effect on catalytic activity of certain important proteins (Brown and Shrift, 1982). Other ways in which selenium induces toxicity in plants are believed to be by interfering with chlorophyll synthesis (Padmaja et al., 1989) as well as with nitrate assimilation (Aslam et al., 1990). There is also evidence that selenium can interfere with production of glutathione, and thus reduce a plant's defense against hydroxyl radicals and oxidative stress (Bosma et al., 1991).

Tolerance by accumulators towards levels of selenium that would result in toxicity in nonaccumulators appears to be largely due to the reduction of intracellular concentrations of selenocysteine and selenomethionine, thus preventing their incorporation into proteins. This is brought about by converting the selenium into nonprotein selenoamino acids, such as selenocystathionine, or into the dipeptide γ-glutamyl-seleno-methyl-selenocysteine (Nigam et al., 1969). There is some evidence that it may, to some extent, be achieved by compartmentation of the element in the form of selenate, or perhaps as nonprotein selenoamino acids, in vacuoles (Terry et al., 2000).

2.3.2.4 Volatilization of Selenium by Plants

Although it is not, strictly speaking, a tolerance mechanism, the ability of plants to convert selenium into volatile compounds that are then released into the atmosphere, thus reducing their selenium load, is an important metabolic activity of a variety of different plant types. The process have been intensively investigated in recent years, mainly in relation to its significance in what is known as phytoremedation of contaminated soil (Bañuelos et al., 1997). Rates of volatilization vary substantially between plant species and are related to a number of factors, including the concentration and chemical form of selenium and of sulfur in the soil, as well as to time of the year. In a laboratory study of the process in different crop species grown in solution culture, the highest rates of volatilization, between 300 and 350 μg Se/m^2 leaf area/day, were in rice, broccoli, and cabbage, while in beet, bean, lettuce, and onion they were >15 μg/m^2/day (Terry et al., 1992). High rates of volatilization have also been reported in the selenium accumulator *A. bisulcatus* (Duckart et al., 1992). In a field study of different plant species, the wetland *Salicornia bigelovii* (pickleweed) was found to have a rate of 420 μg Se/m^2 soil surface/day, 10 to 100 times greater than other plants, including cotton and Eucalyptus (Terry and Lin, 1999).

2.3.3 Selenium in Food Plants

While the mechanisms by which accumulator plants metabolize selenium in a variety of ways, and especially into volatile compounds, is of considerable interest to investigators dealing with the problem of environmental contamination, it is the ability of food plants, the major source of the element in most human diets, to take up this essential nutrient from the soil and store it in their tissues, that is of prime interest to nutritionists.

2.3.3.1 Crops Grown on Low-Selenium Soils

Where soil selenium levels are low, or the element occurs in a form that is not readily available for absorption by the roots, uptake by crops will be limited. In New Zealand, the selenium content of most of the arable land is low and, as a consequence, selenium levels in herbage are also low (Thomson and Robinson, 1980). Until steps were taken to improve soil levels by addition of sodium selenite to fertilizers, grazing on such lands resulted in selenium deficiency diseases in sheep and cattle. A similar situation was a major concern in Finland until it was also overcome by supplementation of fertilizers with selenium (Pykkö et al., 1988). Low-selenium agricultural soils have been reported in other countries also, although usually on a lesser scale than in New Zealand and Finland, with similar effects on animal health. In Australia areas of selenium-deficient soils are found in many agricultural regions and require intervention, either by direct supplementation of animals or by addition of selenium to fertilizers (Langlands, 1987).

Low selenium levels in plant foods used directly for human consumption are implicated in serious health problems in areas of selenium-deficient soils in central and western China and neighboring regions. There, the two best-known selenium deficiency-related conditions in humans—Keshan and Kashin-Beck diseases—are endemic. Dietary intakes of selenium as low as 7 μg/day occur, 10 to 20 times less than intakes in many other countries in which selenium-responsive diseases in humans do not normally occur (Yang, 1991). The cause of the deficiency is reliance by inhabitants of such regions for up to 70% of their food intake on locally produced cereals. These often contain less than 0.02 μg Se/g, reflecting soil levels of about 0.1 μg/g. In contrast, in the USA, where soil levels in the major cereal growing regions are generally high, grains contain on average about 0.30 μg Se/g. This level of intake is more than enough to make a major contribution to meet the dietary requirements for selenium, even though cereals make up only about 30% of the normal American diet (Combs and Combs, 1986).

2.3.3.2 Crops Grown on Adequate-Selenium Soils

The selenium content of food plants grown on soils with an average level of the element in available form which is approximately 0.5 to 1.0 μg/g, according to what is known as the Wells rating scale (Wells, 1967), will generally be in a relatively narrow range of approximately 0.1 to 1.0 μg/kg. The range will vary somewhat between countries, depending on local soil conditions. In Australia, for instance, average selenium levels in wheat of 0.15 μg/g have been reported (Tinggi et al., 1992), compared to North American levels of 0.33 μg/g (Ferretti and Levander, 1974). In vegetables and fruits, Australian figures were 0.001 to 0.022 μg/g, somewhat lower than American findings of 0.004 to 0.063 μg/g in similar foods (Schubert et al., 1987).

2.3.3.3 Crops Grown on High-Selenium Soils

Cereals and other farm crops grown on selenium-rich soils may, under certain conditions, accumulate high levels of the element and even pose a threat of toxicity to consumers. Samples of cereals from seleniferous regions of South Dakota in the USA have been found to contain up to 30 μg Se/g (Byers, 1936). In seleniferous regions of Enshi County in China, rice containing 2.5 μg/g, maize flour 7.5 μg/g, and leafy vegetables up to 7.6 μg/g of selenium have been reported (Yang et al., 1989). However, even on seleniferous soil, not all crops will take up toxic levels of the element. The average selenium content of wheat plants sampled from an area of high-selenium soil in Montana, USA, was 1.9 μg/g, with a maximum of 8 μg/g, even though there were a number of wild accumulator plants containing more than 1,000 μg Se/g (University of California Agricultural Issues Center, 1988). Even in the Chinese study of foods grown on high-selenium soil, several of the plants analyzed had less than 1 μg Se/g (Yang et al., 1989).

Rosenfeld and Beath (1961) in their comprehensive study of the distribution, properties, and health effects of selenium, described several cases of chronic selenium poisoning of people living in South Dakota. In all cases the source of the selenium was home-produced vegetables and other foods. Elimination of these foods from the diet led to recovery. The authors also referred to reports of chronic selenium poisoning in Columbia, South America, caused by consumption of locally produced foods grown in certain seleniferous regions. Soil selenium levels ranged from 12.6 to 20 μg/g and levels in crops were as much as 155 μg/g in wheat and 40 μg/g in barley. The problem, according to the authors, had actually been commented on as long ago as the 16th century when Fra Pedro Simon, a missionary priest, wrote, that "corn as well as other vegetables grow well and healthy but in some regions it is so poisonous that whoever eats it, man or animal, loses his hair. Indian women gave birth to monstrous-looking babies" (Simon, 1560). Rosenfeld and Beath noted that almost 400 years after Simon had made his observations, symptoms of selenosis, including hair and nail loss in humans and hoof damage in animals, continued to be recorded in Colombia: "reports in 1955 from one district described toxic corn and streams that had no animal life. Men and animals using the streams for drinking water showed loss of hair; small animals became sterile, and horses suffered hoof damage" (Rosenfeld and Beath, 1961).

2.3.3.4 The Risk of Selenosis in Humans From Eating Selenium-Rich Crops

The possibility that cereals and other crops grown on high-selenium soils and sold on the market without indication of their place of origin might poses a risk of selenosis to consumers first caused concern several decades ago. This was when information became available on the occurrence of selenium toxicity in farm animals and, to a lesser extent in humans, through consumption of selenium-enriched crops. That concern is still to be met today, as is evidenced by the publicity given to the problem of selenium contamination of farm produce grown in the San Joaquin Valley and other irrigated areas of central California (Bauer, 1997). It is also reflected in the inclusion of maximum permitted levels for selenium in the food standard regulations of many countries. However, extensive investigations have failed to find convincing evidence that selenium toxicity, resulting from consumption of naturally contaminated crops, is a real possibility for humans who consume a reasonably varied diet. As we shall see later, the occurrence of widescale, endemic human selenosis in Enshi County, a high-selenium region in Central China, has been attributed to consumption of a restricted diet of locally produced foods, of which selenium-rich cereals were a major part.

As has been noted by Oldfield (1990), though there are occasional occurrences of chronically toxic levels of selenium (above 5 μg/g) in cereals and other crops grown on seleniferous regions, in general, average figures on plant selenium contents tend to be reassuring. In extensive surveys of many thousands of samples of North American wheat, levels of 1 μg/g, or less, were found, with a maximum of 1.5 μg/g. In global terms these are significant findings, since North American wheat, which is used extensively in many countries, is generally richer in selenium than the grains produced in most other parts of the world.

2.4 Selenium in Animal Tissues

The selenium content of animal tissues reflects that of the foods they consume. Animals raised on low-selenium feeds deposit relatively low concentrations of the element in their tissues and in their products, such as eggs and milk, while those on relatively high-selenium intakes yield products with higher concentrations. Organ meats usually accumulate more selenium than do other tissues, such as muscle (Combs and Combs, 1986). The principle chemical form of selenium in animal tissues is selenocysteine, unlike plant food in which selenomethionine predominates.

Once it has been ingested, the distribution of selenium within the body, of humans as well as of other animals, and also its absorption and excretion, depend on several factors, particularly the chemical form as well as on total amount of the element in the diet. In addition intake can be affected by the presence of certain other components of food, including sulfur, heavy metals, and vitamins (Underwood, 1977). Other factors, including sex, age, condition of health as well as nutritional status, can also affect the level of uptake and distribution in the body.

2.4.1 Absorption, Transport, and Excretion of Selenium

Absorption of selenium occurs mainly at the lower end of the small intestine. All forms of selenium, organic as well as inorganic, are readily absorbed. Overall absorption has been shown, in experimental animals and in humans, to be around 80%. There are differences, however, between levels of absorption, as well as of subsequent utilization, of the different chemical forms of the element. In general, organic compounds, such as selenomethionine, are absorbed more efficiently than are inorganic forms, particularly selenite, with uptake from the gastrointestinal tract of more than 90% of selenomethionine compared to about 60% of selenite (Stewart et al., 1987). Differences in chemical form also affect levels of retention in the body over time. It has been shown, in humans as well as in experimental animals, that selenomethionine is retained more efficiently than selenite or selenate, but is not as efficient in maintaining selenium status (Fairweather-Tait, 1997). Selenomethionine is also better retained in tissues, where it is incorporated into proteins, nonspecifically, in place of methionine, than is selenocysteine (Thomson, 1998).

There is some evidence of differences in the level of absorption of selenium if it is supplied along with food, rather than in isolation as organic or other supplements (Sirichakwal et al., 1985). It has also been reported that selenium is more readily available if it is in plants rather than in animal foodstuffs (Young et al., 1982). Absorption can be affected by a number of dietary factors, in addition to the chemical form of the element. It is enhanced by the presence of protein, vitamin E, and vitamin A, and is decreased by sulfur, arsenic, mercury, guar gum, and vitamin C (Fairweather-Tait, 1997).

The major fate of all selenium absorbed from the diet, whatever its original chemical form or source, is to be incorporated into body proteins. The processes involved can be summarized briefly as follows: the ingested selenium is transported in the blood from the intestine to the liver. There it is reduced to selenide before being transported in the blood, bound to α- and γ-globulins to various organs and target tissues. It is then incorporated into specific selenoproteins, as selenocysteine, and, nonspecifically, as selenomethionine. The highest levels of selenium are deposited in red blood cells, liver, spleen, heart, nails, and tooth enamel. Excretion of absorbed selenium is mainly via the urine, with some loss in sweat, and also in hair. In addition, small amounts are lost through bilary, pancreatic, and intestinal secretions in feces (Linder, 1988).

2.4.2 Enteric Absorption of Selenium

There is uncertainty about the mechanisms of transport of dietary selenium across the intestinal epithelial membrane. Absorption of selenate appears to be by a sodium-mediated carrier transport mechanism shared with sulfur, while selenite uses passive diffusion (Fairweather-Tait, 1997). Both forms of inorganic selenium compete with inorganic sulfur compounds for absorption. In contrast, absorption of selenomethionine is active, using the same enzyme transport system as does methionine, with competition taking place between methionine and its seleno analog (McConnell and Cho, 1965).

Mechanisms of enteric absorption of selenoaminoacids other than selenomethionine are not clear. There is some evidence that the process is not active and is not physiologically controlled. It has been shown, in the case of the hamster, that selenocysteine transport across the duodenum wall will not proceed against a concentration gradient and that it is not inhibited by cysteine. Other findings point to an absence of any homeostatic or physiological control on enteric absorption of either organic or inorganic selenium. However, this view is not supported by reports that selenocysteine, like selenomethionine, may be actively transported in humans by the same transport mechanism as is used by its sulfur analog (Barbezat et al., 1984). It is possible that members of the SLC26 gene family of multifunctional anion exchangers, known to be involved in the transport of sulfate, as well as of other anions, also mediate transport of inorganic selenium in the intestinal brush border (Mount and Romero, 2004).

2.4.3 Transport of Selenium in the Body

Absorbed selenium is transported in the blood mainly bound to protein, following an initial reduction within the erythrocytes to selenide (Dreosti, 1986). The process uses reduced glutathione and involves the enzyme glutathione reductase (Jenkins and Hidiroglou, 1972).

In humans, almost all the protein-bound selenium in blood is reported to be in the very low-density β-lipoprotein fraction, with smaller amounts bound to other proteins (Sandholm, 1974). However, distribution between these proteins appears to depend on the composition of the diet. Whanger et al. (1993) showed that nearly 50% of the selenium in plasma is associated with albumin in people who consume a diet in which selenomethionine is the main form of the element. There is also evidence that different proteins act as selenium carriers in other animal species (Young et al., 1982).

2.4.4 *Selenium Distribution and Retention in the Human Body*

The efficiency of retention of selenium in organs and other tissues appears to depend mainly on its chemical form and subsequent use. Thus selenomethionine is absorbed and retained more efficiently than are selenate and selenite. However, it is not as efficient at maintaining selenium status. The reason for this appears to be that though selenomethionine is retained in muscle and other tissue proteins to a greater extent than are the other forms, this retention is nonspecific, and the selenoamino acid is used immediately as a substitute for methionine in protein structure, not as a component of a functional protein (Thomson, 1998).

The total amount of selenium retained in an adult human body has been shown to range from about 2 to more than 20 mg. The total selenium content of a US adult, whose selenium intake can normally be expected to be high, has been calculated to be approximately 15 mg, with a range of 13 to 20.3 mg (Schroeder et al., 1970), while in New Zealand, where selenium intake is low, the range in women is 2.3 to 10 mg (Griffith et al., 1976).

There is evidence of an order of priority between organs for selenium uptake under different conditions of dietary supply. When intakes are adequate selenium concentrations in liver and kidney will be higher than in other organs. Overall, about 30% of tissue selenium is contained in the liver, 15% in kidney, 30% in muscle and 10% in plasma (WHO/FAO, 2002). At lower intakes, levels in liver and muscle can be markedly reduced, while remaining higher in kidney. It has been suggested that kidney has a 'saturation level' for selenium and a minimum requirement at the expense of other organs at low dietary intakes. This observation has been interpreted as indicating that the kidney plays a special role in selenium balance in the body (Oster et al., 1988).

It may be noted that although selenium concentrations are normally lower in muscle than in kidney and other organs, because of its relative bulk compared to other tissues, skeletal muscle appears to be a major storage compartment for selenium in the body (Whanger et al., 1993).

Using autopsy materials, Oster et al. (1988) determined selenium levels in organs of German adult male accident victims. They compared their results with data reported for other countries, as shown in Table 2.1. The results indicate that

TABLE 2.1 Selenium levels in body organs: International comparisons (μg/g, wet weight)

Country	Liver	Kidney	Muscle	Heart
Canada	–	0.390	0.840	0.370
USA	0.540	1.090	0.240	0.280
Japan	2.300	1.500	1.700	1.900
New Zealand	0.209	0.750	0.061	0.190
Germany	0.291	0.771	0.111	0.170

Adapted from Oster, O., Schmiedel, G., and Prellwitz, W., 1988, The organ distribution of selenium in German adults, *Biol. Trace Elements Res.* **15**, 23–45.

selenium levels in body organs, with the exception of kidneys, appear to be related to the country of residence and hence to dietary intakes. Since dietary selenium intakes are normally high in Japan, USA, and Canada, it can be expected that levels in liver, skeletal, and heart muscle will also be high. In contrast, in Germany, as in several other European countries, and New Zealand, intakes are low, with correspondingly low retention in body organs.

2.4.5 Selenium Levels in Blood

Animal experiments have shown that there is generally a positive correlation between blood selenium levels and dietary intakes (Linberg and Jacobsson, 1970). In humans, blood selenium can vary significantly between different populations, indicating a similar relationship with dietary intakes (Ihnat and Aaseth, 1989).

2.4.5.1 Selenium in Whole Blood

Table 2.2 presents a selection from the literature of data on whole blood selenium levels in subjects in different countries. They are all from persons in good health and exclude anyone suffering from overt selenium excess or deficiency. The reasons for these stipulations are that blood selenium levels are altered in certain disease states.

Selenium levels in whole blood have been shown to alter with change of residence from a high- to a low-selenium area. Thus, blood levels in visitors from the USA where selenium intake is high were found to drop in their initial year of residence in New Zealand where selenium intake is low from >0.15 to <0.10 μg/ml, a level found in permanent residents of the latter country (Rea et al., 1979).

2.4.5.2 Selenium in Serum and Plasma

Plasma and serum contain about 75% of the selenium of whole blood. Levels appear to be directly related to recent dietary intakes. They may also be age related and are altered in various diseases and health conditions (Lombeck et al., 1977). A world reference range, based on data published in the scientific literature for serum selenium levels of healthy adults, of 0.046 to 0.143 μg/ml has been

TABLE 2.2 Whole blood selenium levels (μg/ml) of healthy subjects living in different countries

Country	Reported levels (range or mean ± SD)	Reference
China	0.440–0.027	1
Finland (pre-1984)	0.081–0.056	2
New Zealand	0.072 ± 0.005	3
Sweden	>0.070	4
Australia	0.210–0.110	5
USA	0.300–0.150	6

References:
1. Yang, G., Wang, S., Zhou, R., and Sun, S., 1983, Endemic selenium intoxication of humans in China, *Am. J. Clin. Nutr.* **37**, 872–881.
2. Westermark, T., Rauni, P., Kirjarinta, M., and Lappalainen, L., 1977, Selenium content of whole blood and serum in adults and children of different ages from different parts of Finland, *Acta Pharmacol. Toxicol.* **40**, 465–475.
3. Thomson, C.D., Robinson. M.F., Butler, J.A., and Whanger, P.D., 1993, Long-term supplementation with selenate and selenomethionine: selenium and glutathione peroxidase (EC 1.11.1.9) in blood components of New Zealand women, *Br. J. Nutr.* **69**, 577–588.
4. Dickson, R.C. and Tomlinson, R.H., 1967, Selenium in blood and human tissue, *Clin. Chim. Acta* **16**, 311–7.
5. Judson, G.L., Thomas, W., and Mattschess, K.H., 1982, Blood selenium levels in Kangaroo Island residents, *Med. J. Aust.* **2**, 217.
6. Burk, R.F., 1984, Selenium, in: Black, G. (ed), *Nutrition Reviews: Present Knowledge in Nutrition,* 5th edn., Nutrition Foundation, Washington, DC, pp. 519–527.

proposed by the International Atomic Energy Agency (Iyengar and Woittiez, 1988). This is close to the range of 0.053 ± 0.0207 to 0.161 ± 0.019 μg/ml, derived from another critical survey of published results, which is believed to represent the true values for healthy adults in all but the most exceptional circumstances (Viesieck and Cornelis, 1989). Actual levels of selenium in serum/plasma recorded in residents of several different countries are shown in Table 2.3. The figures have been taken from the extensive data, based on clinical observations

TABLE 2.3 Plasma and serum selenium levels in different countries

Country	Selenium, μg/ml serum/plasma
Austria	0.067 ± 0.025
Australia	0.092 ± 0.015
Canada	0.135 ± 0.013
England	0.088 ± 0.021
France	0.083 ± 0.004
Italy	0.082 ± 0.023
New Zealand	0.065 ± 0.012
South Africa	0.177 ± 0.011
USA	0.140 ± 0.041
Zambia	0.040 ± 0.010

Adapted from Combs, G.F. Jr., 2001, Selenium in global food systems, *Br. J. Nutr.* **85**, 517–547.

reported from more than 70 countries worldwide, from Austria to Zambia, published by Combs (2001).

The apparent effects of disease on serum and plasma selenium levels are illustrated in Table 2.4. There is clearly not a direct relationship between state of health in various disease conditions and blood selenium levels. In some instances there is a reduction from normal levels, while in others the reverse occurs. Such changes are not necessarily a direct effect of a particular disease as such. They may be the result of, for instance, coexisting malnutrition or impaired metabolism. Moreover, it is not easy to interpret reports of clinical findings of changes in trace element levels in body fluids and tissues in conjunction with illnesses. There can be, moreover in some cases, at least a suspicion that not every clinical laboratory is sufficiently conscious of the fact that trace analysis is heavily fraught with technical peril (Versieck and Cornelis, 1989).

TABLE 2.4 Plasma and serum levels (μg/ml) in different disease states

Disease	Selenium level (control)	Reference
Cancer (gastrointestinal)	0.0486 ± 0.015 (0.0543 ± 0.016)	1
Diabetes (children)	0.074 ± 0.008 (0.065 ± 0.008)	2
Myocardial infarction	0.055 ± 0.015 (0.078 ± 0.011)	3
Chron's disease	0.110 ± 0.036 (0.096 ± 0.035)	4
Alcoholic liver cirrhosis	0.058 ± 0.011 (0.080 ± 0.011)	5
Renal disease	0.078 ± 0.016 (0.103 ± 0.018)	6

References:

1. Salonen, J.T., Alfthan, G., Huttunen, J.K., et al., 1984, Association between serum selenium and the risk of cancer, *Am. J. Epidemiol.* **129**, 342–354.
2. Gebre-Medhin, M., Ewald, U., Plantin, L., and Tumevo, T., 1984, Elevated serum selenium in diabetic children, *Acta Paediat. Scan.* **73**, 109–112.
3. Oster, O., Drexler, M., Schenk, J., et al., 1986, Serum selenium concentrations of patients with myocardial infarctions, *Ann. Clin. Res.* **18**, 36–40.
4. Deflandre, J., Weber, G., Delbrouck, J.M., et al., 1985, Trace elements in serum of patients with Chron's disease, *Gastroenterol. Clin. Biol.* **9**, 719–723.
5. Johanssons, U., Johanssons, F., Joelsson, B., et al., 1986, Selenium status in patients with liver cirrhosis and alcoholism, *Br. J. Nutr.* **55**, 227–231.
6. Sprenger, K.B.G., Krivan, V., Geiger, H., and Franz, H.E., 1985, Essential and non-essential trace elements in plasma and erythrocytes in patients with chronic uremic disease, *Nutr. Res.* Suppl. **1**, S-350.

2.4.5.3 Selenium Levels in Other Blood Fractions

Serum and plasma selenium levels are widely used clinically in the assessment of trace element status, although there is evidence that they do not necessarily reflect body stores or dietary intakes. Other blood fractions are also used in clinical investigations and have in some situations advantages over assessment of plasma and selenium (Bibow et al., 1993). Several investigators have reported the use of platelets for this purpose (Levander et al., 1983). Platelets have a relatively high concentration of selenium. They have a short life span and are believed to reflect recent changes in intake and body stores. They can be relatively easily separated from whole blood by gradient density centrifugation, a technique available in many clinical laboratories (Kaspareck et al., 1979).

2.4.6 Selenium Retention and Excretion from the Body

The biological half-life of selenium in the human body has been estimated to be approximately 100 days (Griffith et al., 1976). Actual retention times will depend on a number of factors, including present selenium status, the specific form in which the element is ingested, as well as the state of health of the subject. It has been shown in rats that the apparent whole-body retention of selenium is an average of several discrete processes, as each internal organ probably has its own rate of selenium turnover. For example, the half-life of ^{75}Se in rat kidney was found to be 38 days and 74 days in skeletal muscle, with a whole-body half-life of 55 days (Thomson and Stewart, 1973). It has been shown that the total body retention curve for selenium in humans can be resolved into a number of separate components (Yang et al., 1989).

Selenium is excreted from the body by three distinct routes, in urine via the kidneys, in feces from the gastrointestinal trace, and in expired air via the lungs. The amounts and proportions of each type of excretion depend on the level and form of the element in the diet (Beath et al., 1934).

2.4.6.1 Urinary Excretion of Selenium

The urinary pathway is the dominant excretion route for selenium in humans (Yang et al., 1989). The proportion of intake excreted in this way depends on the level of intake in the diet. When this is high, urinary excretion will also be high (Thomson and Robinson, 1986). At low levels of intake, half or less of the dietary selenium will appear in urine (Robinson et al., 1973). These findings point to the importance of renal regulation of selenium levels in the body. This view is supported by the fact that these levels are not, apparently, homeostatically controlled by the gut (Burk, 1976).

The renal system may have an important role in allowing the body to adapt to low dietary intakes of selenium by reducing excretion under such conditions. It has been shown that women with a low selenium status have low plasma clearance of the element and excrete it more sparingly than do women whose status is high. There is evidence that New Zealanders appear to have adapted to their low-selenium environment by reducing urinary excretion, thus conserving their intake (Robinson et al., 1985). That such adaptation can develop surprisingly rapidly has been shown by results of depletion/repletion studies on healthy young men (Levander et al., 1981).

Several different chemical forms of selenium are found in urine, including selenomethionine, selenocysteine, selenite, selenate, and selenocholine (Robinson et al., 1985). Recently, selenium-containing carbohydrates (selenosugars) were detected in urine of rats fed selenite (Kobayashi et al., 2002). Many studies have reported trimethylselenonium (TMSe) to be the major form of selenium in urine and to account for up to 50% of the total normally present. Levels were believed to increase with higher intakes and it was generally thought to be produced as a way of excreting excess, potentially toxic selenium (Kuehnelt et al., 2005). The availability of improved analytical methods has produced results which changed this generally accepted view of selenium excretion. It is now believed that TMSe is not, under normal conditions, a significant constituent of human urine. However, it is produced in increasing quantities as selenium intake is increased and can be a biomarker of excessive intake (Suzuki et al., 2005). Three selenosugars have been identified in human urine and two of these, selenosugar **1** (methyl-2-acetamido-2-deoxy-1-seleno-β-D-galactopyranoside) and its deacylated analog selenosugar **3** (methyl-2-amino-2-deoxy-1-seleno-β-D-galactopyranoside), are believed to be major constituents. The third, selenosugar **2**, an analog of selenosugar **1**, appears to be a minor constituent. Although the significance of these findings is being investigated, and much more work is still to be done, the results so far obtained suggest that previously accepted pathways for human metabolism of selenium involving TMSe as the excretory end product may need to be reevaluated (Kuehnelt et al., 2005).

2.4.6.2 Fecal Excretion of Selenium

Fecal selenium consists largely of unabsorbed dietary selenium, along with selenium contained in bilary, pancreatic, and intestinal secretions (Levander and Baumann, 1966). It has been postulated that secretion of selenium in bile and its enterohepatic reabsorption may provide a mechanism, in addition to renal control, for conserving body stores. This could have major implications for populations with a low dietary intake (Dreosti, 1986).

Selenium excretion, whether by the urinary or fecal route, is affected by the chemical form of the element in the diet. Significant differences have been found in urinary excretion in rats fed different forms of selenium, as was shown in a series of trials carried out by Robinson's group. One week after feeding rats with selenite, selenocysteine, selenomethionine, "rabbit kidney" selenium, and "fish muscle" selenium, cumulative levels of selenium excreted in urine were 14, 14, 5, 7, and 6% of the absorbed dose, respectively (Richold et al., 1977). There is evidence that the proportion of inorganic to organic selenium that appears in urine is affected by the form of the element provided to the animal, at least when injection, rather than ingestion, is the entry route. When selenomethione was injected into rats, only 3% of the selenium detected in the urine was inorganic, compared to over 35% when selenate was injected (Nahapetian et al., 1983).

Selenium excretion in humans also appears to be affected by the form of the element ingested. Women volunteers who consumed 1 mg of selenium as selenate excreted 81% of the intake in urine, but less than a third of this when selenite was substituted for the selenate (Robinson et al., 1985). Similarly, over a 2-week period, volunteers fed microgram quantities of selenite excreted approximately twice as much total selenium, in urine and feces, as when fed equivalent amounts of selenomethionine (Yang et al., 1989).

2.4.6.3 Pulmonary Excretion of Selenium

Excretion of selenium via the pulmonary route in expired air and via the dermal route in sweat are of minor significance at normal levels of dietary intake. Excretion through the lungs occurs principally when intake is unusually high. Excess selenium is detoxified by successive methylation to form the volatile dimethyl selenide and other methylated species. The garlic-like odor of dimethyl selenide on the breath is characteristic of selenium intoxication (McConnel and Roth, 1966).

2.4.6.4 Losses of Selenium in Hair and Nails

Selenium is also lost to the body to a limited extent in hair and nails. These excretory pathways are of little consequence, from the point of view of homeostasis. However, they do have practical consequences. Selenium levels in nails and hair have been used in several studies as a measure of selenium status (Chen et al., 1980). They are considered to reflect long-term intake and provide a convenient, noninvasive assessment method (Longnecker et al., 1936). However, hair, in particular, must be used with caution, since selenium-containing hair treatments are widely used.

2.4.7 *Selenium Pools and Stores in the Body*

Although there is no evidence of a specific storage form of selenium, analogous to ferritin for iron, there are indications that the human body is capable of storing the element in different body pools. Women, for instance, who moved from the USA where selenium intake is high to New Zealand where selenium intake is low, experienced only a slow drop in blood selenium levels over a year before it reached the local level (Rea et al., 1979).

The storage seems to be due, at least in part, to the nonspecific incorporation of selenomethionine into the primary structure of body proteins and subsequently made available at a rate corresponding to muscle turnover and selenomethionine catabolism (Alfthan et al., 1991). The storage appears to occur in muscle, kidney, and erythrocytes (Whanger et al., 1993).

References

Abrams, M.M., Shennan, C., Zazoski, J., and Burau, R.G., 1990, Selenomethionine uptake by wheat seedlings, *Agron. J.* **82**, 1127–1130.

Andrews, E.D., Hartley, W.J., and Grant, A.B., 1968, Selenium-responsive diseases in animals in New Zealand, *NZ J. Vet. Med.* **16**, 3–17.

Alfthan, G., Aro, A., Arvillomi, H., and Huttunen, J.K., 1991, Selenium metabolism and platelet glutathione peroxidase activity in healthy Finnish men: effects of selenium yeast, selenite and selenate, *Am. J. Clin. Nutr.* **53**, 120–125.

Arvy, M.P., 1993, Selenate and selenite uptake and translocation in bean plants (*Phaseolus vulgaris*), *J. Exp Bot.* **44**, 1083–1087.

Aslam, M., Harbit, K.B., and Huffaker, R.C., 1990, Comparative effects of selenite and selenate on nitrate assimilation in barley seedlings, *Plant Cell. Environ.* **13**, 773–782.

Baker, A.J.M. and Brookes, R.R., 1989, Terrestrial higher plants which accumulate metallic elements – a review of their distribution, ecology and phytochemistry, *Biorecovery* **1**, 81–126.

Bañuelos, G.S., Ajwa, H.A., Mackey, M., et al., 1997, Evaluation of different plant species used for phytoremediation of high soil selenium, *J. Environ. Quality* **26**, 639–646.

Barbezat, G.B., Casey, C.E., Reasbeck, P.G., et al., 1984, Selenium, in: Solomons, N.W. and Rosenberg, I.H. (eds), *Absorption and Malabsorption of Mineral Nutrients*, Liss, New York, pp. 213–258.

Bauer, F., 1997, Selenium and soils in the western United States, *Electronic Green J.* **7**, 1–5, http://egj.lib.uidaho.edu/egj07/bauer.htm

Beath, O.A., 1937, The occurrence of selenium and seleniferous vegetation in Wyoming II. Seleniferous vegetation, *Wyoming Agric. Exp. Station Bull.* **221**, 29–64.

Beath, O.A., Draise, J.H., Eppson, F., et al., 1934, Certain poisonous plants of Wyoming activated by selenium and their association with respect to soil types, *J. Am. Pharmacol. Assoc.* **23**, 94–97.

Bibow, K., Meltzer, H.M., Mundal, H.H., et al., 1993, Platelet selenium as indicator of wheat selenium intake, *J. Trace Elem. Electrolytes Health Dis.* **7**, 171–176.

Bosma, W., Svchupp, R., De Kok, L.J., and Rennenberg, H., 1991, Effect of selenate on assimilatory sulfate reduction and thiol content in spruce needles, *Plant Physiol. Biochem.* **29**, 131–138.

Brown, T.A. and Shrift, A., 1982, Selenium: toxicity and tolerance in higher plants, *Biol. Revs.* **57**, 59–84.

Broyer, T.C., Johnson, C.M., and Hudson, R.P., 1972, Selenium and nutrition of *Astragalus* I: effects of selenite or selenate supply on growth and selenium content, *Plant Soil* **36**, 635–649.

Burau, R.G., McDonald, A., Jacobson, A., et al., 1988, Selenium in tissues of crops sampled from the west side of the San Joaquin Valley, California, in: Tanji, K.K., Valoppi, L., and Woodring, R.C. (eds), *Selenium Contents in Animal and Human Food Crops Grown in California*, University of California Division of Agriculture and Natural Resources, Berkeley, CA, pp. 61–67.

Burk, R.F., 1976, Selenium in man, in: Prasad, A.S. (ed.), *Trace Elements in Human Health and Disease*, Academic Press, New York, pp. 105–133.

Byers, H.G., 1936, Selenium occurrence in certain soils in the United States, with a discussion of certain topics, *US Department of Agriculture Technical Bulletin*, No. 530, USDA, Washington, DC, pp. 1–8.

Chen, X., Yang, G.Q., Chen, J., et al., 1980, Studies on the relation of selenium and Keshan disease, *Biol. Trace Elem. Res.* **2**, 91–107.

Combs, G.F., 2001, Selenium in global food systems, *Br. J. Nutr.* **85**, 517–547.

Combs, G.F. Jr. and Combs, S.B., 1886a, Selenium in foods and feeds, in: Combs, G.F., Jr. and Combs, S.B. (eds), *The Role of Selenium in Nutrition*, Academic Press, New York, pp. 41–54.

Combs, G. and Combs, S., 1986b, *The Role of Selenium in Nutrition*, Academic Press, New York.

Cone, J.E., Martin del Rio, R., and Stadman, T.C., 1976, Selenocysteine in glycine reductase, *Proc. Natl Acad. Sci. USA* **73**, 2659–2663.

Demirici, A., 1999, Enhanced organically bound selenium yeast production by feed-batch fermentation, *J. Agric.Food Chem.* **47**, 2496–2500.

De Souza, M.P., Pilon-Smits, E.A.H., Lytle, C.M., et al., 1998, Rate limiting steps in selenium assimilation and volatilization by Indian mustard, *Plant Physiol.* **117**, 1487–1494

Dreosti, I, 1986, Selenium, *J. Food Nutr.* **43**, 60–78.

Duckart, E.C., Waldron, L.J., and Donner, H.E., 1992, Selenium uptake and volatilization from plants growing in soil, *Soil Sci.* **153**, 94–99.

Eustice, D.C., Kull, F.J., and Shrift, A., 1981, Selenium toxicity: aminoacylation and peptide bond formation with selenomethionine, *Plant Physiol.* **67**, 1054–1058.

Fairweather-Tait, S., 1997, Bioavailability of selenium, *Eur. J. Clin. Nutr.* **51**, S20–S23.

Ferretti, R.J. and Levander, O.A., 1974, Effect of milling and processing on the selenium content of grains and cereal products, *J. Agric. Food Chem.* **22**, 1049–1051.

Flohé, L., Gunzler, W.A., and Schock, H., 1973, Glutathione peroxidase: a selenoenzyme, *FEBS Lett.* **32**, 132–134.

Griffith, N.M., Stewart, R.D.H., and Robinson, M.F., 1976, The metabolism of ^{75}Se-selenomethionine in four women, *Br. J. Nutr*. **35**, 373–382.

Ihnat, M. and Aaseth, J., 1989, in: Ihnat, M. (ed.), *Occurrence and Distribution of Selenium*, CRC Press, Boca Raton, FL, pp. 169–212.

Iyengar, V. and Woittiez, J., 1988, Trace elements in human clinical specimens: evaluation of literature data to identify reference values, *Clin. Chem.* **34**, 474–481.

Jenkins, K.J. and Hidiroglou, M., 1972, Comparative metabolism of ^{75}Se-selenite, ^{75}Se-selenate and ^{75}Se-selenomethionine in bovine erythrocytes, *Can. J. Physiol. Pharmacol.* **50**, 927–935.

Kaspareck, K., Iyengar, G.V., Keiem, J., et al., 1979, Elemental composition of platelets. Part iii. Determination of Ag, Cd, Co, Cr, Mo, Rb, Sb and Se in normal human platelets by neutron activation analysis, *Clin. Chem.* **25**, 711–715.

Kobayashi, Y., Ogra, Y., Ishiwata, K., et al., 2002, Selenosugars are key and urinary metabolites for Se excretion within the required to low-toxic range, *Proc. Natl Acad. Sci. USA* **99**, 15932–15936.

Kuehnelt, D., Kienzl, N., Traar, P., et al., 2005, Selenium metabolites in human urine after ingestion of selenite, L-selenomethionine, or DL-selenomethionine: a quantitative case study by HPLC/ICPMS, *Anal. Bioanal. Chem.* **383**, 235–246.

Langlands, J.P., 1987, Recent advances in copper and selenium supplements in grazing ruminants, in: Farrell, D. (ed.), *Proceedings of Recent Advances in Animal Nutrition Conference*, University New England, Armidale, New South Wales, Australia, May, pp. 1–8.

László, R. and Csába, H., 2004, Iodine and selenium intake from soil to cultivated mushrooms, *2nd Intnational Symposium – Trace Elements in Food, Brussels, Belgium, 7–8 October, Abstracts*, European Commission Joint Research Centre, Brussels, Belgium, p. 21.

Levander, O.A., Alfthan, G., Arvilommi, H., et al., 1983, Bioavailability of selenium in Finnish men as assessed by platelet glutathione peroxidase and other blood parameters, *Am. J. Clin. Nutr.* **37**, 887–897.

Levander, O.A. and Baumann, C.A., 1966, Selenium metabolism VI. Effect of arsenic on excretion of selenium in the bile, *Toxicol. Appl. Pharmacol.* **9**, 106–115.

Levander, O.A., Sutherland, B., Morris, V.C. and King, J.C., 1981, Selenium balance in young men during selenium depletion and repletion, *Am. J. Clin. Nutr.* **34**, 2662–2669.

Linberg, P. and Jacobsson, S.O., 1970, Relationship between selenium content of forage, blood and organs of sheep, and lamb mortality rates, *Acta Vet. Scandinavica* **11**, 49–58.

Linder, M.C., 1988, *Nutritional Biochemistry and Metabolism*, Elsevier, New York, p. 177.

Lindström, K., 1948, Selenium as a growth factor for plankton in laboratory experiments and in some Swedish lakes, *Hydrobiology* **101**, 35–38.

Lindström, K. and Johansson, E., 1995, Improved techniques for analysis of selenium in fresh waters and biological materials, in: *Proc. STDA's Intnl. Symp, 8–10 May*, Brussels, Selenium-Tellurium Development Association, Grimbergen, Belgium, pp. 281–286.

Lombeck, I., Kasparek, K., Harbisch, H.D., et al., 1977, The selenium status of healthy children. I. Serum concentrations at different ages: activity of glutathione peroxidase of erythrocytes at different ages: selenium content of food of infants, *Eur. J. Pediat.* **125**, 81–89.

Longnecker, M.P., Stram, D.O., and Taylor, P.R., 1996, Use of selenium concentrations in whole blood, serum, toenails, or urine as a surrogate measure of selenium intake, *Epidemiology* **7**, 384–390.

McConnell, K.P. and Cho, G.J., 1965, Transmucosal movement of selenium, *Am. J. Physiol.* **208**, 1191–1195.

McConnell, K.P. and Roth, D.M., 1966, Respiratory excretion of selenium, *Proc. Soc. Exp. Biol. Med.* **123**, 919–921.

Marschner, H., 1995, *Mineral Nutrition of Higher Plants*, Academic Press, London, pp. 430–433.

Mikkelson, R.L., Page, A.l., and Bingham, A.T., 1989, Factors affecting selenium accumulation by agricultural crops, *Soil Sci. soc. Am. Special Publications* **23**, 65–94.

Mount, D.B. and Romero, M.F., 2004, The SLC26 gene family of multifunctional anion exchangers, *Pflugers Archives* **447**, 710–721.

Nahapetian, A.T., Janghorbani, M., and Young, V.R., 1983, Urinary trimethylselenonium excretion by the rat: effect of level and sources of ^{75}Se-selenium, *J. Nutr.* **113**, 401–411.

Ng, B.H. and Anderson, J.W., 1979, Light-dependent incorporation of selenite and sulphite into selenocysteine and cysteine by isolated pea chloroplasts, *Phytochemistry* **17**, 2069–2074.

Nigam,S.N., Tu, J-I., and McConnell, W.B., 1969, Distribution of selenomethylcysteine and some other amino acids in species of *Astragalus*, with special reference to their distribution during the growth of *A. bisulcatus*, *Phytochemistry* **8**, 1161–1165.

Novoselov, S.V., Rao, M., Onoshoko, N.V., et al., 2002, Selenoproteins and selenocysteine insertion in the model plant system, *Chlamydomonas reinhardii, EMBO J.* **21**, 3681–3693.

Oldfield, J.E., 1999, *Selenium in agriculture: the early years. A.L. Moxton Honorary Lecture*, Ohio State Uni. Extension Research, http://ohioline.osu/sc167/sc167-04.html

Oldfield, J.E., 1992, *Selenium in Fertilizers*, Selenium–Tellurium Development Association, Grimbergen, Belgium.

Oldfield, J.E., 1990, *Selenium: its Uses in Agriculture, Nutrition and Health and the Environment*, Selenium–Tellurium Development Association, Grimbergen, Belgium.

Oster, O., Schmiedel, G., and Prellwitz, W., 1988, The organ distribution of selenium in German adults, *Biol. Trace Elem. Res.* **15**, 23–45.

Padmaja, K., Prasad, D.D.K., and Prasad, A.R.K., 1989, Effect of selenium on chlorophyll biosynthesis in mung bean seedlings, *Phytochemistry* **28**, 3321–3324.

Patterson, E.L., Milstrey, R., and Stokstad, E.L., 1957, Effect of selenium in preventing exudative diathesis in chicks, *Proc. Soc. Exp Biol. Med.* **95**, 617–620.

Piepponen, S., Liukkonen-Lilja, H., and Kunsi, T., 1983, The selenium content of edible mushrooms in Finland, *Zeitschrift für Lebensmitteluntersuchung und-Forschung* **177**, 257–260.

Pykkö, K., Tuimala, R., Kroneld, R., et al., 1988, Effect of selenium supplementation to fertilizers on the selenium status of the population in different parts of Finland, *Eur. J. Clin. Nutr.* **42**, 571–579.

Rea, H.M., Thomson, C.D., Campbell, D.R., and Robinson, M.F., 1979, Relationship between erythrocyte selenium concentrations and glutathione peroxidase (EC 1.11.1.9) activities of New Zealand residents and visitors to New Zealand, *Br. J. Nutr.* **42**, 201–208.

Richold, M., Robinson, M. F., and Stewart, R.D.H., 1977, Metabolic studies in rats of ^{75}Se incorporated in vivo into fish muscle, *Br. J. Nutr.* **388**, 19–29.

Robinson, M.F., McKenzie, J.M., Thomson, C.D., and van Rij, A.L., 1973, Metabolic balance of zinc, copper, cadmium, iron, molybdenum and selenium in young New Zealand women, *Br. J. Nutr.* **30**, 195–205.

Robinson, J.R., Robinson, M.F., Levander, O.A., and Thomson, C.D., 1985, Urinary excretion of selenium by New Zealand and North American subjects on differing intakes, *Am. J. Clin. Nutr.* **41**, 1023–1031.

Rosenfeld, I. and Beath, O.A., 1961, *Selenium, Geobotany, Biochemistry, Toxicity, and Nutrition*, Academic Press, New York, pp. 7–8.

Rotruck, J.T., Ganther, H.E., Swanson, A.B., et al., 1972, Selenium: biochemical role as a component of glutathione peroxidase, *Science* **179**, 588–590.

Saiki, M.K. and Lowe, T.P., 1987, Selenium in aquatic organisms from subsurface agricultural drainage water, San Joaquin Valley, California, *Arch. Environ. Contam. Toxicol.* **19**, 496–499.

Sandholm, M., 1974, Selenium carrier proteins in mouse plasma, *Acta Pharmacol. Toxicol.* **35**, 427–431.

Schroeder, H.A., Frost, D.V., and Balassa, J.J., 1970, Essential trace elements in man: selenium, J. *Chronic Dis.* **23**, 227–243.

Schubert, A., Holden, J.M., and Wolf, W.R., 1987, Selenium content of a core group of foods based on a critical evaluation of published analytical data, *J. Am. Diet. Assoc.* **87**, 285–299.

Schwartz, K. and Foltz, C.M., 1957, Selenium an integral part of Factor 3 against dietary necrotic liver degeneration, *J. Am. Chem. Soc.* **79**, 3292–3293.

Shrift, A., 1969, Aspects of selenium metabolism in higher plants, *Ann. Rev. Plant Physiol.* **20**, 475–494.

Simon, P.F., 1560, Noticias historiales de las conquistas de tierre en las Indias occidentales, *Biblioteca Autores Colombianos*, Vol. 4, Kelly Publishing, Bogota, Colombia, 1953, pp. 226–254, cited in: Rosenfeld, I. and Beath, O.A., 1961, *Selenium, Geobotany, Biochemistry, Toxicity, and Nutrition*, Academic Press, New York.

Sirichakwal, P.P., Young V.P., and Janghorbani, M., 1985, Absorption and retention of selenium from intrinsically labelled egg and selenite as determined by stable isotope studies in humans, *Am. J. Clin. Nutr.* **41**, 264–269.

Stewart, R.D.H., Griffiths, N.M., Thomson, C.D., and Robinson, M.F., 1987, Quantitative selenium metabolism in normal New Zealand women, *Br. J. Nutr.* **40**, 45–54.

Suzuki, K.T., Kurasaki, K., Okazaki, N., and Ogra, Y., 2005, Selenosugar and trimethylselenonium among urinary metabolites: dose- and age-related changes, *Toxicol. Appl. Pharmacol.* **206**, 1–8.

Suzuki, K.T. and Ogra, Y., 2002, Metabolic pathways for selenium in the body: speciation by HPLC-ICP MS with enriched Se, *Food Add. Contam.* **19**, 974–983.

Terry, N. and Lin, Z.Q., 1999, *Managing High Selenium in Agricultural Drainage Water by Agroforestry Systems: Role of Selenium Volatilization*, Report of the Californian State Department of Water Resources, Sacramento, California, cited in: Terry, N., Zayed, A.M., De Souza, M.P., and Tarun, A.S., 2000, Selenium in higher plants, *Ann. Rev. Plant Physiol. Plant Mol. Biol.* **51**, 401–432.

Terry, N., Carlson, C., Raab, T.K., and Zayed, A.M., 1992, Selenium uptake and volatilization among crop species, *J. Environ. Quality* **21**, 341–344.

Terry, N., Zayed, A.M., De Souza, M.P., and Tarun, A.S., 2000, Selenium in higher plants, *Ann. Rev. Plant Physiol. Plant Mol. Biol.* **51**, 401–432.

Thomson, C.D., 1998, Selenium speciation in human body fluids, *Analyst* **123**, 827–831.

Thomson, C.D. and Robinson, M.F., 1986, Urinary and faecal excretions and absorptions of a large supplement of selenium: superiority of selenate over selenite, *Am. J. Clin. Nutr.* **44**, 659–663.

Thomson, C.D. and Robinson, M.F., 1980, Selenium in human health and disease with emphasis on those aspects peculiar to New Zealand, *Am. J. Clin. Nutr.* **33**, 303–323.

Thomson, C.D. and Stewart, R.D.H., 1973, Metabolic studies of ^{75}Se-selenomethionine and ^{75}Se-selenite in rat, *Br. J. Nutr.* **30**, 139–147.

Tinggi, U., 2005, Selenium toxicity and its adverse health effects, in: Preedy, R. and Watson, R.R. (eds), *Reviews in Food and Nutrition Toxicity*, Taylor & Francis, Boca Raton, FL, pp. 29–55.

Tinggi, U., Reilly, C., and Patterson, C.M., 1992, Determination of selenium in foodstuffs, using spectrofluorimetry and hydride generation atomic absorption spectrometry, *J. Food Comp. Anal.* **5**, 269–280.

Trelase, S.F. and Trelase.H.M., 1939, Physiological differentiation in *Astragalus* with reference to selenium, *Am. J. Bot.* **26**, 530–535.

Turner, D.C. and Stadman, T.C., 1973, Selenium a requirement for glycine reductase activity in *Clostridium sticklandii*, *Arch. Biochem. Biophys.* **154**, 366–381.

Ullrey, D.E., 1981, Selenium in the soil-plant-food chain, in: Spallholz, J.E., Martin, J.L., and Ganther, H.E. (eds), *Selenium in Biology and Medicine*, Avi Publishing, Westport, VA, pp. 176–191.

Underwood, E.J., 1977, *Trace Elements in Human and Animal Nutrition*, 4th edn., Academic Press, London, pp. 302–46.

University of California Agricultural Issues Center, 1988, Selenium, human health and agricultural issues, in: *Resources at Risk in the San Joaquin Valley*, Uni. California, Davis, CA, pp. 1–23.

Versieck, J. and Cornelis, R., 1989, *Trace Elements in Human Plasma or Serum*, CRC Press, Boca Raton, FL, pp. 2–3.

Wells, N., 1967, Selenium in horizons of soil profiles, *NZ J. Sci.* **10**, 142–153.

Werner, A.R. and Beelman, R.B., 2001, Growing selenium-enriched mushrooms as ingredients for functional foods or dietary supplements, *Int. J. Med. Mushrooms* **3**, 112–120.

Whanger, P., Xia, V., and Thomson, C., 1993, Metabolism of different forms of selenium in humans, *J. Trace Elem. Electrolytes Health Dis.* **7**, 121–125.

WHO/FAO, 2002, *Human Vitamin and Mineral Requirements: Report of a Joint WHO/FAO Expert Committee*, World Health Organization/Food and Agricultural Organisation, Rome, pp. 235–255.

Wu, L., Huang, Z.Z., and Burau, R.G., 1988, Selenium accumulation and selenium-salt co-tolerance in five grass species, *Crop Sci.* **28**, 517–522.

Yang, G.Q., 1991, Diet and naturally-occurring human diseases caused by inadequate intake of essential trace elements, in: *Proceedings of the 6th Asian Congress of Nutrition*, Kuala Lumpur, Malaysia, 16–19 Sept, pp. 79–92.

Yang, G., Wang, S., Zhou, R., and Sun, S., 1983, Endemic selenium intoxication of humans in China, *Am. J. Clin. Nutr.* **37**, 872–881.

Yang, G., Zhou, R. Gu, L., et al., 1989, Studies of safe maximal daily dietary selenium intake in a seleniferous area of China. 1. Selenium intake and tissue selenium levels of the inhabitants, *Trace Elem. Electrolytes Health Dis.* **37**, 77–87.

Young, V.S., Nahapetian, A., and Janghorbani, M., 1982, Selenium bioavailability with reference to human nutrition, *Am. J. Clin. Nutr.* **35**, 1076–1088.

Zayed, A.M. and Terry, N., 1994, Selenium volatilization in roots and shoots: effects of shoot removal and sulfate level, *J. Plant Physiol.* **143**, 8–14.

Zayed, A., Lytle, C.M., and Terry, N., 1998, Accumulation and volatilization of different chemical species of selenium by plants, *Planta* **206**, 284–292.

Zayed, A.M., Piton-Smits, E.A.H., De Souza, M.P., et al., 1999, Remediation of selenium-polluted soils and waters by phytovolatilization, in: Terry, N. and Bañuelos, G. (eds), *Phytoremediation of Metal-Contaminated Water and Soils*, CRC Press, Boca Raton, FL, pp. 61–83.

Zinoni, F., Birkmann, K., Stadman, T.C., and Bock, A., 1986, Cotranslational insertion of selenocysteine into formate dehydrogenase from *Eschericia coli* directed by a UGA codon, *Proc. Natl Acad. Sci.* **84**, 4650–4654.

3
Selenium Metabolism

3.1 The Metabolic Roles of Selenium

The primary role of most of the selenium absorbed in the gastrointestinal tract is to be incorporated into proteins, either specifically into a number of different selenoenzymes or nonspecifically into muscle protein. None of the element remains in inorganic and noncomplexed form. Because of its chemical reactivity, it is essential that selenium be handled mainly in a relatively unreactive organic form before its incorporation into catalytically reactive selenoproteins (Arthur, 2003). The mechanisms by which it is incorporated into these proteins are complex, and though a great deal is now known about the process, there are still considerable gaps in our understanding of what is involved, as well as of the functions of many of the different selenoproteins produced. Indeed, in spite of more than 50 years of investigation of selenium metabolism, it is only recently that answers have been found to many uncertainties about the element. What has made this progress possible is an impressive coordination of input from experts in a range of disciplines such as nutrition, human biology, biochemistry, molecular biology, genetics, and other related fields, and, most recently, computing science. A major contribution to progress is being made by the rapidly developing specialization of bioinformatics. Recent advances in genomics have been particularly significant, especially the sequencing of the human genome (Katsanis et al., 2001). A variety of computational biology methods have been used to investigate the human selenoproteome, in which some 25 selenoprotein genes have been identified (Gladyshev et al., 2004).

3.1.1 Selenoproteins

When it was discovered in the 1970s that selenium was a constituent of the antioxidant enzyme glutathione peroxidase (GPX), it was believed that the principal, if not the sole, role of the element was as an antioxidant (Rotruck et al., 1973). Subsequent findings have made it clear that selenium, acting through the expression of a wide range of selenoproteins, has diverse roles in the animal body.

In addition to its antioxidant activities, it is involved in thyroid hormone homeostasis, immunity and fertility, and many other activities. It has been shown to have anticancer properties, to act as a growth factor, and to play important roles in the regulation of synthesis of leukotrienes, thromboxanes, and prostaglandins, and in other metabolic functions (Imai et al., 1998).

All the biological functions attributed to selenium are mediated by selenoproteins. The element is incorporated into the primary structure of these proteins as the amino acid selenocysteine (Sec). More than 40 different selenoproteins have been identified in mammals by sodium dodecyl sulphate-polyacrylamide gel electrophoresis (SDS-PAGE) of ^{75}Se-labeled tissue. Some 20 of these have so far been characterized by purification and cloning (Arthur and Beckett, 1994). Computer searches of the human genome have identified all, or almost all, the genes that encode Sec-containing proteins and have characterized their genomic sequences. These computational investigations have identified 25 selenoprotein genes, as listed in Table 3.1. The names and abbreviations for the different selenoproteins are those used by Gladyshev and his colleagues in their recent reviews (Hatfield and Gladyshev, 2002; Gladyshev et al., 2004). Other names and abbreviations are, however, sometimes used by different authors, leading to a certain amount of confusion among those not familiar with the subject.

The selenoproteins that have been found to be expressed in mammals include several different GPXs, three thyroid hormone deiodinases, and three thioredoxin reductases (TRs). In all of the selenoenzymes so far characterized, selenium is found in the form of Sec at the active site. At physiological pH the selenium in Sec is fully ionized and acts as a very efficient redox catalyst. The selenoproteins with known functions play critical roles in a variety of biological processes, including antioxidant function, thyroid hormone metabolism, and redox balance (McKenzie et al., 2002). In addition to these three "families" of enzymes, a number of other selenoproteins have been identified, with other functions, not all of which have yet been clearly identified.

3.1.1.1 The Glutathione Peroxidases

At least six mammalian GPX isoenzymes have so far been described (Beckett and Arthur, 2005). Each of these appears to be located in a different cellular compartment. They are also impaired to a different degree by selenium deficiency. Thus, depending on the sensitivity of each GPX to selenium deficiency, loss of activity from a particular tissue could cause a specific organ-related condition. This could account for the involvement of selenium deficiency in the pathogenesis of apparently unrelated clinical conditions (Arthur et al., 1987).

"Classical" GPX1, also known as intracellular or cytosolic GPX (cGPX), was the first functional selenoprotein to be clearly characterized. It was originally recognized in 1957, but its selenium dependence was not shown until 1971 (Rotruck et al., 1973). It was found in erythrocytes, where it protected hemoglobin against oxidative damage by hydrogen peroxide (Mills, 1957). The enzyme consists of four identical 22 kDa subunits, each of which contains one Sec residue, with the

TABLE 3.1 Human selenoprotein genes: selenocysteine location and protein length

Selenoprotein	Sec location in protein (protein length)
Thyroid hormone deiodinase 1 (ID1)	126 (249)
Thyroid hormone deiodinase 2 (ID2)	133 (265)
Thyroid hormone deiodinase 3 (ID3)	144 (278)
Glutathione peroxidase 1 (GPX1)	47 (201)
Glutathione peroxidase 2 (GPX2)	40 (190)
Glutathione peroxidase 3 (GPX3)	73 (226)
Glutathione peroxidase 4 (GPX4)	73 (197)
Glutathione peroxidase 6 (GPX6)	73 (221)
Selenoprotein H	44 (122)
Selenoprotein I	387 (397)
Selenoprotein K	92 (94)
Selenoprotein M (SelM)	48 (145)
Selenoprotein N (SelN)	428 (556)
Selenoprotein O	667 (669)
Selenoprotein P (SelP)	59, 300, 318, 330, 345, 352, 367, 369, 376, 378 (381)[a]
Selenoprotein R (methionine-R-sulphoxide reductase; MsrB)	95 (116)
Selenoprotein S	118 (189)
Sep 15 (15 kDa selenoprotein)	93 (116)
Selenophosphate synthetase 2 (SPS2)	60 (448)
Selenoprotein T (Sel T)	36 (182)
Thioredoxin reductase 1 (TR1)	498 (499)
Thioredoxin reductase 2 (TR2)	655 (656)
Thioredoxin reductase 3 (TR3)	522 (523)
Selenoprotein V	273 (346)
Selenoprotein W (Sel W)	13 (87)

Source: Adapted from Gladyshev, V.N., Kryukov, G.V., Fomento, D.E., and Hatfield, D.L., 2004, Identification of trace element-containing proteins in genomic databases, *Ann. Rev. Nutr.* **24**, 579–596; and Hatfield, D.L. and Gladyshev, V.N., 2002, How selenium has altered our understanding of the genetic code, *Mol. Cell. Biol.* **22**, 3565–3576.

[a]All selenoproteins have a single Sec, except for SelP, which has 10 Sec residues.

ionized selenol moiety acting as the redox center in the peroxidase (Forstrum et al., 1978). It is expressed by all cell types in mammals. GPX1 can metabolize a wide range of free hydroperoxides as well as hydrogen peroxide, but not hydroperoxides of fatty acids esterified in phospholipids, such as those in cell membranes (Grossman and Wendel, 1983). The enzyme may also function as a selenium store, a role that could account for its usefulness, at least under certain conditions, as an indicator of selenium status.

GPX2 and GPX3, also known as extracellular GPX, have similar tetrameric structures to GPX1. They are also antioxidants, though they operate in different compartments, with GPX2 in the gastrointestinal tract and GPX3 in plasma (Takahasi and Cohen, 1986). GPX3 is a secreted glycoprotein and is the second most abundant selenoprotein in plasma.

GPX4, also known as phospholipid hydroperoxide GPX (PHGPx), is a protein monomer of 20 to 30 kDa, similar in structure to a single subunit of the other

GPXs. It is found in the same organs as GPX1, but not in the same amounts. In rat liver, for example, there is relatively little, but it is abundant in testis where it may be regulated by gonadotrophins (Roveri et al., 1992). It is more resistant to the effects of selenium deficiency than are other GPXs, which may indicate that GPX4 has a more important antioxidant role than the other enzymes in the family (Arthur, 1992). It has also been suggested that the major nutritional interaction between selenium and vitamin E may be protection of the cell membranes by GPX4 and the vitamin against oxidative damage (Ursini and Bindoli, 1987). In addition to its antioxidative activities, GPX4 is believed to have a number of other roles, for example, in eicosanoid metabolism (Ursini et al., 1997). There is evidence that it is involved in male fertility, having been identified as an enzymatically inactive structural protein of the mitochondrial capsule of spermatozoa where the protein becomes oxidatively cross-linked and inactive (Ursini et al., 1999). It may also be involved in moderating apoptotic cell death (Nomura et al., 2001).

A selenoprotein, similar in composition to GPX4 except in its N-terminal sequence, has been found by ^{75}Se-labeling and separation by SDS-PAGE. It occurs only in testis and spermatozoa of rats after the onset of puberty and is localized in the nuclei of the late spermatids. It has been identified as a specific sperm nuclei GPX (snGPX) and has been shown to act as a protamine thiol peroxidase responsible for disulphide cross-linking and to be necessary for sperm maturation and male fertility (Bene and Kyriakopoulos, 2001).

The function of GPX5 is unclear. GPX6 has been identified by the use of bioinformatic methods to search the human genome. Little is known about its structure or function. It appears to be a homolog of GPX1. It has been detected only in embryos and the olfactory epithelium (Kryukov et al., 2003).

3.1.1.2 The Iodothyronine Deiodinases

The iodothyronine deiodinases play a major physiological role in the body by catalyzing the activation and inactivation of the thyroid hormones, which are responsible for regulating several metabolic processes. The deiodinase family consists of three members that differ in their tissue location, how they are involved in the deiodination of thyroxine, and how, through their combined operation and interaction, they are responsible for the precise and tissue-specific regulation of thyroid hormone metabolism (Bianco et al., 2002). All are integral membrane proteins of 29 to 33 kDa and share 50% sequence identity. Their complex protein structures have been described recently (Callebaut et al., 2002).

The discovery that selenium was involved in iodine metabolism was the first indication that the element had other metabolic roles besides those of a peroxidase which, until then, had appeared to be its sole role. Type 1 deiodinase (IDI) was tentatively identified as a selenoprotein when it was shown that selenium deficiency increased levels of thyroxine (T4), while reducing those of 3,3′,5-triiodothyronine (T3) in rat plasma, and that these changes were due to decreased hepatic deiodinase activity (Beckett et al., 1987). The enzyme was subsequently isolated and its identity as a selenoprotein substantiated by cloning. Its mRNA has been shown to contain a single in-frame UGA codon-specifying Sec at the active site in each substrate-binding subunit (Berry et al., 1991a). IDI is a membrane-bound protein, consisting of a homodimer with two 27 kDa subunits, each of which contains one Sec residue (Berry et al., 1991b). It is located mainly in the thyroid, liver, kidney, and pituitary.

The metabolic role of IDI is to catalyze monodeiodination of the iodothyronines at the 5′-position of the phenolic ring or the 5-position of the tyrosyl ring. The former action results in the formation of the biologically active T3, and the latter, the biologically inactive isomer 3,3′,5-triiodothyronine (reverse T3). Further, deiodination of T3 and reverse T3 leads to the formation of another biologically inactive isomer, 3,3′-diiodothyronine (D2). Thus, the overall role of IDI appears to be to provide active T3 to the plasma, to inactivate T4 and T3, and to eliminate reverse T3 from the circulation (Arthur et al., 1990).

Type 2 deiodinase (ID2) is a membrane-bound Sec-containing protein, with subunits of about 32 kDa. It is expressed predominantly in the brain, brown adipose tissue, pituitary, and placenta. It only catalyzes 5′-monodeiodination and converts T4 to T3 and reverse T3 to T2. Its main role appears to be intracellular production of T3 (Salvatore et al., 1996).

A third iodothyronine deiodinase, type 3 deiodinase (ID3), has also been shown to be a selenoenzyme (Croteau et al., 1995). It is a 32 kDa protein, located mainly in the central nervous system, placenta, and skin. It catalyzes the deiodination of the tyrosyl ring and inactivates thyroid hormones by producing reverse T3 from T4 and T2 from T3. Its role appears to be protection of the developing brain from excessive amounts of T3 (Kaplan, 1986). It also regulates the supply of T4 and T3 from the mother to the fetus (Mortimer et al., 1996).

3.1.1.3 Thioredoxin Reductases

The mammalian TRs are members of the pyridine nucleotide-disulphide family of enzymes that occur in various tissues. They are flavine adenine dinucleotide (FAD)-containing homodimeric selenoenzymes that, in conjunction with thioredoxin (Trx) and NADPH, form a powerful dithiol–disulphide oxidoreductase with multiple roles, known as the TR/Trx system (McKenzie et al., 1996). The significance of TR for the mammalian organism has been shown by an experiment in which targeted disruption of the TR gene in a pregnant mouse resulted in death of the embryo at an early stage of development (Matsui et al., 1996).

Each TR subunit has a single Sec as the penultimate C-terminal amino acid residue (Gladyshev et al.,1996), which is indispensable for their enzymatic activity (Gromer et al., 1998). A number of isoforms of TR have been identified. Thioredoxin reductase 1 (TR1) or cytosolic TR, is a dimer consisting of two identical 56 kDa protein subunits. It was the first TR to be identified as a mammalian Sec-containing TR (Tamura and Stadtman, 1996). Thioredoxin reductase 2 (TR2), or mitochondrial TR, is believed to consist of units of about 56 kDa, with a structure similar to, but not identical with, that of TR1 (Mustacich and Powis, 2000).

Its biological role is not known but it appears to act as a mitochondrial-specific defense against reactive oxygen species produced by the respiratory chain (Lee et al., 1999).

Several other isoforms of TR have been described. One of these, listed as TR3, is similar to TR1 in structure, though it has a long N-terminal extension and a higher molecular mass (Sun et al., 1999). Another form, TR-β has also been described. This has a distinct pattern of tissue expression, with high levels in prostate, testis, liver, uterus, and, small intestine (Arner and Holmgren, 2000). Recent findings, including those obtained by scanning the human genome, point to the existence of further TR species, which may differ in their distribution between tissues and cellular compartments and have specific biological roles (Bene and Kyriakopoulos, 2001).

The TRs affect many different cellular processes. They can catalyze a number of different substrates in addition to Trx, including low molecular weight disulphides and nonsulphides, such as selenate, selenodiglutathione, vitamin K, alloxan, and lipid hyrdoperoxides, as well as dehydroascorbic acid (Holmgren, 2001).

The TR/Trx system is a key player in DNA synthesis, with Trx as a hydrogen donor for ribonucleotide reductase in the initial and rate-limiting step. TR also regulates gene expression through the activation of DNA-binding activity of transcription factors (Berggrem et al., 1996). The system is also involved in several other key functions, including regulation of cell growth, inhibition of apoptosis, regeneration of proteins inactivated by oxidative stress, and regulation of the cellular redox state (Holmgren, 2001). In a cell-free environment, the TR/Trx system can directly reduce hydrogen peroxide, as well as organic and lipid hydroperoxides, and serve as an electron donor to plasma GPX (Björnstedt et al., 1994) and ID1. Considerable interest is currently being shown in the TRs because of their possible relation to a number of diseases in humans and their potential for the development of therapeutic drugs (Gromer et al., 2004).

3.1.1.4 Selenophosphate Synthetase

Selenophosphate synthetase is responsible for the synthesis of selenophosphate, an intermediate in the biosynthesis of Sec. In prokaryotes, the enzyme is identified with the gene product Sel D. Two selenophosphate synthetases have been identified in eukaryotes: Sps 1 and Sps 2. The latter is a Sec-containing protein of about 50 kDa (Low et al., 1995). It has been surmised that if the activity of Sps 2 depends on availability of selenium, the enzymes could have a role as a sensitive autoregulation of selenoprotein synthesis (Guimaraes et al., 1996).

3.1.1.5 Selenoprotein P

Selenoprotein P (Se-P) is a glycoprotein of 43 kDa that contains 10 to 12 Sec residues per molecule. It is the only selenoenzyme that, so far, has been found to contain more than one Sec. The molecule is also rich in histidine and cysteine residues and as a result appears to have strong metal-binding properties. Four isoforms of Se–P have been identified (Ma et al., 2002). Se–P is mainly expressed in liver but is also present in other tissues. It is the major selenoprotein of blood, providing between 60 and 70% of the element in plasma (Read et al., 1990). Its function is still uncertain. It may serve as an antioxidant, especially in extracellular fluid. There is evidence indicating that it can function to protect endothelial cells against peroxidative damage during inflammation, particularly when caused by peroxynitrite, a reactive species formed during the reaction between nitric oxide and superoxide under inflammatory conditions (Arteel et al., 1999). Because of its high selenium content and its extracellular location, it is thought that Se-P may also have a role as a transporter of selenium from the liver to sites where it is required for incorporation into other selenoproteins (Mostenbocker and Tappel, 1982).

3.1.1.6 Other Selenoproteins

Selenoprotein W (Se-W) was first purified from rat skeletal muscle. It is enriched in skeletal and heart muscle, brain, testis, spleen, and some other tissues. It is a low molecular weight cytosolic protein of approximately 10 kDa, with a single Sec residue per molecule (Vendeland et al., 1995). Its biochemical and physiological roles are not known. It appears to be involved in the metabolism of heart muscle, possibly acting in a redox role with glutathione (Gu et al., 1999). In lambs and other farm animals it may be necessary for prevention, in conjunction with vitamin E, of white muscle disease. Levels of Se-W respond rapidly to changes in selenium intake, making it potentially a useful marker of selenium status (Whanger et al., 1993).

15 kDa Selenoprotein (Sel15), a Sec-containing protein that has been detected in both rats and humans, is highly expressed in epithelial cells of the prostate gland (Gladyshev et al., 1998). Since it has been found that the gene for Sel15 is located on a chromosome often affected by cancer (Kumaraswamy et al., 2000), and also that selenium supplementation appears to decrease incidence of prostate cancer (Clark et al., 1998), it is believed that Sel15 may play a role in protection against this form of cancer. In addition to prostate Sel15, a more ubiquitous Sel15 also occurs in mammals (Gladyshev, 2001).

Several other Sec-containing proteins have been identified by bioinformatic methods, but their functions remain unknown. They include an 18 kDa mitochondrial selenoprotein (Kyriakopoulos et al., 1996). They are sometimes described as "orphan selenoproteins" and have been identified by the abbreviations SelR, SelT, SelN, SelX, SelZf1, and SelZf2 (Kryukov et al., 1999; Lescure et al., 1999). Apart from SelR, which has been shown to be a methionine sulfoxide reductase (Kryukov et al., 2002), little is known about these selenoproteins.

Several other selenium-containing proteins, including some less than 10 kDa in size, have been detected by SDS-PAGE and autoradiography. Some of the bands could be further resolved into several spots with different isoelectric points (Kyriakopoulos et al., 2000). Although some of these compounds may be precursors or metabolic products of other selenoproteins, these findings suggest that in addition to the Sec-containing proteins whose existence has so far been confirmed, there are other mammalian selenoproteins still awaiting identification (Bene and Kyriakopoulos, 2001).

3.2 Selenoprotein Synthesis

Our understanding of how selenium is inserted into selenium-containing functional proteins and, not least, of the genetic implications of the processes involved, has progressed at a rapid pace over the past decade. Selenium is present in these proteins in two basic forms (Hatfield and Gladyshev, 2002). One of these, in which the selenium is inserted into the protein posttranslationally as a dissociable cofactor, is extremely rare, found only in a few bacterial molybdenum-containing enzymes, such as an NADP(+)-coupled nicotinic acid hydroxylase in *Clostridium barkeri* (Gladyshev et al., 1996). In all the other functional selenoproteins so far discovered, selenium is inserted cotranslationally into the protein as the amino acid Sec. This process is found in all the major domains of life and is responsible for the majority of the biological effects of selenium (Hatfield and Gladyshev, 2002).

Elucidation of the complex steps involved in the synthesis of Sec and its subsequent incorporation into selenoproteins has been achieved through the collaboration of investigators from a wide range of specialisms, especially molecular biology and genetics (Stadtman, 1990). Their findings, which show that Sec is dramatically different from any of the other amino acids in its mode of incorporation and biosynthetic steps, have, among other significant consequences, dramatically altered our understanding of the genetic code (Hatfield and Gladyshev, 2002).

3.2.1 Selenocysteine: the 21st Amino Acid

Examination of the primary structure of Sec reveals its similarity to two other amino acids, serine and cysteine, as seen in Figure 3.1. This similarity could suggest that its synthesis is brought about by straightforward posttranslational replacement by selenium of serine oxygen or cysteine sulfur. This is not, in fact, what occurs (Burk and Hill, 1993). The synthesis is a cotranslational event, with Sec encoded by a UGA codon. The finding that a codon had specified the insertion into a protein of an amino acid, other than one of the 20 S-amino acids already known to be genetically encoded, was unexpected and remarkable. This was the first time that a nonstandard amino acid had been shown to be incorporated into protein during translation. Sec, according to Stadman (1990), was the 21st amino acid, in terms of ribosome-mediated protein synthesis.

Sec was, for many years, believed to be unique among nonstandard amino acids in being genetically encoded. Recently, however, another nonstandard amino acid, pyrrolysine, has been found to be inserted into protein in response to

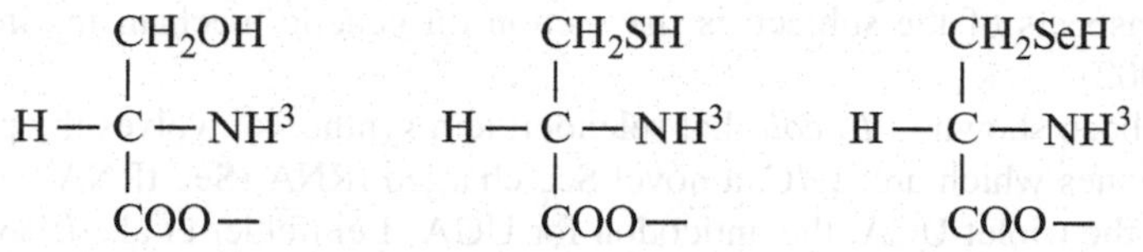

$$
\begin{array}{ccc}
CH_2OH & CH_2SH & CH_2SeH \\
| & | & | \\
H-C-NH^3 & H-C-NH^3 & H-C-NH^3 \\
| & | & | \\
COO- & COO- & COO-
\end{array}
$$

FIGURE 3.1 Structures of serine, cysteine and selenocysteine

a UAG codon and has been designated the 22nd amino acid (Srinivasan et al., 2002). Unlike Sec, however, pyrrolysine is not widely distributed in nature and has been found only in certain eubacteria and archaebacteria (Gladyshev et al., 2004)

3.2.1.1 Dual Function of the UGA Codon

The finding that Sec was genetically encoded was not the only surprising discovery. No less remarkable was the fact that the UGA codon responsible for Sec insertion was known up to that time as a stop codon, signaling, not amino acid insertion, but termination of protein synthesis. It is now known that such a dual function of a codon, though unusual, is not unique. The codon AUG, for instance, which normally codes for the initiation of protein synthesis, also codes for the insertion of methionine at internal positions in the protein (Hatfield and Gladyshev, 2002), while the codon UAG, which, as we have seen, codes for the insertion of pyrrolysine in protein in certain archaea, also functions as a stop codon (Srinivasan et al., 2002).

3.2.2 Selenoprotein Synthesis in Prokaryotes

Although a great deal is now known about the manner in which Sec is synthesized in mammals and how it is incorporated into their proteins, there are still gaps in our knowledge. Much of the information we do have about the synthetic process has been obtained from the study of bacteria, especially *Escherichia coli*. Although there are clear differences between the prokaryotes and eukaryotes, this information does allow us to give an overall, if still incomplete, picture of what occurs in mammals (Hatfield and Gladyshev, 2002).

It would be beyond the scope of this book, however, to attempt to go into all the details of what is known about the processes of selenoprotein synthesis, and that will not be attempted here. For those who wish to follow up these details, several excellent reviews can be consulted. Recommended in particular is that by Driscoll and Copeland (2003), which concentrates largely on the mechanisms and regulation of the synthesis, as well as those by Gladyshev et al. (2004), and Hatfield and Gladyshev (2002), which cover genetic aspects in some detail. A further recommendation, especially for readers who are not too familiar with modern aspects of the subject, is the section on genetic mechanisms in Albert et al. (2002).

It has been shown in *E. coli* that selenoprotein synthesis involves the products of four genes which are: *selC*, a novel Sec-charged tRNA (Sec-tRNA^{Sec}), which contains the triplet UCA, the anticodon for UGA (Leinfelder et al., *1988*); *selA*, the enzyme Sec synthase; *selD*, another enzyme, selenophosphate synthetase (both of these enzymes are essential for the formation of Sec-tRNA^{Sec} from seryl-tRNA^{Sec}); and *selB*, an elongation factor that specifically recognizes Sec-tRNA^{Sec} (Heider et al.,1992).

The first step in the synthesis of Sec is the aminoacylation of the amino acid serine by the enzyme serine synthetase to produce Ser-tRNA^{Sec} (Leinfelder et al., 1990). The serine residue is then used to provide the carbon backbone for Sec. The conversion is brought about by the action of the pyridoxal phosphate-dependent enzyme Sec synthase that changes Ser-tRNA^{Sec} into Sec-tRNA^{Sec} via an intermediate compound, aminoacrylyl-tRNA^{Sec}. This intermediate serves as an acceptor for activated selenium, resulting in the formation of selenocysteyl-tRNA$^{[Ser]Sec}$. The designation tRNA$^{[Ser]Sec}$ indicates that the serine is converted into Sec while attached to the tRNA (Jameson et al., 2002). The two-stage reaction requires ATP (Leinfelder et al., 1988) and involves loss of water (Forschammer and Bock, 1991).

The donor for this reaction has been characterized in prokaryotes as monoselenophosphate that is synthesized from selenium in its reduced selenide form. The selenide is joined to the aminoacrylyl intermediate under the influence of selenophosphate synthetase. The reaction involves hydrolysis of ATP in the presence of magnesium ions. It is likely, but not yet established, that the same donor is employed in eukaryotes (Leinfelder, 1990).

In normal protein synthesis, polypeptide elongation is brought about with the help of an elongation factor, EF-Tu. This forms a ternary complex with GTP and an aminoacylated tRNA which enters the ribosome attached to an mRNA molecule. The mRNA is then pulled through the ribosome and, as its codons encounter the ribosome's active site and a specific codon/anticodon interaction occurs, GTP is hydrolyzed, EF-Tu undergoes a conformational change, and the charged tRNA is freed to add its amino acid in its correct sequence to the growing polypeptide chain. When a stop codon is encountered, elongation of the chain ceases and the finished protein is released.

The process is different in the cotranslational incorporation of Sec. This requires the formation of a quaternary complex between SelB, GTP, Sec-tRNA^{Sec}, and a specific sequence in the selenoprotein mRNA. This sequence is known as the bacterial Sec insertion sequence (bSECIS). It is a stem-loop structure located immediately downstream of the UGA/Sec codon (Huttenhofer et al., 1996). SelB has a unique C-terminal domain, not found in EF-Tu, which mediates its ability to bind to mRNA. This quaternary complex can be considered a "docking device" at the ribosomal site, bringing together the elements necessary for Sec insertion into the nascent polypeptide (Kromayer et al., 1996).

3.2.3 Selenoprotein Synthesis in Eukaryotes

As has been noted, while selenoprotein synthesis in eukaryotes is similar in many respects to the process in prokaryotes, there are some crucial differences. One of these is the location of the SECIS element. In eukaryotes this is found in the 3′untranslated region (3′UTR) of the mRNA and must therefore be effectively acting at a distance, in contrast to prokaryotes in which the sequences are located immediately downstream from the UGA/Sec codon in the open reading frame (Grunder-Culemann et al., 2001). By analogy with the prokaryotic system, a model for the eukaryotic selenoprotein biosynthesis has been proposed which involves a complex of the SECIS element with Sec-tRNA^{Sec} and two proteins, SECIS-binding protein 2 (SBP2) and eukaryotic or mammalian Sec-specific elongation factor (eEFSec), also designated mSelB (Berry et al., 2001). Between them, these two novel proteins are believed to perform functions equivalent to those of SelB in bacteria. Although their structures and precise roles remain to be clarified, it is believed that the two proteins, possibly along with other as yet unidentified proteins, form a large complex that links the SECIS element in the 3′UTR to other elements in the coding region and the ribosome, and allow the UGA codon to be translated as Sec insertion, and not as termination of protein synthesis (Hesketh and Villette, 2002). A simplified outline of the process of selenoprotein synthesis in mammals is shown in Figure 3.2.

3.3 Regulation of Selenoprotein Expression

There is clear evidence, from animal and human studies, that selenoprotein expression is regulated by selenium supply and that selenium deficiency causes a general, though not uniform, decrease in the levels of all selenoproteins (Burk and Hill, 1993). This regulation occurs in a carefully controlled fashion, with prioritization of the available selenium (Hesketh and Villette, 2002). It is believed that there is a hierarchy of selenoprotein expression with respect to maintaining levels of individual selenoproteins and retaining selenium in different organs (Hatfield and Gladyshev, 2002). The effect of deficiency on individual selenoproteins is shown by the finding that while severe deficiency can cause GPX1 activity in rat liver to decrease by 99%, it brings about a fall of 75% in GPX4 activity in the same tissue. Deficiency caused different levels of reduction of activity of the enzymes in different organs of the rats. Compared to the drastic reduction to 1% of control activity in liver, reductions of GPX1 activity in heart, kidney, and lung tissue were about 4 to 9% of levels in selenium-sufficient animals. GPX4 activity was reduced to 25 to 50% in the same tissues and was unaffected in testis (Lei et al., 1995).

Changes in activity of selenoproteins brought about by selenium deficiency are accompanied by changes in abundance of the mRNA of the different proteins. Although changes in mRNA do not always correlate with changes in selenoprotein activity, they do parallel the hierarchy of effects on protein expression.

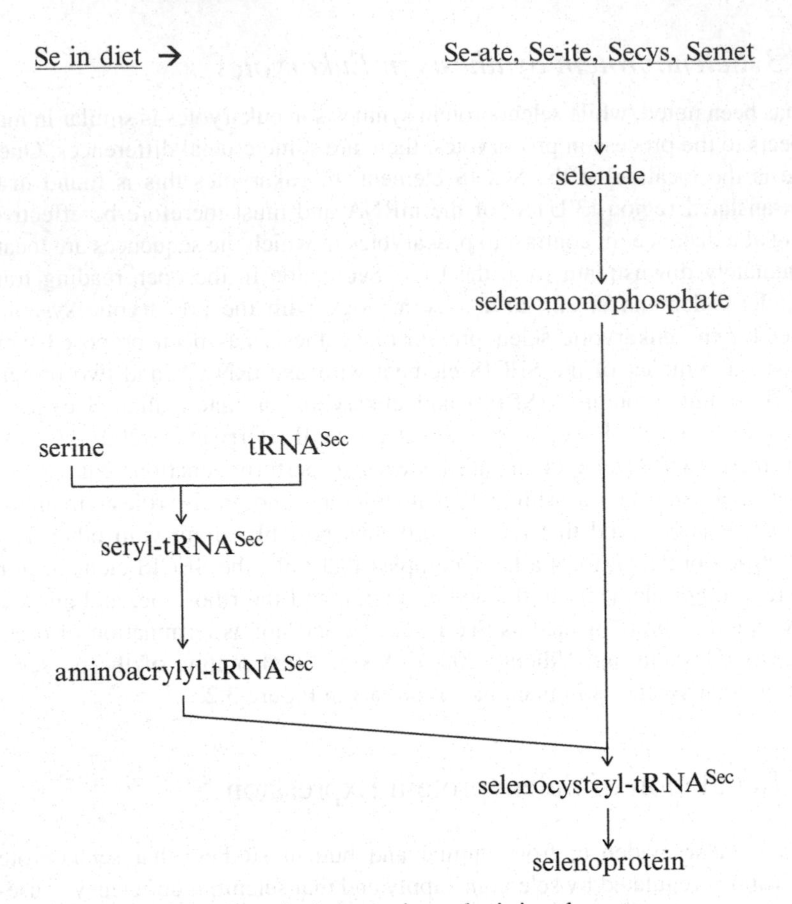

FIGURE 3.2 Schematic outline of selenoprotein systhesis in eukaryotes

Studies on the effects of severe selenium deficiency in rat liver found that GPX1 mRNA abundance was most affected, with a fall of 90%, ID1 mRNA fell by 50%, while there was no significant effect on GPX4 mRNA levels (Bermano et al., 1995). Similar results have been obtained using different tissues and cultured cells. These results indicate that synthesis of individual selenoenzymes and abundance of their mRNA differ in their sensitivity towards selenium supply, both within a single tissue and between tissues (Hesketh and Villette, 2002).

It has been shown, in a study of liver cells from selenium-deficient rats, that the rates of transcription of GPX1, GPX4, and ID1 genes are unaffected by the deficiency, even though there are changes in mRNA abundance and enzyme activity (Bermano et al., 1995). These results have been interpreted as indicating that post-translational mechanisms play an important role in selenoprotein synthesis regulation in response to selenium supply and that this control involves regulation of mRNA stability (Sunde, 2001). This view is supported by the finding that in cell cultures selenium supply affects differentially the stability of GPX1, GPX2, and GPX4 mRNAs (Bermano et al., 1996).

It is believed that the basis of this regulation of selenoprotein synthesis and prioritization of available selenium distribution to different selenoproteins and tissues lies partly in differences in the 3′UTR sequences in the mRNA of the different selenoprotein gene products (Hesketh and Villette, 2002). Every eukaryotic selenoprotein mRNA contains in its 3′UTR a SECIS element, essential for the cotranslational insertion of Sec into the protein (Berry et al., 1991). The element is common to all eukaryotes and allows the translational machinery to recognize UGA codons within the coding sequence as Sec codons and not as a termination signal. Other regions of the 3′UTR, however, are sufficiently different to be able to partly determine the pattern of selenoprotein expression under conditions of limiting selenium supply (Bermano et al., 1995).

Differences in the 3′UTR of the selenoprotein mRNA may be of critical importance in determining the relative extent to which the different mRNAs are translated. This view is supported by several observations, including the finding that when the native 3′UTR of ID-1 and ID-3 was exchanged for those of other selenoproteins, the activities of the enzymes were altered (Berry et al., 1991). Differences in 3′UTR sequences are also believed to be responsible for differences in relative translation rates and mRNA stability between different selenoproteins, probably reflecting difference in ability to form a complex with Sec-tRNA and the proteins forming the SECIS-binding complex (Hesketh and Villette, 2002).

On the basis of these and other findings, a hypothesis has been proposed by Hesketh and Villette (2002) to account for the prioritization of selenium for synthesis of one selenoprotein rather than another under conditions of limiting selenium supply. These authors hypothesize that prioritization depends on small differences in the 3′UTR sequences and 3′UTR-binding proteins. They believe that these lead to differences in the complexes formed by 3′UTR-binding proteins, the SECIS elements and other components of the selenium incorporation machinery. As a result of these differences, the complex formation and the ability of the incorporation machinery to read UGA as a Sec-insertion codon varies with the supply of selenium, and thus Sec production is limited. The hypothesis can be illustrated as follows, taking GPX1 and GPX4 as examples: when selenium is abundant, both GPX1 and GPX4 mRNAs are translated and both selenoproteins are synthesized. However, when selenium is limiting, and assuming that the 3′UTR of the GPX4 mRNA is more effective than that of GPX1 at competing for components of the incorporation machinery, translation of GPX1 is reduced while that of GPX4 is maintained.

3.3.1 Complexities of Regulation of Selenoprotein Synthesis

Although the mechanism proposed by Hesketh and Villette (2002) for the regulation of selenoprotein biosynthesis may appear to be complicated, it is becoming evident that, in reality, the true picture is even more complex. It is now believed that, in addition to selenoprotein mRNA stability and limiting amounts of transitional factors such as SBP2, selenoprotein synthesis is also regulated by stability of Sec-tRNA.

3.3.1.1 A Regulatory Role for $tRNA^{[Ser]Sec}$ in Selenoprotein Synthesis

Two major $tRNA^{[Ser]Sec}$ isoforms have been characterized in mammalian cells. One is designated *mcm*^{5}*U*, the other, *mcm*^{5}*Um*, indicating that the latter has an additional methyl group in the 2′-*O* position of the ribose portion of methylcarboxymethyl-5′-uridine (mcm^{5}U) in the anticodon. The methylation is believed to cause a change in the conformation of $tRNA^{[Ser]Sec}$, from a relatively compact to a more open and possibly more stable conformation (Jameson et al., 2002). The finding that supplemental selenium increases the relative abundance of the methylated isoform, in addition to total $tRNA^{[Ser]Sec}$, indicates that it is this methylated isoform that is translationally active and that selenium-induced tRNA methylation is another mechanism for the regulation of selenoprotein synthesis (Jameson and Diamond, 2004).

3.3.1.2 Single Nucleotide Polymorphisms and Regulation of Selenoprotein Synthesis

Single nucleotide polymorphisms (SNPs, sometimes read as "snips" by the cognoscenti) are genetic sequence variations that occur when a single nucleotide in the genome sequence is altered. SNPs make up about 90% of all human genetic variations and occur every 100 to 300 bases along the 3-billion-base human genome. Two out of every three SNPs involve the replacement of cytosine (C) with thymine (T). Many of these SNPs have no effect on metabolism, but others appear to play a significant role as modifiers of cell function, especially with regard to gene–nutrient interaction.

It is believed, for example, that SNPs may be responsible for differences in the way in which individuals use available dietary selenium for selenoprotein synthesis. Sequence analysis of the GPX4 gene in a Scottish population carried out by Villette et al. (2002) identified a common SNP in a part of the 3′UTR close to the SECIS region. The mutation found was a T/C variation at position 718. The distribution of the SNP was, out of 66 volunteers screened, 34% CC, 25% TT, and 41% TC. The functional significance of this, and other polymorphisms, is not yet fully understood, but it is believed that they are important, especially with regard to differences in the response of individuals to selenium supplementation (Hesketh and Villette, 2002). The T/C718 SNP has been found to be associated with differences in lipoxygenase metabolism, which is consistent with evidence that GPX4 has a role in the 5-lipoxygenase pathway. Significant differences in 5-lipoxygenase metabolites were found in individuals with different C718 genotypes, with C718 showing 36% and 44% increases compared to levels in T718 and T/C718. There was no evidence that differences in selenium status could account for the differences in 5-lipoxygenase products between genotype groups. These results have been interpreted as providing an example of the complex interplay between genetic makeup, nutrition, and physiological status (Villette et al., 2002).

The extent to which genetic variations in components of the cellular machinery may be responsible for the way in which individuals differ in their ability to utilize available selenium for selenoprotein synthesis is being studied in the UK with funding from the Food Standards Agency. A project has been set up to investigate SNPs that occur in SPB2, selenophosphate synthesase, and SelP genes. The aim is to define the extent to which genetic polymorphisms in genes encoding components of the cell machinery for incorporation of selenium determine its bioavailability in the general population (Food Standards Agency, 2004).

Factors other than the supply and availability of dietary selenium can also have implications for the expression of specific selenoproteins. It is known, for example, that oxidative stress leads to induction of TR1 and GPX (Sun et al., 1999). It has also been shown that activation of second-messenger pathways can modify the expression of specific selenoproteins in a tissue-specific manner (Anema et al., 1999).

3.4 Selenium Status

The term "selenium status" is usually used to refer to the effective level of the element in the body in relation to its role in contributing to the maintenance, at optimal level, of the biological functions that are dependent on it. This is not a precise definition, since we are not yet fully aware of all the metabolic functions in which selenium plays a necessary part. Moreover, it is uncertain whether the optimal level referred to means simply prevention of deficiency diseases or reduction of the risk of such chronic diseases as cancer, cvd, and other disorders in the prevention of which selenium may play a part (Nève, 2000).

3.4.1 Assessment of Selenium Status

Diagnosis of trace element deficiency or overloading, as well as monitoring of individuals who are undergoing treatment, requires knowledge of their trace element status. Obtaining this information, reliably and consistently, is not, in the case of selenium, a straightforward task. Trace element status depends on many factors such as dietary intake, absorption, excretion, and, not least, bioavailability of the particular element being investigated (Ermidou-Pollet et al., 2005). Moreover, the effects of low intake may take many years to develop and may not be detectable at early stages of deficiency. In the case of selenium, since it influences a wide range of biochemical processes, levels required for normal health may vary depending on the levels of metabolic activity. Requirements can also be affected by the presence or absence of other trace elements and other nutrients (Arthur et al., 1999).

In spite of reservations about their reliability in all circumstances, a number of different assessment methods are used in practice for the determination of selenium status. At first sight, selenium status would seem to be easy to assess since concentration of the trace element can be determined without difficulty in most biological fluids and tissues. In addition, the selenium-dependent enzyme, GPX, which would seem to be an ideal functional marker of the biologically effective level of the element, can readily be measured in blood and other body fluids. However, problems are encountered with both methods and the question of the best procedures for assessment of selenium status continues to exercise the minds of specialists in the trace element field (Ermidou-Pollet et al., 2005).

Simple measures of dietary intake of selenium, while indicative of the general status of a population, are not sufficient in themselves for determining the status in individuals. Variations in levels of the element between foodstuffs and uncertainty about the availability for absorption of its different forms make it necessary to be able to measure functional levels in the body and not simply gross intake.

In a now somewhat dated, though still pertinent review, Diplock (1993) noted that two criteria have to be taken into consideration when making a judgment about the suitability of a procedure for assessing selenium status. The first is that the methodology for measuring selenium concentrations must be reliable; the second, that it must be established that the variable measured is directly related to the biochemical variables for selenium activity in vivo.

3.4.1.1 Use of Blood Selenium Levels to Assess Selenium Status

With regard to Diplock's first criterion, we have already seen that reliable and reproducible results can be obtained for selenium concentrations in biological tissues using modern analytical equipment and procedures. Determination of selenium levels in whole blood and/or in blood fractions is routinely carried out in clinical laboratories (Medical Toxicology Unit, 2005; Bates et al., 2002). Measurement of selenium levels in serum and plasma is the method most widely reported in the literature for assessing selenium status of populations. However, as such tables show, selenium levels in the blood of healthy subjects vary widely, with a range of 40 to 200 μg/l, between different parts of the world. Thus, results of measurements of blood selenium levels of individuals should be interpreted only with reference to carefully matched controls (Nève, 2000). It must also be recognized, as noted by Diplock (1993), that there may not be a close correlation between levels detected in blood and the true selenium status of individuals, as defined by the functional selenium in an enzyme. It might be, for instance, that some of the element determined in blood is unavailable, unable to be converted into Sec, as would be the case if it were in the form of selenomethionine or complexed with a heavy metal (Whanger and Butler, 1988).

3.4.1.2 Hair, Nail, and Urinary Selenium

Selenium levels in other tissues, besides blood, are of potential values as biomarkers of selenium status and are used by some investigators for this purpose. They have the advantage of not requiring any invasive techniques, and sample collection can be carried out by relatively unskilled collectors who do not have access to refrigeration for sample storage. Consequently, the method is particularly appropriate in epidemiological investigations, especially in remote regions.

Finger- and toenail selenium levels have been proposed as a useful indicator of long-term human selenium status and have been employed for this purpose in several studies. These include a large-scale study of Finnish men (Ovaskainen et al., 1993) and a more recent investigation into the relationship of low selenium status and the occurrence of preeclampsia in British women (Rayman et al., 2003). In the latter study, toenail clippings were prepared, and analyzed by NAA, in accordance with an IAEA (1978) protocol for hair analysis. Toenail clippings from an impressive 62,641 women who participated in the Harvard University Nurses Health Study were collected and analyzed in an investigation of a possible relationship between cancer incidence and selenium intake (Garland et al., 1995).

Although evidence has been published showing a strong correlation between hair and whole blood selenium, and hair analysis has been used in several studies of selenium status in China and elsewhere (Chen et al., 1980), doubts have been expressed about the reliability of the method (Dreosti, 1981). There is a need for standardization of the technique and the possibility of external contamination of the hair before it is removed from the heads of subjects, from the environment, and from the use of selenium-containing shampoo preparations must be taken into consideration (Reilly and Harrison, 1979).

3.4.1.3 Use of Functional Indicators of Selenium Status

Although at present there is no ideal functional indicator that can be used to assess selenium status, a number of different procedures are used in practice. Measurement of activity of the plasma GPX (EC 1.11.1.9) is the most widely used procedure and, in spite of some problems, still continues to serve well in clinical practice. The assay is relatively easily performed and is adaptable to an automated procedure. A significant positive correlation between GPX activity and selenium concentrations in the body has been shown in populations with a large range of individual selenium intakes. However, this correlation is only found at relatively low levels of intake. At higher intakes, the relationship becomes less significant and even disappears in the upper ranges, apparently as a saturation level is reached, above which no additional enzyme is synthesized (Nève, 2000). According to Diplock (1993), there is a good correlation between blood selenium and GPX activity up to approximately 1.0 μmol/l (79 μg/l). Thus, GPX activity can be taken as an appropriate indicator of human selenium status only in populations with a relatively low exposure to dietary selenium. Whether the saturation level is 79 μg/l, as Diplock (1993) suggests, or 1.0 mg/l, or a higher figure as believed by other investigators (Valentine et al., 1980) it still uncertain.

Arthur (1999), in a review of functional indicators of iodine and selenium status, has noted that there is uncertainty about how measurements of plasma GPX relate to other biochemical functions of selenium, such as thyroid metabolism or possible redox control of transcription factors. While different GPXs are often the most sensitive indicators of dietary selenium intake and have been used successfully in studies of animals with a similar genetic background and dietary intake, their use in humans is complicated by a number of factors. These include differences between individuals that increase variability of selenoenzyme activities from person to person, variability due to individual differences in selenium intake, and the possibility that other dietary factors, such as vitamin E and iodine, may influence enzyme activity (Arthur et al., 1999).

The activities of several other selenoproteins, apart from the various isoforms of GPX, could potentially serve as functional markers of selenium status. Among those that have been identified for this purpose are iodothyronine deiodinase, TR, Se-P, and Se-W (Nève, 2000). So far none of these have been used in routine investigations and clinical practice, and much still remains to be learned about their potential as functional markers.

As has been pointed out by Arthur (1999), it is important to remember that more than 30 selenoproteins have been identified in human tissues, many, if not all, of which could be used as functional markers. Yet, because of the diversity of function of these selenoproteins, conclusions drawn from measurement of one of them may not apply to all biological functions that are dependent on selenium. Thus, it may prove impossible to find one status indicator that is useful for every circumstance. Rather, a series of markers, each applicable to a particular problem related to suboptimal selenium status may be required. These markers, Arthur suggests, might be: (1) plasma or whole blood selenium concentrations; (2) plasma GPX activities; (3) erythrocyte GPX activities; (4) GPX activities in other blood fractions (platelets, lymphocytes, and neutrophils); and (5) ID levels.

3.4.1.4 Other Potential Markers of Selenium Functional Status

It is most probable that current developments in genetics and molecular biology will lead to the recognition of new and highly specific markers of selenium status. There is now a range of technologies, generally collectively known as transcriptomics, which is being used to transform the scope for exploration of complex interactions between dietary components and gene expression in human cells. One of these procedures, microarray technology, has made it possible to obtain an overview of interactions between dietary components and gene expression at a partial or even complete genome level (Elliott, 2005). It is a powerful and sophisticated investigative tool which, to the dismay of many traditional nutritionists, requires a high degree of expertize in the fields of molecular biology and statistics, as well as advanced technological skills and, not least, the use of expensive and technically demanding instrumentation. However, there can be little doubt that transcriptomics and its technologies will be increasingly used in the study of human nutrition. The recent report by Broome et al. (2004) on their identification of specific cytokine genes that change in response to selenium supplementation and thus may be potential indicators of selenium-sensitive aspects of immune function shows the use to which microarray technology is being put and indicates its potential for delivering the universally acceptable and accurate method of assessing selenium status, which is currently lacking.

References

Anema, S.M., Walker, S.W., Howie, A.F., Arthur, J.R., Nicol, F., and Beckett, G.J., 1999, Thioredoxin reductase is the major selenoprotein expressed in human umbilical-vein endothelial cells and is regulated by protein kinase C, *Biochem. J.* **342**, 111–117.

Arner, E.S.J. and Holmgren, A., 2000, Physiological functions of thioredoxin and thioredoxin reductase, *Eur. J. Biochem.* **276**, 6102–6109.

Arteel, G.E., Briviba, T., and Sies, H., 1999, Protection against peroxynitrite, *FEBS Lett.* **445**, 226–230.

Arthur, J.R., 1999, Functional indicators of iodine and selenium status, *Proc. Nutr. Soc.* **58**, 507–512.

Arthur, J.R. 2003, Selenium supplementation: does soil supplementation help and why? *Proc. Nutr. Soc.* **62**, 393–397.

Arthur, J.R. and Beckett, G.J., 1994, Newer aspects of micronutrients in at risk groups. New metabolic roles for selenium, *Proc. Nutr. Soc.* **53**, 615–624.

Arthur, J.R., Brown, K.M., Nicol, F., and Pickard, K., 1999, Assessment of selenium status, *Clin. Chem. Lab. Med.* **37**, Special Suppl., S89.

Arthur, J.R., Morrice, P.C., Nicol, F., et al., 1987, The effects of selenium and copper deficiencies on glutathione peroxidase in rat liver, *Biochem. J.* **248**, 539–544.

Bates, C.J., Thane, C.W., Prentice A., Delves, H.T., and Gregory, J., 2002, Selenium status and associated factors in a British National Diet and Nutrition Survey: young people aged 4–18 y, *Eur. J. Clin. Nutr.* **56**, 873–881.

Beckett, G.J., Beddows, S.L., Morrice, P.C. et al., 1987, Inhibition of hepatic deiodination of thyroxine is caused by selenium deficiency in rats, *Biochem. J.* **248**, 443–447.

Bene, D. and Kyriakopoulos, A., 2001, Mammalian selenium-containing proteins, *Ann. Rev. Nutr.* **21**, 453–473.

Bermano, G., Arthur, J.R., and Hesketh, J.E., 1996, Role of the 3′untranslated region in the regulation of cytosolic glutathione peroxidase and phospholipid-hydroperoxide gene expression by selenium supply, *Biochem. J.* **320**, 891–895.

Bermano, G., Nicol, F., Dyer, A., Sunde, R.A., et al., 1995, Tissue-specific regulation of selenoenzyme gene expression during selenium deficiency in rats, *Biochem. J.* **311**, 425–430.

Berry, J., Banu, L., Chen, Y.Y. et al., 1991a, Recognition of UGA as a selenocysteine codon in type I deiodinase requires sequences in the 3′ untranslated region, *Nature* **353**, 273–276.

Berry, M.J., Banu, L., Chen, Y.Y., Mandel, S.J., et al., 1991, Recognition of UGA as a selenocysteine codon in type 1 deiodinase requires sequences in the 3′ untranslated region, *Nature* **353**, 273–276.

Berry, M.J., Kieffer, J.D., Harvey, J.W. and Larsen, P.R., 1991b, Selenocysteine confers the biochemical properties characteristic of type I iodothyronine deiodinase, *J. Biol. Chem.* **266**, 14155–14158.

Berry, M.J., Tujebajeva, R., Copeland, P.R. et al., 2001, Selenocysteine incorporation directed from the 3′UTR: characterization of eukaryotic EFsec and mechanistic implications, *Biofactors* **14**, 17–24.

Bianco, A. C., Salvatore, D., Gereben, B. et al., 2002, Biochemistry, cellular and molecular biology, and physiological roles of iodothyronine selenodeiodinases, *Endocrine Revs.* **23**, 38–89.

Björnstedt, M., Xue, J., Huang, W. et al., 1994, The thioredoxin and glutathione systems are efficient electron donors to human plasma glutathione peroxidase, *J. Biol. Chem.* **269**, 29382–29384.

Bratter, P., Negretti de Bratter, V.E., Jaffe, W.G., et al., 1991, Selenium status of children living in seleniferous regions of Venezuela, *J. Trace Elem. Electrolytes Health Dis.* **5**, 269–270.

Broome, C.S., McArdle, F., Kyle, J., et al., 2004, An increase in selenium intake improves immune function and poliovirus handling in adults with marginal selenium status, *Am. J. Clin. Nutr.* **80**, 154–162.

Burk, R. and Hill, K.E., 1993, Regulation of selenoproteins, *Ann. Rev. Nutr.* **13**, 65–81.

Callebaut, I., Curcio-Morelli, C., Momon, J.P. et al., 2002, The iodothyronine deiodinases are thioredoxin-fold family proteins containing a glycocide hydrolase clan GH-A like structure, *J. Biol. Chem.* **278**, 36887–36896.

Chen, X., Yang, G., Chen, J.S., et al., 1980, Studies on the relations of selenium to Keshan disease, *Biol. Trace Elem. Res.* **2**, 91–104.

Clark, L.C., Dalkin, B., Krongrad, A., et al., 1998, Decreased incidence of prostate cancer with selenium supplementation: results of a double-blind prevention trial, *Br. J. Urol.* **81**, 730–734.

Croteau, W., Whittemore, S.L., Schneider, M.J. and St. Germain, D.L., 1995, Cloning and expression of a cDNA for a mammalian type III iodothyronine deiodinase, *J. Biol. Chem.* **270**, 16569–16575.

Diplock, A.T. 1993, Indexes of selenium status in human populations, *Am. J. Clin. Nutr.* **57**, 256S–258S.

Dreosti, I., 1981, Laboratory methods for mineral nutritional assessment in man, *Trans. Menzies Foundation* **3**, 123–136.

Elliott, R.M., 2005, Transcriptomics: the use of new technologies to complement traditional approaches, in: *12th International Symposium on Trace Elements in Man and Animals—TEMA 12*, June 19–23, 2005, University of Ulster, Coleraine, Northern Ireland, Abstracts A4.

Ermidou-Pollet, S., Silagyi, M., and Pollet, S., 2005, Problems associated with the determination of trace element status and trace element requirements—a mini-review, *Trace Elem. Electrolytes* **22**, 105–113.

Food Standards Agency 2004. Genotypes underlying functional bioavailability of selenium, http://www.food.gov.uk/science/research/researchinfo/nutritionresearch/optimalnutrition/n05programme/n05listbio/n05041/

Forchhammer, K., and Bock, A., 1991, Selenocysteine synthase from *Escherichia coli*. Analysis of reaction sequence, *J. Biol. Chem.* **266**, 6324–6328.

Forstrom, J.W., Zakowski, J.J. and Tappel, A.L., 1978, Identification of the catalytic site of rat liver glutathione peroxidase as selenocysteine, *Biochem. J.* **17**, 2639–2644.

Garland, M., Morris, J.S., Stampfer, M.J., et al., 1995, Prospective study of toenail selenium levels and cancer among women, *J. Natl Cancer Inst.* **87**, 497–505.

Gladyshev, V.N. 2001, Identity, evolution and function of selenoproteins and selenoprotein genes, in: Hatfield, D.L. (ed.), *Selenium, its Molecular Biology and Role in Human Health*, Kluwer, Boston, MA, pp. 99–114.

Gladyshev, V.N., Jeang, K.T. and Stadtman, T.C., 1996, Selenocysteine identified as the penultimate C-terminal residue in human T-cell thioredoxin reductase corresponds to TGA in the human placental gene, *Proc. Natl. Acad. Sci. USA* **93**, 6146–6151.

Gladyshev, V.N., Jeang, K.T., Wootton, J.C., and Hatfield, D.L. 1998, A new human selenium-containing protein. Purification, characterization, and cDNA sequence, *J. Biol. Chem.* **273**, 8910–8915.

Gladyshev, V.N., Kryukov, G.V., Fomenko, D.E., and Hatfield, D.L., 2004, Identification of trace element-containing proteins in genomic databases, *Ann. Rev. Nutr.* **24**, 579–596.

Gromer, S., Wissing, J., Behene, D., et al., 1998, A hypothesis on the catalytic mechanisms of selenoenzyme thioredoxin reductase, *Biochem. J.* **332**, 591–592.

Gromer, S., Urig, S. and Becker, K., 2004, The thioredoxin system-from science to clinic, *Med. Res. Revs.* **24**, 40–89.

Grossman, A. and Wendel, A., 1983, Non-reactivity of the selenoenzyme glutathione peroxidase with enzymatically hydroperoxidized phosphorlipids, *Eur. J. Biochem.* **135**, 549–552.

Grunder-Culemann, E., Martin, G.W., Tujebajeva, R., et al., 2001, Interplay between termination and translation machinery in eukaryotic selenoprotein synthesis, *J. Mol. Biol.* **310**, 699–707.

Gu, Q-P., Beilstein, M.A., Barofsky, F., Ream, W., and Whanger, P.D., 1999, Purification, characterization and glutathione binding to selenoprotein W from monkey muscle, *Arch. Biochem. Biophys.* **361**, 25–33.

Guimaraes, M.J., Peterson, D., Vicari, A., et al., 1996, Identification of a novel selD homolog from eukaryotes, bacteria, and archea: Is there an autoregulatory mechanism in selenocysteine metabolism? *Proc. Natl. Acad. Sci. USA* 93, 15086–15091.

Hatfield, D.L. and Gladyshev, V.N., 2002, How selenium has altered our understanding of the genetic code, *Mol. Cell Biol.* **22**, 3565–3576.

Heider, J., Baron, C. and Bock, A., 1992, Coding from a distance: dissection of the mRNA determinants required for the incorporation of selenocysteine into protein, *EMBO J.* **11**, 3759–3766.

Hesketh, J.E. and Villette, S., 2002, Intracellular trafficking of micronutrients: from gene regulation to nutrient requirements, *Proc. Nutr. Soc.* **61**, 405–414.

Holmgren, A., 2001, Selenoprotein of the thioredoxin system, in: Hatfield, D. (ed.), *Selenium: its Molecular Biology and Role in Human Health*, Kluwer, Boston, MA., pp. 178–198.

Huttenhofer, M., Westhof, E. and Bock, A., 1996, Solution structure of mRNA hairpins promoting selenocysteine incorporation in *Escherichia coli* and their base-specific interaction with special elongation factor selB, *RNA*, **2**, 354–366.

IAEA, 1978, Report IAEA/RI/50: Activation analysis of hair as an indicator of contamination of man by environmental trace element pollutants, International Atomic Energy Agency, Vienna.

Imai, H., Narashima, K., Arai, M., et al., 1998, Superexpression of leukotriene formation in RBL-2Hl cells that overexpressed phospholipid hydroperoxide glutathione peroxidase, *J. Biol. Chem.* **273**, 1990–1997.

Jameson, R.R. and Diamond, A.M., 2004, A regulatory role for Sec tRNA$^{[Ser]Sec}$ in selenoprotein synthesis, *RNA* **10**, 1142–1152.

Jameson, R.R., Carlson, B.A., Butz, M., Esser, K., et al., 2002, Selenium influences the turnover of selenocysteine tRNA$^{[Ser]Sec}$ in Chinese hamster ovary cells, *J. Nutr.* **132**, 1830–1835.

Kaplan, M.M., 1986, Regulatory influences on iodothyronine deiodination in animal tissues, in: Hennemann, G. (ed.), *Thyroid Hormone Metabolism*, Dekker, New York, pp. 231–253.

Katsanis, N., Worley, K.C., and Lupski, J.R., 2001, An evaluation of the draft human genome sequence, *Nature Genet.* **29**, 88–91.

Kromayer, M., Wilting, R., Tormay, P. and Bock, A., 1996, Domain structure of the prokaryotic selenocysteine-specific elongation factor selB, *J. Mol. Biol.* **262**, 413–420.

Kryukov, G.V., Castellano, S., Novoselov, S.V., et al., 2003, Characterization of mammalian selenoproteomes, *Science* **300**, 1439–1443.

Kryukov, G.V., Kryukov, V.M., and Gladyshev, V.N., 1999, New mammalian selenocysteine-containing proteins identified with an algorithm that searches for selenocysteine insertion sequence elements, *J. Biol. Chem.* **274**, 33888–33897.

Kryukov, G.V., Kumar, R.A., Koe, A., and Gladyshev, V.N., 2002, Selenoprotein R is a zinc-containing stereo-specific methionine sulfoxide reductase, *Proc. Natl Acad. Sci. USA* **99**, 4245–4250.

Kumaraswamy, E., Malykh, A., Korotkov, K.V., et al., 2000, Structure-expression relationships of the 15-kDa selenoprotein gene. Possible role of the protein in cancer etiology, *J. Biol.Chem.* **275**, 35540–35547.

Kyriakopoulos, A., Hammel, C., Gessner, H., and Behne, D., 1996, Characterization of an 18 kDa-selenium-containing protein in several tissues of the rat, *Am. Biotech. Lab.* **14**, 22.

Kyriakopoulos, A., Röthlein, D., Pfeifer, H., et al., 2000, Detection of small selenium-containing proteins in tissues of the rat. *J. Trace Elem. Med. Biol.* **14**, 170–183.

Lee, R., Kim, J., Kwon, K., et al., 1999, Molecular cloning and characterization of a mitochondrial selenocysteine-containing thioredoxin reductase from rat liver, *Proc. Natl. Acad. Sci. USA* **274**, 4722–4734.

Lei, X.G., Evenson, J.K., Thompson, K.M., and Sunde, R.A., 1995, Glutathione peroxidase and phospholipid hydroperoxide glutathione peroxidase are differentially regulated in rats by dietary selenium, *J. Nutr.* **125**, 1438–1446.

Leinfelder, W., Forchhammer, K., Veprek, B., et al., 1990, In vitro synthesis of selenocysteinyl-tRNA (UCA) from seryl-tRNA (UCA): involvement and characterization of the selD gene product, *Proc. Natl. Acad. Sci. USA* **87,** 543–547.

Leinfelder, W., Forchhammer, K., Zinoni, F., et al., 1988, *Escherichia coli* genes whose products are involved in selenium metabolism, *J. Bacteriol.* **170**, 540–546.

Lescure, A., Gautheret, D., Carbon, P., and Krol, A., 1999, Novel selenoproteins identified in silico and in vivo by using a conserved RNA structural motif, *J. Biol. Chem.* **274**, 38147–38154.

Low, S.C., Harney, J.W. and Berry, M.J., 1995, Cloning and functional characterization of human selenophosphate synthetase, an essential component of selenoprotein synthesis, *J. Biol. Chem.* **270**, 21659–21664.

Ma, S., Hill, K.E., Caprioloi, R.M., and Burk, R.F., 2002, Mass spectrometric characterization of full-length rat selenoprotein P and three isoforms shortened at the C terminus. Evidence that three UGA-codons in the mRNA open reading frame have alternative functions of specifying selenocysteine insertion or translation termination, *J. Biol. Chem.* **277**, 12749–12754.

Matsui, M., Oshima, M., Oshima, H., et al., 1996, Early embryonic lethality caused by targeted disruption of the mouse thioredoxin gene, *Dev. Biol.* **178**, 179–185.

McKenzie, R.C., Arthur, J.R., and Beckett, G.J., 2002, Selenium and the regulation of cell signalling, growth, and survival: molecular and mechanistic aspects, *Antiox. Redox Signal* **4**, 339–351.

Medical Toxicology Unit, Guy's and St Thomas' Hospitals, 2005, Selenium. http://www.medtox.org/lab/assay.asp? ID = 138.

Mills, J.C., 1957, Hemoglobin catabolism. I. Glutathione peroxidase, an erythrocyte enzyme which protects haemoglobin from oxidative breakdown, *J. Biol. Chem.* **229**, 189–197.

Mortimer, R.H., Galligan, J.P., Canell, G.R. et al., 1996, Maternal to fetal thyroxine transmission in the human term placenta is limited by inner ring deiodination, *J. Clin. Endocrinol. Metab.* **81**, 2247–2249.

Mostenbocker, M.A. and Tappel, A.L., 1982, A selenocysteine-containing selenium-transport protein in rat plasma, *Biochim. Biophys. Acta* **719**, 147–153.

Mustacich, D. and Powis, G., 2000, Thioredoxin reductase, *Biochem. J.* **346**, 1–8.

Nomura K, Imai, H., Komura, T. and Nakagawa, Y., 2001, Involvement of mitochondrial phospholipid hydroperoxide glutathione peroxidase as an antiapoptic factor, *Biol. Signals Recept.* **10**, 81–92.

Nève, J., 2000, New approaches to assess selenium status and requirements, *Nutr. Rev.* **58**, 363–369.

Ovaskainen, M-J., Virtamo, J., Alfthan, G., et al., 1993, Toenail selenium as an indicator of selenium intake among middle-aged men in an area of low soil selenium, *Am. J. Clin. Nutr.* **57**, 662–665.

Rayman, M.P., Bode, P., and Redman, C.W.G., 2003, Low selenium status is associated with the occurrence of the pregnancy disease preeclampsia in women from the United Kingdom, *Am. J. Obstet. Gynecol.* **189**, 1343–1349.

Read, R., Bellew, T., Yang, J.G., et al., 1990, Selenium and amino acid composition of selenoprotein P in rat serum, *J. Biol. Chem.* **265**, 17899–17905.

Reilly, C. and Harrison, F., 1979, Zinc, copper, iron and lead in scalp hair of students in Oxford, *J. Hum. Nutr.* **33**, 250–254.

Rotruck, J.T., Pope, A.L., Ganther, H.E., et al., 1973, Selenium: biochemical role as a component of glutathione peroxidase, *Science* **179**, 588–590.

Roveri, A., Casaco, A., Mairoini, M. et al., 1992, Phospholipid hydroperoxide glutathione peroxidase of rat testis, *J. Biochem.* **267**, 6142–6146.

Salvatore, D., Bartha, T., Harvey, J.W. and Lassen, P.R., 1996, Molecular, biological and biochemical characterization of the human type 2 selenode-iodinase, *Endocrinol.* **137**, 3308–3315.

Srinivasan, G., James, C.M. and Krzycki, J.A., 2002, Pyrrdysine encoded by UGA in Archaea: charging of a UGA-decoding specialized tRNA, *Science* **296**, 1459–1462.

Stadtman, T.C., 1990, Selenium biochemistry, *Ann. Rev. Biochem.* **59**, 111–127.

Sun, Q.A., Zappacosta, F., Jeang, K.T., Lee, B.J., et al., 1999, Redox regulation of cell signalling of selenocysteine in mammalian thioredoxin reductases, *J. Biol. Chem.* **274**, 24522–24530.

Sunde, R.A., 2001, Regulation of selenoprotein expression. in: Hatfield, D.L. (ed.), *Selenium: Its Molecular Biology and Role in Human Health*, Kluwer, Boston, pp. 81–98.

Takahashi, K. and Cohen, H.J., 1986, Selenium-dependent glutathione peroxidase protein and activity: immunological investigations of cellular and plasma enzymes, *Blood*, **68**, 640–645.

Tamura, T. and Stadtman, T.C., 1996, A new selenoprotein from human lung adenocarcinoma cells: purification, properties, and thioredoxin activity, *Proc. Natl. Acad. Sci. USA* **93**, 1006–1011.

Thomson, C.D., Rea, H.M., Doesburg, V.M., and Robinson, M.F., 1977, Selenium concentrations and glutathione peroxidase activities in whole blood of New Zealand residents, *Br. J. Nutr.* **37**, 457–465.

Ursini, F. and Bindoli, A., 1987, The role of selenium peroxidase in the protection against oxidative damage of membranes, *Chem. Phys. Lipid.*, **44**, 225–276.

Ursini, F., Heim, S., Keiss, M, et al., 1999, Dual function of the selenoprotein PHGPx during sperm maturation, *Science*, **285**, 1393–1396.

Ursini, F., Maiorino, M and Roveri, A., 1997, Phospholipid hydroperoxide glutathione peroxidase more than an antioxidant enzyme? *Biomed. Environ. Sci.* **10**, 327–332.

Valentine, J.L., Kang, H.K., Dang, P.M., and Schluchter, M., 1980, Selenium concentrations and glutathione peroxidase activities in a population exposed to selenium via drinking water, *J. Toxicol. Environ. Health* **6**, 731–736.

Vendeland, S.C., Beilstein, M.A., Chen, C.L., et al., 1995, Rat skeletal muscle selenoprotein W: cDNA clone and mRNA modulation by dietary selenium, *Proc. Natl Acad. Sci. USA* **92**, 8749–8753.

Villette, S., Kyle, J.A.M., Brown, K.M., et al., 2002, A novel single nucleotide polymorphism in the 3′ untranslated region of the human glutathione peroxidase 4 influences lipoxygenase metabolism, *Blood Cells Mol. Dis.* **29**, 174–178.

Whanger, P.D. and Butler, J.A., 1988, Effects of various dietary levels of selenium as selenite or selenomethionine on tissue selenium levels and glutathione peroxidase activity in rats, *J. Nutr.* **118**, 846–852.

Whanger, P.D., Vendeland, S.C., and Beilstein, M.A., 1993, Some biochemical properties of selenoprotein W, in: Anke, M., Meissner, D., and Mills, C.F. (eds), *Trace Elements in Man and Animals—TEMA 8*, Verlag Media Touristik, Gersdorf, Germany, pp. 119–126.

4
Selenium in Health and Disease I: The Agricultural Connection

4.1 Selenium and Agriculture

The earliest reported investigations of the role of selenium in health and disease were carried out in relation to agriculture and animal production. Even today, our growing understanding of the element's biological functions continues to rely to a significant extent on the work of agricultural and veterinary scientists. The stimulus that initially set these investigators on their way was largely an economic one—recognition that selenium toxicity was responsible for considerable losses to farmers in areas where the element occurred in high concentrations in soil. Before very long it came to be recognized that it was not just selenium toxicity but, on an even more widespread scale, selenium deficiency that caused problems for agriculture.

It was several decades after the pioneering investigations of agricultural scientists into the problems of selenium deficiency and toxicity in farm animals that the significance of their findings for human health began to be suspected. Parallels between selenium-related conditions in animals and in humans were recognized and some treatments that were effective in agricultural practice were found to have applications also in human nutrition and medicine.

4.2 Selenium Toxicity in Farm Animals

As we have seen earlier, what appears to have been selenium toxicity, or selenosis, in horses was recorded as long ago as the 13th century by Marco Polo in China. In Columbia, South America, in the 16th century a missionary, Pedro Simon (1560), recorded that in some areas corn was so poisonous that it caused loss of hair and other abnormalities in farm animals. Investigations four centuries later identified the cause of the poisoning as selenium taken up by plants from the highly seleniferous soils of that part of Colombia (Rosenfeld and Beath, 1964).

Similar incidents of selenosis in farm animals were recorded over the following centuries in Venezuela, Spain, Ireland, Germany, and other countries in which there are areas of seleniferous soils. Neither Polo nor the farmers who lost their cattle through this mysterious illness had any real idea of its cause. They probably accepted their losses as unfortunate accidents or "acts of God." Their way of preventing the disease was to avoid their "poisoned fields" and move their animals to safer pastures—a protective method which is probably the most effective even today. It was not until the 20th century that the role of selenium in these poisonings began to be understood, mainly through the investigations of scientists working in Agricultural Experiment Stations of the USA (Oldfield, 2005).

When, in the 19th century, expansion of the cattle trade to meet the demands of Europe for meat to feed its ever-expanding cities encouraged American farmers to move west to the Great Plains to find new grazing lands, a problem occurred. The settlers found that not all the new lands were good for grazing. In what became known as the "bad lands" of South Dakota and neighboring states, certain plants grew which, if eaten by farm animals, caused hoofs to drop off, hair to fall away, and even death. The settlers gave the name "locoweed" to these poisonous plants, from the Spanish *loco* (meaning "crazy"), which seemed to describe the abnormal behavior of the poisoned animals (USDA, 2005a). Not just one or two animals, but whole herds were affected. This was a problem that threatened the future of range livestock production in the affected areas. In 1908 in Wyoming, for example, the deaths of 15,000 sheep from this cause were reported (Wyoming State Board of Sheep Commissioners, 1908).

There had been earlier reports of large-scale poisonings, in this case of horses, in the same region of the USA. They occurred in cavalry mounts that had been put out to graze on native forage plants at Fort Randall, near the Nebraska–South Dakota state line. The horses developed symptoms that included hoof drop and loss of mane and tail, and many died (Madison, 1860). It has been suggested that the disastrous defeat of General George A. Custer at the battle of the Little Big Horn in Montana in 1876 was at least partly due to consumption of locoweed by the horses of the beleaguered cavalry as well as those of the relief column, which consequently failed to reach them in time (Jukes, 1983).

Reports of similar poisonings in horses and other domestic animals continued to appear over the following years, right into the next century. They occurred in scattered areas of South Dakota, Nebraska, Wyoming, Utah, and other western states where new farmland was being opened (Wolf et al., 1963). The condition in the animals was characterized by general dullness, lack of vitality, emaciation, stiffness, and lameness. Horses lost hair from their mane and tail, and cattle from the switch. Hoofs became loose and often sloughed off. There were also reports of teratogenic effects and reduction in reproductive performance.

4.2.1 Alkali Disease and Blind Staggers

The new settlers whose animals developed symptoms of poisoning found that this often occurred when their herds were placed on particular tracts of land where the soil was alkaline. They believed that certain plants that grew there took up "alkali" from the soil and as a result the herds developed "alkali disease." Another name they used was "blind staggers," which described the tottering steps of their "locoed" livestock.

The disease occurred in differing degrees, from a mild, chronic condition to an acute form resulting in death, sometimes within a few hours of consuming the poisonous plants. The primary targets of acute selenium toxicity in animals are the cardiovascular, gastrointestinal, and possibly hemopoietic systems, with occasionally neurological lesions, at least in swine (Raisbeck, 2000). In acute poisoning, movement of the animal became abnormal. It would walk a short distance and then assume a characteristic stance, with lowered head and drooped ears. Vomiting, spasms, and, within a few days, death from respiratory failure followed. In less severe subacute poisoning, the illness lasted over weeks or months. The animals showed a number of symptoms, including blindness and paralysis and suffered abdominal pain, with respiratory failure resulting in death. In some cases, loss of appetite as well as extreme pain in the hoofs made the animals unwilling to move about to secure water and food, so that they died of thirst and starvation (McDowell, 1992).

It was not until the 1930s that the connection between selenium and alkali disease/blind staggers was established. Orville Beath, an agricultural chemist at the Wyoming Agricultural Experiment Station, identified a group of native plants capable of causing blind staggers in livestock. These were species of *Astragalus*, milk vetch, which grew in parts of Wyoming where the soil was known to be seleniferous (Beath et al., 1934). Beath and his colleagues had followed up a report that selenium had been found in unusual quantities in wheat, which had poisoned cattle in South Dakota (Franke, 1934). They had looked for, and found, the same element in *Astragalus* and were convinced that they had at last found the cause of blind staggers and alkali disease: consumption by livestock species of native plants that grow on seleniferous soils and accumulated selenium in their tissues to toxic levels.

Attempts by Beath and others to find the particular form of selenium in plant tissues that caused poisoning were not successful. They also failed to reproduce typical symptoms of the condition by administering inorganic compounds of selenium in the animals' feed. It was suggested by some investigators that perhaps it was not selenium, but rather a toxic alkaloid that was responsible for symptoms commonly associated with blind staggers (Magg and Glen, 1967). The possibility that the condition is caused by factors other than excessive selenium intake has been suggested by other investigators also (O'Toole and Raisbeck, 1995). The finding that the mold *Fusarium* is associated with Degnala disease, a condition occurring in Indian water buffalo and which has symptoms resembling those of selenosis, suggests that mycotoxins may play a part in alkali disease (McDowell, 1992).

The picture is further complicated by other observations. It was found, for instance, that a high-protein diet could protect animals against a potentially toxic intake of selenium, especially if the protein was rich in lysine (Jaffe, 1973). The presence, in the diet, of a number of different inorganic elements, including arsenic, silver, and mercury, was found to modify the toxicity of selenium (Levander and Baumann, 1966). It is significant that in a study of the occurrence of selenosis on Irish farms, high levels of molybdenum have been found in association with the selenium and molybdenum-induced copper deficiency in affected cattle (Rogers et al., 1990). There was also some evidence that animals can adapt to higher than average levels of selenium intake (Jaffe and Mondragon, 1969).

Experience has shown that an oral selenium dose of 1 to –5 mg/kg body weight is probably toxic and that acute selenosis can be caused by an intake of 400 mg/kg. A lower dose between 5 and 40 mg over a period of several weeks or months can result in chronic poisoning (USDA, 2005b). In experimental animals selenium toxicity has been shown to occur at different levels of intake. An LD50 of 0.455 mg Se/kg has been reported in lambs, compared to 4.8 to 7.0 in rats and 1.0 in rabbits (Tinggi, 2005).

In spite of many years of investigation, the mechanism by which selenium exerts its toxic effects in animals has still to be clarified and, as commented by Raisbeck (2000), some aspects of the natural history of selenosis remain confused in modern texts. While there are indications from clinical and morphological lesions that glutathione depletion and secondary lipid peroxidation are important in its pathogenesis, how this occurs is uncertain. It has been suggested that selenium may block the function of SH groups involved in oxidative metabolism within cells (Martin, 1978). There is also evidence that the element may interfere with protein synthesis by affecting the redox state of elongation factor 2 (Vernie et al., 1975).

4.2.2 Selenosis in Farm Animals Outside the USA

Although selenosis in farm animals has not been a major problem for animal producers outside the USA, it is nevertheless a matter of concern for agriculture in some countries. Outbreaks of blind staggers and alkali disease in livestock have been reported, usually on a relatively small scale, in a number of countries, as shown in Table 4.1. The earliest modern report of selenosis in cattle outside the USA seems to have been of an isolated case in Limerick in Ireland (Walsh et al., 1951). In more recent years, several outbreaks of selenosis have been reported in domestic water buffalo, as well as in cows, in India (Subramanian and Muhuntha, 1993). In Australia poisoning of horses by the selenium-accumulating plants, *Morinda reticulata* and *Neptunia amplexicaulis*, has been found to occur in Queensland in a few isolated areas of the tropical interior in the north of the state (Knott and McCray, 1958). In addition, in Australia, and in some other countries, a few cases of acute and chronic selenium intoxication in pigs and other farm animals resulting from overdosing with selenium supplements have been reported (Hill et al., 1985).

4.2.2.1 Selenosis in Irish Farms

In spite of its small size and the absence of any large-scale incidents of selenosis in farm animals, seleniferous soils and their consequences for the livestock industry in Ireland have received attention from agricultural scientists for more than a

TABLE 4.1 Reports of selenosis in livestock in different countries

Country	Reference	Date of occurrence
Ireland	1	1890
Mexico	2	1940
Canada	2	1941
Australia	3	1954
India	4	1975

References:
1. Fream, W., 1890, The herbage of pastures, *J. Roy. Agr. Soc. England* **1**, 384–394.
2. Williams, K.T., Lakin, H.W., and Byers, H.G., 1941, Selenium occurrence in certain soils in the United States with a discussion on related topics. Fifth Report, US Department of Agriculture Technical Bulletin 785, 1–69.
3. Knott, S.G. and McCray, C.W.R., 1958, Selenium poisoning in horses in North Queensland, *Qld J. Agric. Sci.* **15**, 43–58.
4. Arora, S.P., Parvinder, K., Kirwar, S.S., et al., 1975, Se levels in fodder and its relationship with Degnala disease, *Ind. J. Dairy Sci.* **28**, 249–253.

century. One of the earliest published reports of selenosis in stock was of an outbreak that occurred near Dublin in the late 1880s (Fream, 1890). Seleniferous soils are found only in isolated pockets around the country, and probably affect not more than a total of 50 farms, unlike selenium deficiency, which is widespread (Rogers et al., 1990). However, where seleniferous areas exist, soil levels of selenium can be dramatic. Some of the most highly seleniferous soils in the world have been found in the counties of Limerick, Tipperary, and Meath, with levels up to 1,250 mg/kg, ten times higher than in the most highly seleniferous soils of the USA (Oldfield, 1999). Unlike seleniferous soils in South Dakota and elsewhere in the USA, the actual toxic areas in Ireland are very limited in size and are confined to specific areas, often just one field, or even part of a field, usually as sporadic localized pockets. Moreover, on many farms, selenium-deficient soils are found within a relatively short distance of these selenium "hot-spots" (Rogers et al., 1990).

The origin of the selenium may be traced to leaching from selenium-rich parent materials and subsequent deposition in low-lying areas, such as old glacial lakebeds and river flood plains. The most important parent rocks are black shales and limestones, which are often interbedded in the shale (Rogers, 2000). Many of these selenium-containing rocks are also molybdenum-rich, as are the seleniferous soils made from them. The highest levels of soil selenium are found in low-lying peaty bogs of neutral to alkaline pH. These conditions favor formation of selenate, which is readily assimilated by plants (Fleming and Walsh, 1957). Apart from some extreme concentrations noted above, selenium levels in toxic fields in Ireland average 21 mg/kg, with a range of 3.2 to 130.0 mg/kg. Symptoms displayed by farm animals, particularly horses, grazing on these toxic areas are similar to those seen in the seleniferous regions of the USA, including lameness, damaged hoofs, reluctance to move, and hair loss. The disease is sporadic, occurring in some years, usually in the autumn, and not in others. While grazing of selenium-enriched pasture plants, and consumption of contaminated hay and silage, is recognized as a cause of selenosis, soil ingestion is also a factor. If allowed to range freely, stock tend to avoid toxic areas, possibly because they find selenium-accumulating herbage unpalatable. Transfer from toxic areas has been found to be the most practical way of preventing selenosis. Even if animals have already been affected and are showing signs of lameness, removal to "clean" fields usually results in spontaneous recovery within a relatively short time.

4.3 The other Face of Selenium—an Essential Nutrient

In a review of selenium and animal production in Australia, Peter and Costa (1992) made the interesting comment that concentration on the toxic effects of ingested selenium was probably the major factor that delayed consideration of the element's essentiality to animals. They believed that, even after selenium's essential role became known, the toxicity caused by excess of the element continued to affect attitudes towards its use in animal production and possible function in biological systems. This concern over toxicity still persists to some extent today, not least in relation to human health.

4.3.1 Selenium as an Essential Nutritional Factor

The research that eventually led to the discovery of selenium as an essential nutritional factor originated in studies of brewer's yeast as a protein supplement carried on in Europe during World War II (Wolf et al., 1963). It was found by German researchers that if rats were fed a yeast-based diet, they developed liver necrosis. They could be protected against this disease if wheat germ and wheat bran, which contained α-tocopherol (vitamin E) were added to their diet (Schwarz, 1944).

American scientists who later attempted to repeat these experiments failed to produce the necrotic liver syndrome by feeding rats on brewer's yeast. Schwartz, who had performed the original experiments in Germany and was now working at the National Institutes of Health at Bethesda, Maryland, did succeed in reproducing his earlier results when he fed rats on torula yeast, rather than brewer's yeast. He concluded that the American yeast contained a component, which he called Factor 3, that was able to protect against the development of liver necrosis, but was absent in European brewer's yeast as well as in torula yeast. Two other protective factors against liver necrosis had already been identified: vitamin E and, mistakenly, L-cysteine, which was known as Factor 2 (Schwarz, 1951).

Schwarz and his colleagues continued to investigate liver necrosis and the factors involved in its prevention. Six years later he was able to announce that they had identified selenium as the key component in Factor 3 (Schwarz and Foltz, 1957). This discovery represented an important milestone in our understanding of the biological significance of selenium. For the first time, the element which until that time had been known only as a toxin, responsible for the poisoning of livestock and posing in some places a serious economic threat to agriculture, was now shown to play a positive and presumably essential role in animal health.

The floodgates were opened and in rapid succession additional discoveries were made which revealed the important biological role of selenium in living organisms. Many of these early discoveries proved to have considerable practical consequences for agriculture. In the year that Schwarz announced that selenium could protect against liver necrosis in rats, it was reported that it could also control growth depression, mortality, and exudative diathesis (ED) in chickens (Patterson et al., 1957). Its essential role in swine was also soon established (Eggert et al., 1957). Subsequently, it was found that certain enzootic myopathies in cattle and sheep, which responded to vitamin E treatment, could also be controlled by selenium, and that the element was often even more effective than α-tocopherol (Andrews et al., 1968). Further findings, e.g., that a single dose of selenite given to vitamin E-replete sows increased farrowing percentages (Levander, 1986), helped to confirm that selenium was an essential nutrient in its own right and not merely an adjuvant to vitamin E (Oldfield, 2003).

The precise relationship of selenium to vitamin E, however, was a puzzle to these early investigators and, indeed, has not yet been fully elucidated. What was established early on was that selenium is necessary for growth and fertility in animals and for the prevention of various diseases that show a variable response to vitamin E (Underwood, 1977). However, although selenium was shown to be more effective in producing a cure in some cases, in others, such as encephalomalacia in chicks, which responded to vitamin E, it had no effect (Scott, 1962). Although selenium and vitamin E were clearly related in their actions and had collaborative roles in metabolism, they did not function merely as substitutes for each other.

The report by Schwarz of the nutritionally beneficial effects of selenium was rapidly followed by the recognition among agricultural scientists that a range of vitamin E-related selenium-responsive conditions occurred in farm animals, sometimes on a very wide scale, in many countries. This finding appeared to provide the long-sought answer to the problem of certain diseases of unknown aetiology that failed to respond to vitamin E or other treatments.

This was particularly welcome in New Zealand where large tracts of agricultural soil were selenium-deficient, and stock losses, which were now seen to be related to selenium deficiency, were of considerable economic importance (Andrews et al., 1968). Soon steps were taken, by government and other research organizations in New Zealand and elsewhere, to determine the extent of the problem and to find means of overcoming it. In the USA, where up to that time selenium had been seen only as a problem to agriculture because of its toxicity, the widespread occurrence of selenium deficiency was quickly recognized, and determined efforts made to cope with the problem. Other countries, including Ireland and Australia, where the economic consequences of selenium deficiency in farm animals were considerable, also mobilized their scientific resources to investigate the problem.

4.4 Selenium-Responsive Conditions in Farm Animals

Table 4.2 lists some of the conditions in animals that are recognized as being related to selenium deficiency. Some of them occur on a wide scale in several countries and have caused problems in agriculture for many years. Several of them respond also to vitamin E, but not as effectively as to selenium. In some cases, though selenium deficiency is a major factor, it is not necessarily the only cause. Other factors may also play a part, and selenium supplementation may not always be the best solution to the problem.

4.4.1 White Muscle Disease

White muscle disease (WMD), a nutritional muscular dystrophy, is a degenerative disease (myopathy) of the striated muscles. It gets its name from a characteristic lightening of the color of muscle, which is sometimes accompanied by deposits of calcium. When heart muscles are affected, sudden exertion can cause heart failure and death. If muscles of the limbs are involved, the animal becomes stiff and has difficulty in getting up and down and in walking, hence the other name of the condition given by sheep farmers is "stiff lamb disease" (Oldfield, 1990).

WMD is probably the most widely recognized and economically important of the selenium-deficient conditions in livestock. It affects many different species, primarily lambs and calves, also horses, goats, poultry, as well as nonfarm animals such as rabbits, deer, and rats (Wolf et al., 1963). Its symptoms were described in calves in Europe as early as 1880, long before its cause was identified (Underwood, 1977). An extensive international survey of the use of selenium in agriculture carried out by Wolf and his colleagues some 40 years ago found that WMD occurred in all the major sheep-producing countries, such as Australia, Canada, New Zealand, Argentina, as well as in Britain, South Africa, Scandinavia, Germany, France, Switzerland, Italy, Japan, Ireland, and elsewhere.

TABLE 4.2 Selenium-responsive conditions in farm animals

Condition	Animals affected	Tissues involved
White muscle disease (myopathy)	Cattle, sheep, poultry, pigs, horses, etc.	Skeletal, heart, and gizzard muscle
Exudative diathesis	Poultry	Capillary walls
Pancreatic degeneration	Poultry	Pancreas
Liver necrosis	Pigs	Liver
Ill-thrift	Cattle, poultry, sheep	Muscle mass
Still birth, embryonic resorption	Sheep	Embryos
Esophagogastric ulcers	Pigs	Esophagus stomach
Sperm immobility	Sheep	Sperm

Source: Based on Oldfield, J.E., 1990, *Selenium: Its Uses in Agriculture, Nutrition and Health and the Environment*, Selenium-Tellurium Development Association, Grimbergen, Belgium; and Oldfield, J.E., 2005, Selenium in Nutrition: the Early Years, *A.L. Moxon Honorary Lectures, Special Circular 167–99*, Ohio State University, http://ohioline.osu.edu/sc167/sc167_04.html.

It was estimated that at that time in New Zealand alone some 10 to 15 million sheep, or 20 to 30% of the total stock, were at risk of developing WMD or some other selenium-deficient condition (Wolf et al., 1963). However, in other countries, WMD is sporadic, with less than 1% of herds affected in some years (McDowell, 1992). WMD continues to be reported in many countries and in a variety of animal species: e.g., goats in Mexico (Ramirez-Bribiesca et al., 2005); horse foals in the USA (Lofstedt, 1997); lambs in Serbia (Olivera et al., 2004), Turkey (Or et al., 2003), and India (Gupta and Gupta, 2002); and camels in East Africa (Faye and Bengoumi, 1994).

WMD occurs in two clinical patterns: the first is a congenital form in which calves, foals, lambs, and young of other animals are stillborn or die within a few days of birth after sudden physical exertion such as nursing or running. The second form, "delayed WMD," develops after birth, usually between week 3 and 6, though it may be delayed for longer. The animals display the typical stilted gait and arched back of stiff lamb disease. In foals the disease has been reported as presenting either as an acute, fulminant syndrome, which is rapidly fatal, or as a subacute syndrome characterized by profound muscular weakness. Foals with the subacute form may survive if they are supplemented early with selenium, but even in this form of the disease, mortality rates range from 30 to 45% (Lofstedt, 1997). In all cases WMD is associated with a low intake of dietary selenium. It is believed that an increased peroxidative challenge in muscle is involved in its pathogenesis. It has been shown that calves fed on a diet depleted in vitamin E and/or selenium have decreased activity in heart and limb muscles of the antioxidant enzyme glucose-6-phosphate dehydrogenase, but not of other enzymes with antioxidant functions (Kennedy et al., 1993).

Not all nutritional myopathies in farm animals are selenium-responsive. A myopathy due to vitamin E deficiency can occur in both selenium-adequate and selenium-deficient areas (Peter and Costa, 1992). Another, more unusual, myopathy is lupinosis-associated myopathy (LAM). This is sometimes seen in sheep grazing on lupin stubble infected by the fungus *Phomopsis leptostromiformis*. LAM does not respond either to selenium or to vitamin E treatment, although there is some evidence that both nutrients may be associated with it (Allen et al., 1992).

4.4.2 Exudative Diathesis

Exudative diathesis (ED) is a disease of selenium-deficient chicks. It is also seen in turkey poults and young ducks. In the chick, it usually occurs in 3- to –6-week-old birds and shows initially as an edema on the musculature of the breast, wings, and neck. There is a pathological increase in capillary permeability resulting in subcutaneous hemorrhages (Jenkins et al., 1993). Because of the blood in the fluid, the abdomen and other regions of the bird take on a bluish-green coloration. The growth rate of the birds is slowed and they lose condition, develop leg weakness, and eventually die (Salisbury et al., 1962). The disease often develops concurrently with other selenium deficiency-related conditions, such as WMD. ED has occurred most commonly in commercial flocks fed on low selenium grain (Bains et al., 1975).

It was shown as early as in 1957 that selenium played a part in preventing ED (Patterson et al., 1957). It can also be prevented by supplementation with vitamin E. However, if the animals are severely selenium deficient, vitamin E supplementation is ineffective, whereas addition of as little as 0.5 mg/kg of selenium to the diet prevents the disease (McDowell, 1992). Some protection against ED in chicks can be provided by the addition of certain flavonoids to their diet. Both rutin and silymarin have been found to reduce the incidence and severity of the disease. Flavonoids have been shown to be successful in reducing vascular disorders in humans by strengthening fibrous membranes. It is suggested that they act in a similar manner in ED and thus reduce membrane permeability (Jenkins et al., 1993).

4.4.3 Hepatosis Dietetica

Hepatosis dietetica (HD), also known as liver necrosis or toxic liver dystrophy, is a selenium-responsive disease that affects pigs fed on a low vitamin E/low selenium diet. It occurs most commonly when the animals are 3 to 15 weeks old and can result in a high death rate. HD closely resembles the liver necrosis in the rats studied by Schwarz (1951). Severe necrotic lesions are seen at post mortem. Body fat has a yellowish color (yellow fat) due to deposition of a waxy pigment, and there may also be generalized subcutaneous edema. The mortality and liver lesions can be prevented by providing selenium supplements (Moir and Masters, 1970).

4.4.4 Pancreatic Degeneration

Nutritional pancreatic atrophy is a condition that can occur in poultry fed rations severely depleted in selenium. It is an uncomplicated effect of selenium deficiency and can develop even when vitamin E levels are high. It causes degeneration of the pancreas, with development of fibrosis, and leads to reduction in the amounts of lipase, trypsinogen, and chymotrypsinogen produced. It affects absorption of fat, including vitamin E, and results in poor growth and feathering (McDowell, 1992). Supplementation with selenium is effective and within a few weeks of the beginning of treatment the pancreas returns to its normal appearance (Gries and Scott, 1972).

4.4.5 Ill Thrift

Unthriftiness or ill thrift is a serious condition, which was reported to occur extensively in animals grazing on improved pastures in New Zealand and Australia (McDonald, 1975). It is seen particularly in lambs and yearlings, but also occurs in a less severe form in older sheep as well as in beef and dairy cattle on selenium-deficient soils. Symptoms vary from a mild, subclinical condition to a severe state, with a rapid loss of weight and even death. In sheep there is also a decrease in wool quality and quantity (Drake et al., 1960). It can be readily treated with selenium supplements. Improvements in weight and wool quality in sheep and in growth rates in calves following this treatment can be dramatic (Wilson, 1964).

4.4.6 Impaired Reproduction

Reproductive performance is adversely affected in many species of economically important livestock by selenium deficiency (Underwood, 1977). The production and hatchability of fertile eggs and the viability of newly hatched chicks have been found to be reduced by a low selenium intake. Fertility in ewes and calving in cows are improved by selenium supplementation. A reduction of retained placenta from 17.5% to zero was shown in dairy cows given both selenium and vitamin E (McDowell, 1992). In sheep, in particular, reproductive disorders generally occur in association with other selenium-responsive conditions such as WMD and ill thrift.

4.4.7 Impaired Immune Response

Selenium is essential for the efficient and effective operation of many aspects of the immune system. The exact manner in which the element is involved in the very complex collection of processes that act together to give protection against attacks by pathogens and malignancy is as yet far from fully understood (Arthur et al., 2003). There is evidence that selenium is involved in both the innate, non adaptive system, which includes barriers to infection and nonspecific effector cells such as macrophages, and in the acquired adaptive immune system, in which both T and B lymphocytes form the major effector cells that mature on exposure to immune challenges (Turner and Finch, 1991).

In investigations of the associations between selenium and the immune system, a good deal of attention has been given to the effect of the micronutrient on neutrophil function. Phagocytic neutrophils from selenium-deficient cattle have been shown to have reduced ability to kill ingested cells of *Candida albicans* (Boyne and Arthur, 1979). This has been interpreted as indicating that, in the absence of protection by adequate levels of GPX, the oxygen-derived free radicals produced by neutrophils in the respiratory burst to kill the invading organisms can damage the phagocytic cells themselves (Arthur et al., 1981). The process is believed to involve a delicate balance between production of sufficient radicals to kill the invaders and the neutrophils' ability to protect themselves against the radicals they produce. In many animal species, selenium deficiency does not directly lead to a reduction in neutrophil numbers, but it does affect aspects of their function. This function has been associated with cytosolic GPX (GPX1). Neutrophil production has been shown to be the same in selenium-deficient and selenium-replete mice. Examination of the rate of radical production by the neutrophils from the two sets of mice found that the initial rate of production was the same in both selenium-deplete and -replete animals. However, only the neutrophils from the latter were able to continue producing radicals for >10 and ≤45 min. Thus, ability to continue producing free radicals depends on increased selenium status and GPX activity in the neutrophils. It was concluded from these studies that more than one selenium-dependent function or intracellular compartment is involved in regulating the ability of immune cells to kill ingested organisms. It is possible that other selenoenzymes, including phospholipid hydroperoxide GPX as well as cytosolic and mitochondrial TR may be involved, along with GPX1, in these changes in candidacidal activity (Arthur et al., 2003).

As has been commented by Turner and Finch (1991), most of the earlier investigations of the immunological effects of selenium concluded that IgM and IgG antibody responses could be boosted most effectively by using levels of supplements considerably in excess of those required for normal growth and nutrition. Subsequent studies have found that these results depend on species, age, sex, and antigen. For example, whereas selenium supplementation in young mice was shown to enhance antibody production against sheep red blood cell antigen (Mulhern et al., 1985), the same level of supplementation was inhibitory in male, but not in female, chicks (Marsh et al., 1981). Considerable differences in lymphocyte reactivity to phytolectin mitogens have been shown in different animal species in response to selenium deficiency. In addition to species differences, the use of mitogen probes has also shown that adult ruminants appear to be unusually resistant to the immunological effects of selenium deficiency compared to young animals (Turner and Finch, 1991).

Such findings serve to underline the complexity of the immune system and the continuing need for further research to resolve many problems that still remain regarding the relation between selenium and immunity. Much has still to be learned, for example, about the significance of species differences, supplement dose amounts, growth stages, and antigen types. To complicate matters, there is the observation by Boyne and Arthur (1979) that selenium deficiency may, in some circumstances, be preferable to supplementation. Their finding that selenium-deficient rats survived longer after an injection of *Salmonella typhimurium* than did selenium-supplemented animals is of significance in this regard. They comment that when selenium is given to a bacterially infected, selenium-deficient animal, the treatment may have undesirable consequences if the organism's growth and yield of endotoxin are stimulated so effectively that the resistance of the host is overwhelmed.

Selenium and vitamin E appear to play similar roles in immune function and for this reason are often given to farm animals as a mixed supplement. Their effects have been shown to be additive. In weaning pigs, for instance, humural antibody production in response to sheep red blood cells increases when either selenium or α-tocopherol is given on their own and is further increased when both nutrients are given together (Peplowski et al., 1980). Combined selenium and vitamin E deficiency has been found to affect the ability of dogs to produce antibodies to distemper virus (Sheffy and Schulz, 1978).

4.5 Subclinical Selenium Deficiencies

While clinical effects associated with frank selenium deficiency in animals are reasonably well defined and can be identified by their visible symptoms, subclinical effects of marginal deficiency are much more difficult to detect. These are associated with depressed growth and production and other conditions such as impaired immune response. Although the effects may be transient and not result in clear-cut symptoms, the overall implications for livestock can be considerable (Langlands, 1987).

When treatment of frank selenium deficiency in farm animals was introduced on a wide scale in New Zealand, Australia, and other countries, there were frequent reports that, in addition to the expected effect of alleviating clearly recognized symptoms of, for example, WMD, unexpected dividends in productive and reproductive performance were obtained (Oldfield, 1992). Even in some cases where there was no history of frank deficiency, selenium supplementation was seen to bring about considerable benefits. This was shown in the 1950s by New Zealand investigators who produced increases in body weight and wool yield in sheep, with no previous indications of any selenium-responsive disorders, when they were provided with selenium supplementation.

In Australia, scientists at the Division of Animal Production of the Commonwealth Scientific and Industrial Research Organization (CSIRO) found that when sheep with low blood-selenium levels, though showing no signs of overt deficiency, were treated with selenium, in addition to increases in live weight, fleece weight and quality also improved significantly (Langlands et al., 1991a). It was also found that selenium supplementation increased the numberof lambs weaned per ewe and that lamb survival rate also improved (Langlands et al., 1991b). Live weight at birth also increased significantly (Langlands et al., 1991c).

These investigations of subclinical selenium deficiency in farm animals carried out by Langlands and his colleagues have been described by Oldfield (1992) as remarkable because they explore the uncertain area of marginal deficiency and provide evidence that selenium supplementation may be useful here too, as it is in areas of frank deficiency. He also points out that the number of animals worldwide whose selenium intake is marginal is very much greater than that of those with frank deficiency.

4.6 Selenium Supplementation of Livestock

Since the recognition of the essential nature of selenium and its role in the prevention of a variety of economically significant diseases in farm animals, selenium supplementation of livestock has become normal practice in agriculture.

A variety of different methods are used as supplementation strategies. These can be classified into three groups:

1. Application of the element directly to pastures
2. Free choice supplementation
3. Direct administration to animals

Direct application of selenium to agricultural land was pioneered on a large scale in New Zealand, where soil selenium deficiency is a major problem. The practice has been followed in many other countries with a similar problem, notably in Finland. There, the addition of selenium to agricultural fertilizers is a legal requirement. Elsewhere the practice is encouraged but is not mandatory. Selenium is added to normal fertilizers, usually as sodium selenate, either encapsulated in clay as a water-soluble prill or sprayed as an aqueous solution onto the fertilizer granules. It has been shown to be an effective and reliable method for boosting selenium levels in pasture plants as well as in cereals and other crops (Oldfield, 1993).

In free-access methods, sodium selenate or selenite is incorporated into salt blocks or licks of different compositions. These are placed where they can be accessed by free-ranging animals. In the UK a selenite-enriched molasses-based feed, which can be distributed in suitable containers, is widely used with dairy and beef cattle herds. Typically these feeds are vitamin and mineral mixes, made attractive to the animals by the molasses.

Dietary supplementation of rations with selenium is now standard agricultural practice in many countries. Because of concerns about possible adverse health effects of increased selenium intakes to consumers of milk and other animal products, the amounts of selenium that may be added to the feed are limited by government regulations in many countries. Permitted levels vary between countries, with a range of 0.1 to 0.5 mg/kg in diets and 25 to 90 mg/kg in salt/mineral mixes (Oldfield, 1990). In the USA use of selenium compounds as additives in animal rations was prohibited until 1974 on the grounds that the element was carcinogenic. This prohibition was subsequently removed by the Food and Drug Administration (FDA) (1993).

Several different techniques have been developed for administering supplementary selenium directly to livestock. Aqueous solutions of selenium salts, given orally in the form of drenches, is a widely used method, since it is relatively easy to administer and the materials used are inexpensive. Sodium selenite and selenate, as well as the barium salts, can be administered by subcutaneous and intramuscular injection. Injection bypasses the rumen and thus avoids the possibility of reduction of the soluble selenium to unavailable selenide.

A slow release technique, based on the one developed in Australia in the 1960s for cobalt supplementation, is widely used, especially by sheep farmers in the antipodes. The selenium is incorporated into heavy pellets, containing up to 95% iron. These are administered orally and, because of their density, lodge in the reticulum or rumen where they slowly dissolve and release selenium. In addition to the heavy pellets, glass boluses and miniature osmotic pumps are also available as rumen inclusions.

References

Allen, J.G., Steele, P., Masters, H.G., and Lambe, W.J., 1992, Lupinosis in sheep, *Aust. Vet. J.* **69**, 75–80.

Andrews, E.D., Hartley, W.J., and Grant, A.B., 1968, Selenium-responsive diseases in animals in New Zealand, *NZ Vet. J.* **16**, 3–17.

Arthur, J.R., Boyne, R., and Okolow-Zubkowska, M.J., 1981, The production of oxygen-derived radicals by neutrophils from selenium-deficient cattle, *FEBS Letts* **135**, 187–190.

Arthur, J.R., McKenzie, R.C., and Beckett, G.J., 2003, Selenium in the immune system, *J. Nutr.* **133**, 1457S–1459S.

Bains, B.S., Mackenzie, M.A., and Mackenzie, R.A., 1975, Selenium deficiency in a commercial poultry operation, *Aust. Vet. J.* **55**, 140–145.

Beath, O.A., Draizze, J.H., Eppson, H.F., et al., 1934, Certain poisonous plants of Wyoming activated by selenium and their associations with respect to soil types, *J. Am. Pharmacol. Assoc. Sci. Edu.* **23**, 94–97.

Boyne, R. and Arthur, J.R., 1979, Alterations in neutrophil function in selenium deficient cattle, *J. Compar. Pathol.* **89**, 151–158.

Drake, C., Grant, A.B., and Hartley, W.J., 1960. Selenium in animal health 2. The effects of selenium on unthrifty weaned lambs, *NZ Vet. J.* **8**, 7–10.

Eggert, R.O., Patterson, E., Akers, W.J., and Stokstad, K.L.R., 1957, The role of vitamin E and selenium in the nutrition of the pig, *J. Anim. Sci.* **16**, 1037.

Faye, B. and Bengoumi, M., 1994, Trace element status in camels—a review, *Biol. Trace Elem. Res.* **41**, 1–11.

Fleming, S.A. and Walsh, T., 1957, Selenium occurrence in certain Irish soils and its toxic effects on animals, *Proc. Roy. Irish Acad.* **58B**, 151–166.

Food and Drug Administration, 1993, Food Additives permitted in feed and drinking water of animals; selenium; stay of the 1987 amendments; final rule. *Federal Register* **58**, No. 175, 47962–47973.

Franke, K.W., 1934, A new toxicant occurring naturally in certain samples of plant foodstuffs. 1. Results obtained in preliminary feeding trials, *J. Nutr.* **8**, 597–608.

Fream, W., 1890, The herbage of pastures, *J. Roy. Agr. Soc. England* **1**, 384–394.

Gill, G.P.S., Roy, K.S., and Uppal, V., 2003, Histopathological study after selenium toxicity in buffalo calves, *Ind. J. Anim. Sci.* **73**, 131–135.

Gries, C.L. and Scott, M.L., 1972, Pathology of selenium deficiency in the chick, *J. Nutr.* **102**, 1287–1292.

Gupta, U.C. and Gupta, S.C., 2002, Quality of animal and human life as affected by selenium management of soils and crops, *Comm. Soil Sci. Plant. Anal.* **33**, 2537–2555.

Hill, J., Allison, F., and Halpin, C., 1985, An episode of acute selenium toxicity in a commercial piggery, *Aust. Vet. J.* **62**, 207–209.

Jaffe, W.G., 1973, Selenium in food plants and feed. Toxicology and nutrition, *Qualitas Plantarum. Plant Foods Human Nutr.* **23**, 191–204.

Jaffe, W.G. and Mondragon, M.C., 1969, Adaptation of rats to selenium intake, *J. Nutr.* **97**, 431–436.

Jenkins, K.J., Hidiroglou, M., and Collins, F.W., 1993, Influence of various flavonoids and simple phenolics on development of exudative diathesis in the chick, *J. Agric. Food Chem.* **41**, 441–445.

Jukes, T.H., 1983, Nuggets on the surface: selenium an "essential poison". *J. Appl. Sci.* **5**, 233–234.

Kennedy, D.G., Goodall, E.A., and Kennedy, S., 1993, Antioxidant enzyme activity in the muscles of calves depleted of vitamin E or selenium or both, *Br. J. Nutr.* **70**, 621–630.

Knott, S.G. and McCray, C.W.R., 1958, Selenium poisoning in horses in North Queensland, *Qld J. Agric. Sci.* **15**, 43–58.

Langlands, J.P., 1987, Recent advances in copper and selenium supplementation of grazing ruminants, in: *Proc. Advances in Animal Nutrition Conference*, University of New England, May 2–4, University of New England, Armidale, NSW, Australia.

Langlands, J.P., Donald, G.E., Bowles, J.E., et al., 1991a, Subclinical selenium insufficiency 1. Selenium status and the response in liveweight and wool production of grazing ewes supplemented with selenium, *Aust. J. Exp. Agr.* **31**, 25–31.

Langlands, J.P., Donald, G.E., Bowles, J.E., et al., 1991b, Subclinical selenium deficiency 2. The response in reproductive performance of grazing ewes supplemented with selenium, *Aust. J. Exp. Agr.* **31**, 33–35

Langlands, J.P., Donald, G.E., Bowles, J.E., et al., 1991c, Subclinical selenium insufficiency 3. The selenium status and productivity of lambs born to ewes supplemented with selenium, *Aust. J. Exper. Agr.* **31**, 37–43.

Levander, O.A., 1986, Selenium, in: Mertz, W. (ed.), *Trace Elements in Human and Animal Nutrition*, Academic Press, New York, pp. 209–219.

Levander, O.A. and Baumann, C.A., 1966, Selenium metabolism VI. Effect of arsenic on the secretion of selenium in the bile, *Toxicol. Appl. Pharmacol.* **9**, 106–115.

Lofstedt, J., 1997, White muscle disease of foals, *Vet. Clin. North Am – Equine Pract.* **13**, 169–171.

Madison, T.C., 1860, Sanitary report—Fort Randall, in: Coolidge, R.H. (ed.), Statistical Report on the Sickness and Mortality in the Army of the United States, January 1855 to January 1860, US Congress 36th, 1st Session, Senate Exchange Document, as cited in Rosenfeldt, I. and Beath, O.A. (1964), Selenium Geobotany, Biochemistry, Toxicity and Nutrition, Academic Press, New York, p. 7.

Magg, D.D. and Glen, M.W., 1967, Toxicity of selenium: farm animals, in: Muth, O.H., Oldfield, J.E., and Heswig, P.H. (eds), *Selenium in Biomedicine*, AVI, Westport, CT, pp. 127–140.

Marsh, J.A., Dietert, R.R., and Combs, G.F., 1981, Effect of dietary selenium and vitamin E on the humoral immunity of the chick, *Proc. Soc. Exp. Biol. Med.* **166**, 228–236.

Martin, J.L., 1978, Nutrition toxicities in animals and man: selenium, in: Rechcigl, M. (ed.), *CRC Handbook Series in Nutrition and Food*, Vol. 1, CRC Press, Boca Raton, FL, pp. 309–317.

McDonald, J.W., 1975, Selenium-responsive unthriftiness of young Merino sheep in central Victoria, *Aust. Vet. J.* **51**, 433–435.

McDowell, L.R., 1992, *Minerals in Animal Nutrition*, Academic Press, New York, pp. 325–327.

Moir, D.C. and Masters, H.G., 1970, Selenium deficiency and hepatosis dietetica in pigs, *Aust. Vet. J.* **55**, 360–366.

Mulhern, S.A., Taylor, G.I., Macgruder, L.E., and Vessey, A.R., 1985, Deficient levels of dietary selenium suppress the antibody response in first and second generation mice, *Nutr. Res.* **5**, 201–210.

Oldfield, J.E., 1990, *Selenium: Its Uses in Agriculture, Nutrition and Health and Environment*, Selenium–Tellurium Development Association, Grimbergen, Belgium.

Oldfield, J.E., 1992, Subclinical selenium deficiencies in livestock, *Bull. Se-Te Dev. Assoc.* Sept., Selenium-Tellurium Development Association, Grimbergen, Belgium, pp. 5–6.

Oldfield, J.E., 1993, *Selenium in Fertilizers*, Selenium–Tellurium Development Association, Grimbergen, Belgium.

Oldfield, J.E., 1999, *Selenium World Atlas*, Selenium–Tellurium Development Association, Grimbergen, Belgium, p. 39.

Oldfield, J.E., 2003, Some recollections of early swine research with selenium and vitamin E, *J. Anim. Sci.* **81** (E. Suppl. 2), E145–E148.

Oldfield, J.E., 2005, Selenium in nutrition: the early years. *A.L. Moxton Honorary Lectures Special Circular 167–99*, Ohio State University, http://ohioline.osu.edu/sc167/sc167_04.html.

Olivera, P., Jovanovic, B., Gvozdic, D., and Stojic, V., 2004, Selenium status of sheep and their lambs in the Northern Serbian Province of Vojvodina, *Acta Vet.-Beograd.* **54**, 403–409.

Or, M.E., Dodurka, H.T., and Kayar, A., 2003, The diagnostic importance of erythrocyte glutathione peroxidase (GSH-Px) activity and some serum parameters in lambs with white muscle disease, *Turk. J. Vet. Anim. Sci.* **27**, 1–6.

O'Toole, D. and Raisbeck, M.F., 1995, Pathology of experimentally induced chronic selenosis (alkali disease) in yearling cattle, *J. Vet. Diagn. Invest.* **7**, 364–367.

Patterson, E.L., Milstrey, R., and Stokstad, E.L.R., 1957, Effect of selenium in preventing exudative diathesis in chicks, *Proc. Soc. Exp. Biol. Med.* **95**, 617–620.

Peplowski, M.A., Mahan, D.C., Murray, F.A., et al., 1980, Effect of dietary and injectable vitamin E and selenium in weanling swine antigenically challenged with sheep red blood cells, *J. Anim. Sci.* **51**, 344–349.

Peter, D.W. and Costa, N.D., 1992, Selenium in animal production in Australia, *Proc. Nutr. Soc. Aust.* **17**, 99–108.

Raisbeck, M.F., 2000, Selenosis, *Vet. Clin. North Am. Food Anim. Pract.* **16**, 465–480.

Ramirez-Bribiesca, J.E., Tortora, J.L., Huerta, M., et al., 2005, Effect of selenium-vitamin E injection in selenium-deficient dairy goats and kids on the Mexican plateau, *Arquivo Brasileiro de Medicina Veterinaria Zootecnia* **57**, 77–84.

Rogers, P.A.M., Arora, S.P., Fleming, G.A., et al., 1990, Selenium toxicity in farm animals: treatment and prevention, *Irish Vet. J.* **43**, 151–153.

Rosenfeld, I. and Beath, O.A., 1964, *Selenium Geobotany, Biochemistry, Toxicity and Nutrition*, Academic Press, New York, p. 7.

Salisbury, R.M., Edmondson, J., Poole, W.S.H., et al., 1962, Exudative diathesis and white muscle disease in poultry in New Zealand, *Proc. 12th World Poultry Cong.*, University of Sydney, Australia, pp. 379–84.

Schwarz, K., 1944, Selen, *Zeitschrift f. Physiologische Chemie* **281**, 109–112.

Schwarz, K., 1951, A hitherto unrecognized factor against dietary necrotic liver degeneration in American yeast (factor 3), *Proc. Soc. Exp. Biol. Med.* **78**, 852–854.

Schwarz, K. and Foltz, C.M., 1957, Selenium as an integral part of Factor 3 against dietary necrotic liver degeneration, *J. Am. Chem. Soc.* **79**, 3292–3293.

Scott, M.L., 1962, Antioxidants, selenium and sulphur amino acids in the vitamin E nutrition of chicks, *Nutr. Abs. Rev.* **32**, 1–8.

Sheffy, B.E. and Schulz, R.D., 1978, Influence of vitamin E and selenium on immune response mechanisms, *Cornell Vet.* **68**, 89–93.

Simon, P., 1560. Noticias historiales de las conquistas de tierre firme en las Indias, *Biblioteca Autores Colombianos*, Vol. 4, Kelly Publishing, Bogota, Colombia, pp. 226–254, cited in Roselfeld, I. and Beath, O.A., 1964, *Selenium Geobotany, Biochemistry, Toxicity and Nutrition*, Academic Press, New York.

Subramanian, R. and Muhuntha, A., 1993, Soil–fodder–animal relationship of selenium toxicity in buffaloes, in: Anke, M., Meissner, D., and Mills, C.F. (eds), *Trace Elements in Man and Animals—TEMA 8*, Verlag Media Touristik, Gersdorf, Germany, pp. 498–501.

Tinggi, U., 2005, Selenium toxicity and its adverse health effects, in: Preedy, R. and Watson, R.R. (eds), *Reviews in Food and Nutrition Toxicity*, Taylor & Francis, Boca Raton, FL, pp. 29–55.

Turner, R.J. and Finch, J.M., 1991, Selenium and the immune response, *Proc. Nutr. Soc.* **50**, 275–285.

Underwood, E.J., 1977, *Trace Elements in Human and Animal Nutrition*, 4th edn., Academic Press, New York, pp. 303–345.

USDA, 2005a, *Locoweed (Astragalus and Oxytropis spp.)*, United States Department of Agriculture Poisonous Plant Research Laboratory, http://www.pprl.ars.usda.gov/locoweed.htm.

USDA, 2005b, *Selenium accumulating plants*, United States Department of Agriculture Poisonous Plant Research Laboratory, http://www.pprl.usu.edu/selenium_accumulators.htm.

Vernie, L.N., Bont, W.S., Ginjaar, H.B., and Emmelot, P., 1975, Elongation factor 2 as the target of the reaction product between sodium selenite and glutathione (GSSeSG) in the inhibition of amino acid incorporation in vitro, *Biochim. Biophys. Acta* **416**, 283–292.

Wilson, G.F., 1964, Responses in dairy calves to mineral supplements, *NZ J Agric. Res.* **7**, 432–433.

Walsh, T., Fleming, S.A., O'Connor, R., and Sweaney, A., 1951, Selenium toxicity associated with an Irish soil series, *Nature (Lond.)* **168**, 881–882.

Wolf, E., Kollonitsch, V., and Kline, C.H., 1963, A survey of selenium treatments in livestock production, *Agric. Food Chem.* **11**, 355–360.

Wyoming State Board of Sheep Commissioners, 1908, *10th Annual Report, Cheyenne, Wyoming*, cited in: Rosenfeld, I. and Beath, O.A. (eds), *Selenium Geobotany, Biochemistry, Toxicity and Nutrition*, Academic Press, New York, p. 7.

5 Selenium in Health and Disease II: Endemic Selenium-Related Conditions in Humans

5.1 Selenium Toxicity

It was inevitable that once the importance of selenium in animal health had been recognized, the question would be asked whether the element was also of significance to humans. The possibility began to be considered seriously following the identification in the early 1930s of selenium toxicity in livestock in seleniferous areas of some of the states in the Midwest. If cattle could be poisoned by eating selenium-rich plants, including grain, perhaps a similar effect occurred in farmers and their families who raised these animals and consumed locally produced foods.

5.1.1 Selenium Toxicity in Humans in Seleniferous Regions of North America

In 1934 a survey of a rural population living on farms in South Dakota with a history of selenosis in livestock was undertaken by the US Public Health Service (Smith et al., 1936). The health status of each member of the families was recorded, along with their intakes of locally grown foods. Urine samples were collected and analyzed for selenium.

No clear symptoms of selenium poisoning were found, even in individuals with high levels of selenium in their urine. However, a number of vague indications of ill health and a higher than normal incidence of bad teeth, damaged nails, and other less clearly defined conditions were observed, especially in those with the highest urine selenium levels. Results of a more detailed survey carried out in the following year were interpreted as indicating that though none of the observed symptoms could be regarded as specific for selenium poisoning, some at least could be considered to be related to selenium ingestion (Smith and Westfall, 1937).

The investigation found that the average intake of selenium in the diet in the area surveyed was as much as 10 to 200 μg/kg body weight, equivalent to 700 to 1,400 μg/day for a 70 kg adult.

In subsequent years several other reports were published on selenium intake and its effects on health of residents of South Dakota and neighboring states where significant seleniferous regions occurred. While no cases of frank selenosis were found, overall findings were interpreted as indicating that selenium poisoning was, in fact, common in those regions and posed a health problem (Lemley, 1943). However, possibly owing to the difficult wartime conditions that prevailed, little appears to have been done at that time by the Public Health Service to find a solution to the problem (Kilness, 1973).

Another US government agency, the FDA, had begun at about the same time to take a serious interest in the possible health implications of high levels of selenium in human food (Nelson et al., 1943). Researchers at the Agency's laboratories had found evidence that consumption of selenium-rich wheat, as well as a selenium-containing pesticide, could cause liver cancer in rats. The pesticide was potassium ammonium sulfoselenide, marketed under the trade name Selocide as a systemic insecticide (Gnadinger, 1933). On the basis of these findings, the FDA decided to classify selenium as a carcinogen, and its use as a supplement in animal rations, and later in human diets, was officially restricted. This decision caused considerable difficulties over the following years for animal as well as human nutritionists who believed that selenium supplementation had an important role to play in the promotion of health (Frost, 1972). As was argued by Frost and Ingvoldstad (1975), it was the FDA's classification of selenium as a carcinogen, rather than the findings of what were apparently selenium-related toxic symptoms among rural communities in South Dakota, that was responsible for what they called *selenophobia*, an exaggerated fear of selenium as a toxin, which helped to concentrate interest among health professionals for several decades on the negative rather than the positive aspects of the element.

5.1.2 Human Selenosis in Latin America

The Great Plains were not the only parts of America where selenium-related toxicity symptoms were observed in residents of seleniferous regions. In the early 1970s there were reports of selenosis in Venezuela (Jaffe et al., 1972). Children living in a seleniferous area were found to have symptoms, which included dermatitis, loose hair, and damaged nails, accompanied by elevated serum and urine selenium levels. One group had a mean serum level of over 1.3 mg/l. Twenty years later the survey was repeated. Elevated levels of selenium in serum were again found, though symptoms of selenosis were observed in only a few children (Bratter et al., 1991).

Selenium poisoning in some areas of tropical America has been associated with consumption of nuts of a species of Lecythidaceae, a large family of forest trees. They include *Bertholletia excelsa*, the tree that produces the well-known Brazil nut, and *Lecythis elliptica* on which the sapucaia nut grows. Brazil nuts are rich in edible oils and protein and can make an important contribution to the diet, especially of some of the forest-dwelling inhabitants of the Amazon region. In addition, the trees are selenium accumulators and can concentrate it in the nuts to very high levels, in some cases to more than 500 µg/g (Sector and Lisk, 1989). While in theory consumption of even one Brazil nut with this level of selenium concentration could be lethal, especially for a child, there do not appear to be any reported deaths from this cause. However, death has been caused by the nuts of the related *Lecythis ollaria*. Consumption of these nuts, which are also known as "Coco de Mono" or "monkey coconut," has been known to cause symptoms of chronic selenium poisoning, including hair loss, nail damage, and a foul breath (Kerdel-Vegas, 1966).

As long ago as the 16th century it had been reported that a disease, with symptoms very similar to those described in 20th-century Venezuela, occurred among humans as well as animals in Colombia (Simón, 1953). The report was written by a Spanish Franciscan missionary, Father Pedro Simón, who had observed, in some parts of the country, symptoms of disease in domestic animals and humans that included hair and nail loss, hoof drop in cattle, as well as malformation in children, infertility, and "monster births." Simon attributed the condition to consumption of poisonous corn and other vegetables grown in the area. Three hundred years later, the symptoms, which had continued to be observed in parts of Colombia, were recognized as being the result of selenium poisoning (Rosenfeld and Beath, 1964).

5.1.3 Endemic Selenosis in China

Reports of large-scale endemic selenium intoxication of humans in China began to appear in the world scientific literature in the early 1980s. Among the earliest of these reports was that of Guangi Yang and his colleagues at the Chinese Academy of Preventive Medicine (Yang et al., 1983). This presented information on a human disease of unknown origin, characterized by loss of nails and hair, which had first come to the attention of health authorities in Enshi County, Hubei Province, in the early 1960s. This is a remote, mountainous region in the midwest of China, about 1,100 km west of Shanghai.

At its peak the illness affected on average nearly half the inhabitants of villages in the area, with an incidence of over 80% in one. In victims, tissues most affected were hair, nails, skin, nervous system, and teeth. Hair became dry, lost color, and was easily broken off at the base. A rash developed on the scalp and skin lesions appeared elsewhere on the body. Nails were brittle and fell out, and on regrowth were rough and fell out again. A high proportion of those affected had mottled teeth, in some cases with erosion and pitting.

In the most seriously affected villages, abnormalities of the nervous system were observed. Initially this showed as peripheral anesthesia and pain in the extremities. A few patients had parasthesia and one hemiplagic died. Disturbances of the digestive tract also occurred.

It was found that vegetables and grains consumed by the villagers contained unusually high concentrations of selenium. These were considerably higher than those in similar foods produced in nonseleniferous regions. In the case of cereals, for instance, there was a difference of approximately 200-fold between samples from Enshi County and from a normal soil region. Even more spectacular was the difference of more than 45,000-fold between selenium levels in green turnips from Enshi and another region in which selenium deficiency was widespread. Since the normal diet of inhabitants of the seleniferous region was very restricted in variety and consisted mainly of locally produced foods, intake of selenium was high. This was calculated to be an average of 4.99 mg, with a range of 3.20 to 6.99 mg/day, more than 40 times the usual intake of members of the investigating team who normally lived in the selenium-adequate Beijing region.

As might be expected, as a result of their very high regular intake, Enshi County residents had unusually high levels of selenium in their blood, hair, and urine. In one case, a level of 7.5 μg/ml was recorded in whole blood, about 1,000 times the average found in a selenium-deficient area of neighboring Shanxi province. The report made the interesting comment that the occurrence of such extremely high-tissue-selenium levels pointed to the possibility that an adaptive mechanism toward chronically high selenium levels was in action in the residents of the seleniferous region.

The source of the high levels of selenium in foods and consequently in the diet of villagers was traced to the high levels of biologically available selenium in the soil of the area. Total selenium levels in soil collected in Enshi County averaged 7,870 ± 69 μg/kg, of which 354 ± 45 μg/kg was water-soluble. In contrast, the mean level in soil from a nonseleniferous region was 84 ± 11 μg/kg for total and 2.8 ± 0.3 μg/kg for water-soluble selenium.

The ultimate source of the high levels of selenium in the soil of Enshi County was believed to be selenium-rich coal outcrops in the area. In Ziyang County, Shaanxi Province, there is another region in which selenosis occurs among local residents. Here too, crops enriched in selenium which are grown on seleniferous soil are consumed. The soil is derived from highly seleniferous slate, shale, and volcanic tuff, and contains as much as 10 to 30 mg/kg of selenium.

In Enshi County, as well as enriching agricultural soil with selenium, the locally mined coal is believed to contribute to the occurrence of selenosis in another way also, through the smoke it emits when burned. Burning of raw coal in unvented domestic stoves is believed to have widespread and serious effects on the health of considerable numbers of people in parts of China because of the high levels of selenium, as well as, in some regions, of arsenic and other toxic elements, in the smoke (Finkleman et al., 1999). In addition to contamination of food and water, the selenium-rich fumes are also inhaled, contributing to the high levels of intake by occupants of poorly ventilated homes. This remains a serious problem in parts of Southwest China where nearly 500 cases of endemic selenium intoxication due to this cause were reported in 1999 (Zheng et al., 1999).

5.1.4 Other Consequences of Large-Scale Selenium Intake

Several other conditions have been reported to be associated with high intakes of selenium by people living in seleniferous regions. Evidence to support the associations is not always very strong and often the situation is complicated by other concurrent factors.

5.1.4.1 Dental Caries

One of the symptoms reported by the Chinese investigators of selenium toxicity in Hubei Province was dental decay (Yang et al., 1983). It has also been reported in other incidents of selenosis. In the early studies of seleniferous regions in South Dakota and neighboring states of the Midwest, Smith and his fellow investigators noted a high prevalence of dental caries among their subjects (Smith et al., 1936). The results of subsequent studies by Hadjimarkos et al. (1952) in the same areas were interpreted as showing that the prevalence of dental caries was directly related to the high selenium levels in urine found in children. However, the findings of another study in Wyoming, which also pointed to an association between dental caries and selenium intake, were complicated by the presence of high levels of fluoride in local water supplies (Tank and Storvick, 1960).

In the Chinese investigation (Yang et al., 1983) nearly one third of those affected by high selenium intakes had mottled teeth, some showing pitting or erosion. However, as in the Wyoming study, since there was fluorosis also in the region, the investigators could not decide whether the tooth decay was caused by fluorine or selenium, or by a combination of the two. Hadjimarkos had, in fact, pointed out that dental caries is a multifactorial disease and that it is erroneous to compare and interpret differences in the prevalence of caries seen in children living in different parts of the USA on the basis of dietary selenium alone (Hadjimarkos, 1973).

5.1.4.2 Amyotrophic Lateral Sclerosis (Motor Neuron Disease)

Another condition, which has been attributed by some investigators to a high intake of selenium, is amyotrophic lateral sclerosis (ALS). It is also known as Lou Gehrig's disease and is the most common type of motor neuron disease. ALS is a rare condition, with, for example, one or two cases per 100,000 diagnosed annually in the UK. The disease usually affects people over the age of 50 and is most common in men. It is a disease of the nervous system in which degeneration of nerve cells of the brain and spine occurs, with progressive wasting of the body and spastic paralysis.

In the late 1970s an unusual cluster of four cases of ALS were reported in male farmers living in a seleniferous region of South Dakota (Kilness and Hochberg, 1977). The findings were interpreted by the investigators as indicating a possible relationship between high selenium intakes and the disease. The report produced immediate and vigorous debate in the letter pages of the *Journal of the American Medical Association*. The findings were criticized on the grounds that the level of incidence found in South Dakota was not greater than in nonseleniferous areas (Schwarz, 1977), and it was claimed that the cluster was more likely to be indicative of a chance occurrence than of an association with high selenium intakes (Kurland, 1977). Further investigations produced conflicting results, some pointing toward an association, others apparently not. The controversy appeared to have been ended in favor of the doubter by the results of another study which found that, out of 20 ALS patients, 19 had lower than average urinary selenium levels (Norris and Sang, 1978). However, 15 years later it was reopened by a report of a Japanese investigation that looked at ALS in people consuming fish containing high levels of both selenium and mercury. The results appeared to indicate that there was a correlation between a high intake of selenium and incidence of ALS among fish consumers (Moriwako, 1993).

The debate continues, with the results of some recent studies once more suggesting that trace metals, including selenium, are implicated in the pathogenesis of sporadic motor neuron disease (SMND). However, in several cases the results have been contradictory. One study, which looked at levels of both toxic and trace elements in the blood of SMND patients, found that none of the range of metals tested, except for cadmium, was significantly raised (Pamphlett et al., 2001). A population-based study, which used toenail clippings to determine environmental exposure to a range of trace elements, also found no evidence that trace elements played a major role in the etiology of sporadic ALS (Bergomi et al., 2002). However, the investigators did not totally reject the possibility of an association between the disease and at least some trace elements. They noted that their results for selenium, as well as for zinc and copper, needed to be evaluated with caution because of the limitations of toenails as biomarkers of chronic exposure to these metals.

5.1.4.3 Defective Reproduction

There are some indications that a high dietary intake of selenium may result in infertility and be teratogenic. Some findings suggest that impaired reproduction may be a consequence of selenium intoxication in farm and other animals (Mahan and Peters, 2004), including fish (Palace et al., 2004). Convincing evidence for similar effects in humans is lacking. There are anecdotal reports of infertility and the birth of "monsters" in seleniferous regions of South America in the 16th century (Rosenfeld and Beath, 1964). However, a late 20th-century investigation by Jaffe and Velez (1973) failed to find any evidence of a correlation between selenium intake and congenital malformations in seleniferous areas of Venezuela. It has been claimed that occupational exposure to selenium has caused spontaneous abortions in pregnant factory workers who were involved in the preparation of selenium-containing microbiological media, though it is not clear that selenium was the actual cause of the problem (Robertson, 1970).

5.2 Endemic Diseases Related to Selenium Deficiency in Humans

As had been the case with selenium toxicity, so it was to be with the discovery of selenium deficiency-related diseases in humans. The finding of such conditions in farm animals directed the attention of investigators to the possibility that humans might also be at risk from an inadequate intake of the element. Nevertheless, although the essentiality of selenium for animals had been established by the late 1950s, it was several years before the first tentative steps were taken to establish a similar role for selenium in humans. Many investigators and government health authorities continued to focus attention on the toxic nature of the element rather than on its possible positive nutritional role.

Frost (1972), one of the pioneers of studies of the role of selenium in human health, in his provocative review entitled *The two faces of selenium*, summed up the situation as he saw it at a time when the FDA still banned all agricultural use of the element, in spite of its proved nutritional role in animals. Although he was hopeful that the use of selenium supplements in animal rations would eventually be approved, he feared that a similar use in human diets was many years away. However, he noted that in spite of erroneous fears and misconceptions, knowledge of the biochemical and nutritional role of selenium continued to advance. He referred to studies by Marjanen (1969) in Finland that had found indications that deficiency of selenium in the national diet might underlie the high cancer and cardiac mortality rates observed in Finns. This observation was, in the light of subsequent events in that country, highly significant.

Frost also referred to studies in New Zealand that also pointed towards the positive role of selenium in human health. Results of an investigation of the levels of incidence of sudden infant death syndrome (SIDS) or cot death, which were unusually high in the country, were interpreted by some physicians as indicating that the condition was related to a deficiency in the infants' diet of both selenium and vitamin E (Money, 1970). This question will be discussed more at length in a later section. Here it will be sufficient to note, as did Frost, that the New Zealand Department of Health responded to this report by issuing an instruction to physicians asking them to keep records of details of the diet of SIDS victims they attended (Thompson and Paul, 1971). Frost commented that the overall tone of the government instruction illustrated the customary official attitude toward selenium. This was, he wrote, shown by one sentence in particular which stated: "selenium being a toxic substance which is not known to be essential in human nutrition, is not at present recommended for supplementation" (Frost, 1972).

At about the same time as these New Zealand studies were being carried out, investigations were also underway in the USA into the possibility that cancer mortality might be inversely related to selenium levels in the diet (Shamberger and Frost, 1969). However, none of these studies were enough to convince the majority of health officials and researchers that selenium deficiency might indeed have a role to play in the causation of human disease. It took a finding of international significance to bring about acceptance of the view that inadequate dietary selenium was a potentially serious health problem and that life-threatening conditions of selenium deficiency did indeed occur on a large scale, at least in some parts of the world.

5.2.1 *Keshan Disease*

In 1935 an outbreak of an unknown disease with a sudden onset of precardial oppression and pain, nausea, and vomiting, in some cases ending in death, was reported to have occurred in an isolated area of what was then Japanese-occupied Manchuria. This was Keshan County, Heilongjiang Province in modern northeastern Peoples Republic of China (Yang et al., 1984). Since the etiology of the disease was unknown, it was given the name Keshan disease (KD) after the place where it was first observed. Later, though the disease was found to occur also in other parts of China, as well as of neighboring countries, its name was not changed.

This was probably not the first time that the disease had been recorded. As early as 1907 outbreaks of an illness with similar symptoms had been reported in Manchuria (Gu, 1993), but the 1935 outbreak was apparently far more severe than the earlier incidents, and was described as plague-like in its extent (Ge and Yang, 1993).

KD attracted a great deal of attention in the mid-1930s in the region and medical investigation teams were organized to deal with it. However, for a variety of reasons, not least of which was the war, progress was limited and the outbreak does not appear to have been reported in overseas scientific literature at the time. Following the arrival of political stability, active investigation into KD was resumed. Medical interest was further stimulated by the discovery of several other locations besides Keshan county where the disease occurred. In the late 1950s and the 1960s considerable progress was made in discovering the distribution, implications, and possible causes of KD. Management strategies were developed and practical treatments investigated. Of particular importance to this progress was the establishment in China of dedicated groups, such as the Department of Keshan Research of Jilin University and the KD Research Group of the Chinese Academy of Medical Sciences at Beijing.

The work of these groups did not come to wide international attention for several decades, though many reports, written in Chinese, had been published in the intervening years and in 1973 the *First National Symposium of the Etiology of Keshan Disease* had been held in Beijing. It was only in 1979 that Chinese scientists first reported their findings in a major overseas journal and the importance of their work began to be recognized internationally (Keshan Disease Group, 1979). Since then there has been a continuous stream of publications by Chinese investigators and their collaborators from the world scientific community, and the extent and importance of selenium research in China is now well recognized.

5.2.1.1 Regional Studies of Keshan Disease in China

Distribution of KD is in a belt-like zone more than 4,000 km in length, through mainland China, from the Amur River border separating Heilongjiang Province from Russia in the northeast to Yunnan Province touching Miramar, Laos, and Vietnam in the southwest. The disease occurs generally in hilly regions, with heavily eroded soils. It has been recorded in 14 of the 22 provinces of China (Ge and Yang, 1993).

There is a marked seasonal fluctuation in the incidence of KD, with a peak occurrence during winter at the northern end of its spread and during summer in the south. Epidemics occur irregularly from year to year with, in recent years, a sharp decline in numbers affected compared to earlier outbreaks.

Women of childbearing age and children 2 to 10 years of age are the most susceptible to the disease. It occurs preferentially in families of peasant farmers rather than of factory or other nonagricultural workers. Its onset can be abrupt in otherwise healthy people without any preexisting cardiac disorders or infections. Since it was found that KD can occur in families within 3 months of their moving from a nonendemic to an endemic area, while people who have been affected by the disease and later move to a nonendemic region show no signs of fresh damage to their heart muscle, it was concluded that KD is a biogeochemical condition caused, probably, by multiple factors.

5.2.1.2 Features of Keshan Disease

The main features of KD include acute or chronic cardiac insufficiency, cardiac enlargement, congestive heart failure, cardiac arrhythmias, and ECG changes. However, there is no unique symptom or specific sign that can be used to identify the disease clearly. Histopathologically, KD is characterized by multifocal necrosis and fibrous replacement of the myocardium. Multifocal myocardial necrosis (MMN) is considered to be the main and most characteristic feature of KD. MMN is, however, also seen in some other pathological conditions, including cystic fibrosis (Nezelof et al., 2002).

KD is classified into four types: acute, subacute, chronic, and latent. Depending on which type is present, symptoms can vary from dizziness, malaise, loss of appetite, and nausea in acute cases to restlessness and slight dilation of the heart in the subacute type. The latter is the most common form of the disease, especially in children. Patients with the latent type may be unaware that they are affected. It may show up only as an incidental finding in a routine physical examination, or, unfortunately, in an autopsy. However, this insidious form is normally accompanied by dizziness, fatigue, and palpitations after physical activity (Ge and Yang, 1993).

5.2.1.3 Etiology of Keshan Disease

The etiology of KD is still uncertain. The absence of an animal model that can match all the symptoms seen in humans has made it difficult to research the origins of the disease. However, on the basis of epidemiological as well as laboratory and other studies, it is accepted by most investigators that KD has a dual etiology, involving both a nutritional deficiency of selenium and a viral infection. Xie and his coworkers (Xie et al., 1964), in their pioneering investigations in the early 1960s, came to the conclusion that the disease was the result of a combination of several factors, one of which is selenium deficiency. This view is strengthened by the finding that similarly low levels of selenium intake in Zaire, Africa, do not cause cardiomyopathy, implying that additional factors, besides selenium deficiency, are involved in the pathogenesis of KD (Vanderpas et al., 1990). There is little doubt of the connection with the element, as indicated by findings of very low dietary selenium intakes of its victims and the effectiveness of selenium supplementation in alleviating the condition (Tan et al., 2002). However, whether selenium is the only trace element involved has been questioned and it has been suggested that deficiencies of molybdenum, boron, and other nutrients may also play a part in the pathogenicity of KD (Fang et al., 2002). This view would seem to be supported by the fact that the disease occurs in isolated rural areas, with eroded and often nutritionally deficient soils, and the diet of those affected is usually restricted to a small range of locally produced foods. Deficiencies of both magnesium and thiamin have been found to be widespread and possibly contribute to the occurrence of the disease (Yang et al., 1984).

The investigations of Beck and her colleagues into the relationship of selenium deficiency to viral infection has added weight to the view of Ge et al. (1987) that KD is an infectious myocarditis caused by a virus. These workers had isolated strains of enteroviruses, including coxsackie B4, from some patients with KD. When these viruses were injected into mice fed on a low-selenium diet based on grain from a KD area, extensive damage to heart muscle occurred. Supplementation of the deficient mice with selenium before inoculation with the virus was found to reduce the severity of the heart lesions. They concluded that selenium had a protective effect against the virus, which, in selenium-deficient patients, was able to cause damage to heart muscle. These findings were confirmed by the results of later studies, which found that selenium deficiency increased the histopathological damage to the heart caused by CVB3/20, a strain of coxsackievirus (Beck et al., 1994).

Further investigations by Beck and her colleagues have produced strong evidence of a close relationship between selenium deficiency and viral infection. They found that an amyocarditic strain of coxsackievirus B3 became virulent when it was injected into selenium-deficient mice. This change in virulence was accompanied by changes in the genetic structure of the virus so that its genome came to resemble closely that of known virulent types of the same strain of virus. Similar changes in virulence and genomic composition of the coxsackievirus have been found to occur in knockout mice that did not have a functioning GPX enzyme (Beck et al., 2003).

The importance of these discoveries was highlighted by a subsequent finding that a mild strain of influenza virus also exhibited increased virulence when given to selenium-deficient mice. This increased virulence was accompanied by multiple changes in the viral genome in a segment previously thought to be relatively stable. The significance of the work of Beck and her colleagues, in relation to the possible role of malnutrition in contributing to the emergence of novel viral diseases, is considerable, and suggests that other epidemic diseases, besides KD, may also have a combined nutritional/viral etiology (Beck et al., 2003).

Several other hypotheses have also been proposed to account for the etiology of KD. The possibility of chronic poisoning by environmental pollutants such as nitrite and barium, or by mycotoxins in food, has been suggested (Qing and Fan, 1991). In support of the possible role of nitrite is the finding that, in experimental animals, addition of sodium nitrite to the diet can cause a decrease in myocardial GPX and that this can be prevented by both vitamin E and selenium (Qing and Fan, 1991).

There seems to be little other evidence in support of the view that KD is caused by a toxin, whether organic or inorganic. As Xie et al. (1964) observed, none of the different hypotheses then being put forward could explain adequately the etiology of KD. Their own view, that the disease is a result of a combination of several factors, not least of which is selenium deficiency, remains the most convincing hypothesis.

5.2.2 Selenium Status of Residents of Keshan Disease Areas

Extensive surveys carried out in the 1970s showed that selenium deficiency was widespread in humans living in KD-affected areas and that there were significant differences in selenium status between populations of KD and nonKD areas (Wang et al., 1979). The mean blood selenium level of those in the affected areas was found to be 0.021 ± 0.001 μg/ml, compared to 0.095 ± 0.088 μg/ml for those in nonendemic areas. The KD levels were lower than those then reported for healthy people in any other country in the world.

Hair selenium levels also differed between residents of endemic and nonendemic regions. While an average of 0.074 ± 0.050 μg/g selenium was recorded in scalp hair of residents of the KD areas, in nonKD areas it was 0.343 ± 0.173 μg/g, a highly significant difference. It was also shown that hair and blood selenium levels, within a practical range of 0.002 to 0.266 μg/ml for blood and 0.023 to 0.890 μg/g for hair, were highly correlated.

In a survey carried out in 1975 on children in Sichuan Province, one of the KD-endemic areas, whole blood GPX activities were measured. They were found to be significantly lower in the KD than in the nonKD areas. When KD-affected children were treated with sodium selenite for 1 year, their GPX activities increased and approached those of children in the nonendemic areas.

Urinary excretion of selenium was also found to differ significantly between residents of KD and nonKD areas. In the case of rural children, average 12 h night urine excretion was 0.69 ± 0.18 μg in KD areas and 1.50 ± 0.13 μg in the nonKD areas. It was noted at the same time that children living in Beijing excreted 11.9 ± 1.34 μg selenium in the same time. This major difference in excretion was attributed to the more varied diet and the much larger intake of animal foods of urban compared to rural children, both KD and nonKD (Yin et al., 1979).

The Chinese studies found that the selenium content of staple foods in KD areas and consequently daily selenium intakes of local people was very low. The average concentration of selenium in maize, for example, in affected areas was 0.005 ± 0.002 μg/g compared to 0.036 ± 0.056 μg/g in unaffected areas. Similarly, the average level in rice was 0.007 ± 0.003 μg/g in KD areas compared to 0.024 ± 0.038 μg/g in nonKD areas. The contrast was even greater between levels in Chinese rice and rice grown in some other countries, as seen in Table 5.1. Clearly, such low levels of selenium in rice as in other staple foods that made

TABLE 5.1 Selenium in rice from Keshan disease–affected and nonaffected countries

Country	Se concentration (mean), μg/g	Reference
Australia	0.08 ± 0.01	1
China, KD area	0.007 ± 0.003	2
China, nonKD area	0.024 ± 0.038	2
France	0.29 ± 0.003	3
Japan	0.043 ± 0.027	4
Thailand	0.054 (polished, raw)	5
Thailand	0.046 (polished, jasmine variety)	5
USA	0.078 (range 0.039–0.10)	6

References:

1. Tinggi, U., Reilly, C., and Patterson, C.M., 1992, Determination of selenium in foodstuffs using spectrofluorimetry and hydride generation atomic absorption spectrophotometry, *J. Food Comp. Anal.* **5**, 269–280.
2. Yang, G., Ghen, J., Wen, Z., et al., 1984, The role of selenium in Keshan disease, *Adv. Nutr. Res.* **6**, 203–231.
3. Simonoff, M., Hamon, C., Moretto, P., et al., 1988, Selenium in foods in France, *J. Food Comp. Anal.* **1**, 295–302.
4. Yoshida, M. and Yasumoto, K., 1987, Selenium content of rice grown in various sites in Japan, *J. Food Comp. Anal.* **1**, 71–75.
5. Sirichakwal, P.P., Puwastien, P., Polngam, J., and Kongkachuichai, R., 2005, Selenium content of Thai foods, *J. Food Comp. Anal.* **18**, 47–59.
6. Wolf, W.R., Holden, J.M., Schubert, A., et al., 1992, Selenium content of selected foods important for improved assessment of dietary intake, *J. Food Comp. Anal.* **5**, 2–9.

up the bulk of the normal diet of Keshan sufferers accounted for their poor selenium status, as indicated by the low levels of the element measured in their blood, hair, and urine.

Consumption of a different type of rice was shown to have a significant effect on dietary intake of selenium, even within a KD area. It was found that in Heilongjiang Province, where many Koreans nationals live, acute KD did not occur in the Koreans, apparently because the type of rice they consumed contained 0.02 ± 0.003 μg/g of selenium, in contrast to the Chinese who suffered from KD and whose rice had only 0.0032 ± 0.0002 μg selenium/g (Yang, 1983).

5.2.3 Interventions in the Management of Keshan Disease

Following the successful outcome of earlier, limited, interventions, in which sodium selenite was given as a dietary supplement to KD sufferers, several larger studies were carried out by the Chinese investigators. One was the Five Counties Study of 1976–1980 in which observations on the effects of sodium selenite were extended to include approximately 1.5 million children. The counties were in the Sichuan Province, in the southern section of the KD belt, an area that had the highest incidence of KD in China (Xia et al., 1990).

All children, aged 1 to 12 years, in some of the most severely affected communes, were treated with selenium, while children from nearby communes served as untreated controls. The results are summarized in Table 5.2. As this shows,

TABLE 5.2 Keshan disease incidence rates in selenium-treated and untreated children in five Chinese counties, 1976–1980

	Treated children			Untreated children		
Year	Subjects	Cases	Incidence/1,000	Subjects	Cases	Incidence/1,000
1976	45,515	8	0.17[a]	243,649	488	2.00[a]
1977	67,754	15	0.22[b]	222,944	350	1.57[b]
1978	65,953	10	0.15[c]	220,599	373	1.69[c]
1979	69,910	33	0.47[d]	223,280	300	1.34[d]
1980	74,740	22	0.29[e]	197,096	202	1.07[e]
Total	323,872	88	0.27[f]	1,107,568	1,713	1.55[f]

Source: Data adapted from Yang, G., Chen, J., Wen, Z., et al., 1987, The role of selenium in Keshan disease, *Adv. Nutr. Res.* **6**, 203–231.
[a–e] Means with the same subscripts are significantly different ($P < 0.001$).
[f] Means are significantly different ($P < 0.00001$).

each year the incidence of KD among treated children was significantly lower than among the control children, with, over the 5 years of the trial, a reduction to 0.27 cases per 1,000 following treatment, compared with 1.55 per 1,000 in the untreated children, a highly significant difference.

Large-scale interventions have been carried out successfully in several other provinces right through the KD belt. All the interventions showed the same trend, with a consistent difference in morbidity between selenium-treated and control groups, especially in the more severely affected areas. These trials have shown that oral administration of a sodium selenite supplement is an effective procedure for reducing the incidence, morbidity, and fatality of KD.

In addition to the use of sodium selenite tablets, control of KD has also been achieved by supplying selenized salt for use by local residents, even in some of the most severely affected KD areas. The salt is prepared by adding sodium selenite to domestic salt (sodium chloride) at the rate of 15 mg selenite/kg salt. The effect of this intervention has been remarkable. For example, in Mianning County, one of the most severely affected KD counties, where since mid-1983 all salt sold has been fortified, per capita selenium intake rose from 11 μg/day to 80 μg/day in less than 2 years.

The incidence of KD has been observed to decrease significantly over the years since these interventions began to be made, with a particularly sharp fall in the early years of the programs. The situation has continued to improve up to the present time, probably not simply due to availability and use of selenium supplements, but also as a result of improved living and economic conditions, not least with the availability of a more varied and better diet, better sanitation and housing, and increased medical attention. However, though KD is no longer a serious endemic problem in China, it still occurs. As a group of Chinese investigators of KD and other endemic diseases commented in a recent paper, though 50 years of research has already gone into the problem, there is still much to be done (Lin et al., 2004). While it is clear that selenium supplementation has largely eliminated endemic KD in China, there are concerns that marginal selenium deficiency still causes cardiac problems (Wu et al., 1997). A considerable amount of research is, indeed, still being carried out in China, examples of which include investigation of the role of enteroviruses in KD (Li et al., 2000), as well as of the relation of antioxidants and fatty acid status to mortality from the disease (Hensrud et al., 1994).

5.2.4 *Keshan Disease in Russia*

Doubts have been expressed by some experts in the field as to whether KD occurs outside China (Alfthan and Nève, 1996). However, there have been reports of a disease, with KD-like symptoms and related to selenium deficiency, in other countries. In 1987 a research team from the Medical Institute of Chita in southern Siberia in the former USSR investigated an outbreak of what was apparently KD in Transbaikalia (Ankina, 1992), a mountainous region in the neighborhood of Lake Baikal, bordering on Mongolia. Symptoms observed were similar to those described in KD sufferers in China, and a selenium deficiency-related cardiomyopathy was diagnosed. Those affected were mainly 12- to –17-year-old adolescents and women of childbearing age. They lived in rural areas where soil and water were low in selenium. Selenium deficiency-related conditions, such as WMD, were also seen in local farm animals. Analysis of locally grown foods found that they were low in selenium. Dietary intakes by local residents were on average 45 μg/day for adults and 20 μg/day for children. Although these are not as low as those recorded in KD areas of China, the Russian investigators also reported that they had found low blood GPX activity and high levels of malonaldehyde, indicative of increased tissue oxidation, in the Transbaikalian patients.

A survey carried out in the same area only 4 years later found, surprisingly, that the selenium status of local residents was "fairly good" and that there were no symptoms of heart disease caused by selenium deficiency. While selenium levels in locally produced foods were still low, levels in bread, which was a major item in the diet of residents of the villages investigated, were considerably higher. This was, apparently, due to the fact that imported high-selenium US wheat was used for baking. As the authors of the report pointed out, were it not for the use of US flour, the selenium intake of the population would be reduced to a very low level if only locally produced foods were consumed (Aro et al., 1994).

Selenium deficiency-related cardiomyopathy, typical of KD, has also been reported to occur in other parts of Russia. It has been found in 2- to –15-year-old children whose daily dietary intake of selenium is 12 to 40 μg. Oral supplementation with sodium selenite has been found to be effective in treating the condition (Voshchenko et al., 1992).

5.3 Kashin–Beck Disease

Kashin–Beck disease (KBD), which is sometimes known as Urov disease, is another endemic condition believed to be selenium-related. It occurs in areas that often overlap with the KD belt through China (Moreno-Reyes et al., 1998). KBD is an osteoarthropathy characterized by chronic disabling degeneration and necrosis of the joints and the epiphysial-plate cartilages of the arms and legs. It becomes evident in childhood and adolescence and leads to varying degrees of disability throughout adult life, with possible stunting. Clinically, weakness is followed by joint stiffness and pain. Advanced cases show typical signs of enlargement of joints and deformity of limbs (Diplock, 1987).

The disease occurs in some 300 counties in 15 provinces and autonomous regions of China, predominantly in hilly and mountainous districts. Incidence of the disease has been reported to be particularly high in Tibet, where KD appears to be still evolving, in contrast to northern and central parts of China where its frequency has been found to be decreasing (Mathieu et al., 1997). It is also reported in Russia, Japan, and Korea (Research Group of Environment and Endemic Diseases, 1990). The disease was first discovered in 1849 by the Russian physician I.M. Urenskii in the basin of the River Urov in Transbaikalia, Eastern Siberia. In 1854 H.I. Kashin studied the disease in the same area. More detailed investigations were made in the first decade of the 20th century by E.V. Beck. The two names of the disease, Urov and Kashin–Beck, were coined, respectively, after the locality of its first discovery and to honor the pioneering research of its early investigators.

KD was still being reported as endemic in Transbaikalian Russia at the end of the 20th century, but with much smaller numbers of individuals affected than in parts of China (Aro et al., 1994). In that country, as many as two million people were believed to be affected, with a local incidence as high as 30 to 40% in heavily affected areas (Ge and Yang, 1993).

There appears to be little doubt that KBD is of environmental origin. Since, like KD, it occurs in areas of low-selenium soil, and is not found in selenium-adequate regions, it has been linked by many of its Chinese investigators to pronounced selenium deficiency (Dongxu, 1987; Zhilun et al., 1993). However, KBD is not identical to KD, in spite of the indications of low selenium status is those suffering from both diseases. Moreover, unlike the case of KD, the efficacy of selenium supplementation in the prevention of KBD has never, according to some investigators, been satisfactorily demonstrated (Allander, 1994), though this view is not supported by recent findings (Vanderpas and Nève, 1999).

5.3.1 The Etiology of Kashin–Beck Disease

The etiology of KBD is still far from clear. Apart from selenium deficiency, a number of other possible causative factors have been put forward by various investigators. It has been hypothesized that the presence of high levels of humic substances, in particular fulvic acid (FA), in drinking water in KBD areas may be a contributing factor (Jiang and Xu, 1989). FAs are water-soluble components of soil whose chemical structure is still not fully known. They are a group of yellow-brown water-soluble aromatic polymers that can be extracted from the soil. The different members of the group are closely related in structure, with numerous functional groups, particularly –COOH, OH, and C=O. They appear to differ from one another in molecular weight, number of functional groups, and degree of polymerization. The exact structure of individual FAs is unclear. Animal experiments have shown that oxy- and hydroxy-groups in an FA may generate free radicals, which can interfere with the cell membrane and result in enhancement of lipid peroxidation, especially when GPX activity is reduced (Peng et al., 1999). Hydroxylation of collagen molecules leads to irregular bone formation and reduction in its mechanical strength, both features of KBD (Yang et al., 1992).

There are also indications that mycotoxin contamination of cereals by strains of the mould *Fusarium*, which is often found in grain grown in KBD areas, may bring about changes in collagen structure (Chasseur et al., 1997). It has been shown that toxin extracted from *Fusarium tricinatum* is able to cause a decrease in collagen microfibrils in chicken embryo chondriocytes. The decrease is reversed by the addition of sodium selenite to the culture, suggesting that the role of selenium in preventing KBD may be linked to its inhibitory effect on *Fusarium* toxin (Lin et al., 1992).

Other factors may also be involved in the etiology of KBD, which, like KD, probably has multiple interrelated causes. Nutritional imbalances and deficiencies of selenium as well as other inorganic nutrients, such as phosphates and manganese, may be involved (Levander, 1987). It is possible that nutritional deficiency, especially of selenium, in conjunction with the stress of poor diet, harsh living conditions, and the intense cold experienced in the prolonged winter of many KBD-endemic areas, may contribute to the onset of the disease. In support of this view is the remarkable decrease in KBD incidence in affected areas since the 1970s, which has occurred progressively in parallel with improvements in the general nutritional status, economic conditions, and medical services of the Chinese rural population (Ge and Yang, 1993).

5.4 Combined Endemic Selenium and Iodine Deficiencies

Observations made by Nève and his colleagues during their extensive studies of KBD in Tibet have thrown light on a possible additional, and very significant, factor in the etiology of the disease, namely iodine deficiency (Moreno-Reyes et al., 1998). Results of an earlier study of hypothyroid cretenism in northern Zaire (now the Republic of the Congo) in Central Africa had indicated that the condition was related to coexisting iodine and selenium deficiencies (Vanderpas et al., 1990). Their finding in Tibet that selenium and iodine deficiencies occur in the same region and that goiter can affect people with both KD and KBD (Ma et al., 1993) led them to investigate the relationship between the two elements in the etiology of both goiter and KBD.

5.4.1 Selenium, Kashin–Beck Disease, and Goiter

Nève and his colleagues (Moreno-Reyes et al., 1998) looked at the incidence of KBD in a total of 575 children 11 to 15 years of age in 12 villages in the neighborhood of Lhasa. One of the villages, selected as the control, with 73 of the children, had never been reported to have had the disease. In the other villages, KBD incidence ranged from 13 to 100%. In all the villages, including the control, a very severe selenium deficiency was diagnosed by low serum values (a mean value of close to 10 μg/l, with a value of less than 5 μg/l in 38% of the subjects) and low GPX activity. Remarkably, in the control village, serum selenium levels were even slightly lower than in the KBD villages, and GPX activity was also lower in the KBD-free children. A multivariate analysis of the results showed that selenium status alone was not associated with KBD (Moreno-Reyes et al., 1998).

When iodine status and incidence of iodine deficiency-related disorders were investigated in the 12 villages, it was found that 46% of the children had goiter. The incidence of goiter was higher in the KBD villages than in the KBD-free control village. In addition, seven of the subjects in the KBD villages had cretinism, and none in the control village. Children in the KBD villages also had a relatively high serum thyrotropin concentration and lower serum thyroxine and T3 compared to those in the KBD-free village. Urinary iodine concentration was also significantly lower in children with KBD than in those without the disease, both in KBD and the control villages. An association between iodine deficiency and KBD was demonstrated by multivariate analysis of the results.

The investigators concluded that KBD is the result of a combination of iodine and selenium deficiencies. Deficiency of iodine alone does not cause KBD; nor is the disease a symptom of endemic goiter. Although hypothyroidism due to iodine deficiency does affect growth and bone development, it does not cause chondronecrosis typical of KBD. It is possible, according to Moreno-Reyes et al. (1998), that the combined deficiencies affect the growth-plate cartilage in two ways: a reduction in thyroid hormone production both at the thyroid level (due to the iodine deficiency) and at the local level (related to a reduction in the selenium-dependent enzyme iodothyronine deiodinase), and a deficit in antioxidant protection (due to reduced GPX activity).

The results of further trials of combined iodine and selenium supplementation to combat KBD in Tibet and other parts of China have lent support to the view that iodine deficiency is a major etiological cofactor in the cause of KBD. This may account for the finding that over the past several decades, since large-scale iodine supplementation has been introduced in China to combat goiter, there has been a decrease in the incidence of KBD (Nève, 1999).

5.4.2 The Role of Selenium Deficiency in Endemic Goiter

The occurrence of goiter in mountainous regions of Europe has been recorded in medical literature since classical times (Porter, 1997). The Roman writer Juvenal in the 1st century AD noted the frequency of swollen necks in people living in the Alps; in England the condition was known for hundreds of years and was common in the Peak District where it was known as "Derbyshire neck." Paracelsus in the 16th century commented on the occurrence of goiter, along with cretinism, in mountainous areas of Central Europe. Many different remedies were tried, including "the royal touch," which was popular in the reign of King Charles 1 in 17th-century England. The Medieval physician, Arnold of Villanova, did, however, come close to a real remedy when he recommended the use of burnt sponge ash and seaweed, both of which contain iodine. Nearly 200 years ago, in 1812, the English physician, William Prout, used iodine to treat his goiter patients. In 1891 another English physician, George Redmayne Murray (1865–1939), reported that the condition of a myxedematic women had been improved by an injection of an extract of thyroid gland taken from a sheep. Not long afterwards iodine was found to be present in the thyroid gland and it began to be accepted that iodine deficiency was responsible for overgrowth of the thyroid gland. Eventually goiter was largely eliminated from its endemic areas of Europe, by iodine supplementation of the diet, particularly by the use of iodized salt. The extension of this method to other far more extensive regions of endemic goiter, subsequently discovered in the Himalayas and other mountainous regions, led to dramatic results.

Although, however, the introduction of iodized salt as a preventive of goiter was a highly successful intervention, it became clear subsequently that iodine was not the complete answer to the problem. There followed wide-ranging investigations, involving the complementary efforts of many researchers with different basic orientations and different interests, working over many years, which has finally led to "a remarkable attainment which deserves scientific recognition" (Nève, 1992).

A significant early step in these investigations was taken by a group of Norwegian researchers, who were investigating levels of trace elements in body tissues, when they found that there was a much higher level of selenium in the thyroid gland than in other organs and tissues (Aaseth et al., 1990). They also produced evidence that they believed pointed toward an epidemiological relationship between serum selenium concentrations and the risk of thyroid cancer (Glattre et al., 1989). However, they failed to find clear evidence that selenium had a beneficial effect against cancer, but speculated that the element might have a role to play in decreasing iodination of possible carcinogens in the gland.

Another important step was taken by a Belgian-Zairean team, which was investigating endemic goiter in the Congo, then known as Zaire, in Central Africa (Corvilan et al., 1993). They were particularly concerned about cretinism, a syndrome of mental and growth retardation. It is seen in different forms in areas of endemic goiter in different parts of the world. In Latin America and Papua New Guinea it is associated with goiter and is known as neurological cretinism. In Zaire, in contrast, cretins are normally hypothyroid, with a negative correlation between size of the thyroid and severity of the cretinism. This form is known as myxedematous endemic cretinism.

The investigators hypothesized that in myxedematous cretinism the thyroid was destroyed before or around the time of birth, or in some cases, later in infancy. The causes of the destruction were not clear. Thiocyanate overload, resulting from consumption of cyanide-containing foods, including cassava (*Manihot esculantia*), although known to aggravate iodine deficiency, was not believed to explain thyroid atrophy in the cretins (Delange and Ermans, 1971).

It was noted that in the island of Idjwi, an area of high incidence of endemic goiter in Kivu Province, Zaire, the distribution of goiter and cretinism closely matched the geological map. In the north, where underlying rock was granite, severe endemia occurred; in the south where the rocks were basaltic, the endemia was mild. Analyses showed that the northern granite and the soil related to it were severely deficient in both iodine and selenium, whereas the basaltic soils in the south were deficient only in iodine (Corvilan et al., 1993).

The investigators believed that they now had evidence that an inadequate dietary supply of selenium was implicated, along with iodine deficiency, in the myxedematous cretinism in the north of Idjwi Island. Their observation provided the first clue that selenium intake may modulate the effects of iodine deficiency in humans (Arthur et al., 1999).

A hypothesis developed by the investigators to account for these observations (Goyens et al., 1987) can be summarized as follows: when iodine is limited, thyroid hormone synthesis is impaired and concentrations of thyrotrophin, the thyroid stimulating hormone (TSH) of the pituitary gland, rise in an effort to increase iodine uptake. This leads to increased production of hydrogen peroxide (H_2O_2), which is required for thyroid hormone production. The H_2O_2 is used by thyroid peroxidase to oxidize iodide in a reaction leading to its incorporation into thyroglobulin and production of T3 and T4. Under normal conditions any excess H_2O_2 is detoxified by enzymes such as GPX and catalase. However, under conditions of concurrent selenium and iodine deficiencies, there would be a reduction in supply of selenoprotein enzymes and thus an accumulation of H_2O_2 to toxic levels. As a result, peroxidative damage to the thyroid gland occurs accompanied by development of other features of myxedematous cretinism.

Although the proposers of this hypothesis did not claim that their findings in Zaire proved that selenium deficiency has a direct role in the development of endemic goiter or cretinism, they did claim that the evidence they had found was compatible with that role. However, it is doubtful whether a loss of thyroidal GPX activity can on its own account for the development of myxedematous cretinism. It has been shown that thyroidal GPX activity in rats subjected to very severe selenium deficiency, or combined iodine and selenium deficiencies, continues to be at least 50% of the level in normal animals. Since decreases in liver GPX activity of up to 99% normally fail to bring about serious health disturbances in rats, it is unlikely that a 50% loss of thyroidal GPX activity would be responsible for peroxide-mediated damage to the thyroid gland (Arthur et al., 1990b).

More recent findings have also failed to provide convincing support for the hypothesis. These point toward other compounding factors that are responsible for the endemic cretinism seen in some iodine-deficient regions. In parts of Africa where there is a similar degree of selenium deficiency, but iodine deficiency is even more severe than in Zaire, myxedematous cretinism does not occur (Ngo et al., 1997). In Tibet there are severe concurrent iodine and selenium deficiencies, but very little myxedematous cretinism, while neurological cretinism predominates (Moreno-Reyes et al., 1998). Thus, combined iodine and selenium deficiency does not appear to explain adequately the elevated frequency of myxedematous cretinism in central Africa, and the possible role of other additional factors, such as thiocyanates, must again be considered (Arthur et al., 1999).

5.4.3 Thyroid Biochemistry and Selenium

What we now know about the role of several different selenoproteins in the metabolism of the thyroid gland provides confirmation that selenium has a major role to play in relation to goiter and its different manifestations. The precise details of that role are still the subject of investigation by several different research groups. What is clear is that the enzyme, IDI, which converts T4 to T3 by monoiodination, a crucial step in thyroid metabolism, is a selenoprotein (Arthur et al., 1990a). In addition, two other deiodinases, IDII and IDIII, are also essential for the interconversion of active and inactive forms of the thyroid hormone. They both have been shown to be selenoproteins (Croteau, 1996; Larsen, 1996). The importance of these enzymes for normal thyroid hormone metabolism is indicated by the maintenance of IDII and IDIII activities, even in severe selenium deficiency (Mitchell et al., 1997).

Several other selenoenzymes have been shown to be involved in thyroid hormone metabolism, if not as centrally as the deiodinases, nevertheless with considerable significance. These include the GPXs, which provide intra- and extracellular protection against H_2O_2 and lipid peroxides, which can damage the thyroid gland and interfere with its functions (Arthur et al., 1996). The selenoprotein flavoenzyme TR is believed to contribute to cellular antioxidation (Howie et al., 1998), while SeP may provide extracellular antioxidant action (Burk et al., 1995). Thus, TR, SeP, and possibly other selenoproteins, in addition to the GPXs, can be seen as having a role in the protection of the thyroid gland from H_2O_2, and, along with the regulation of T3 levels by the three deiodinases, are the functions of selenium that are most likely to underlie the interactions of the element with iodine (Arthur et al., 1999).

5.4.3.1 Selenium Supplementation and Iodine Deficiency: a Caution

The complexity of the interaction of selenium and iodine in thyroid metabolism is highlighted by the fact that selenium can have both beneficial and adverse effects on subjects with iodine deficiency. While selenium deficiency exacerbates hypothyroidism due to iodine deficiency, it has also been shown that a concurrent selenium deficiency has a sparing effect on plasma T4 concentrations, and thus may provide protection in the fetus against the development of neurological cretinism (Contempre et al., 1991).

It has been shown that when selenium supplements are given to normal children and to endemic cretins, serum selenium levels and GPX activity are normalized in both (Corvilan et al., 1993). However, while plasma T4 levels are also reduced in the two groups, the fall in the cretins is considerably greater than in normal children. TSH concentrations also increase significantly in the cretins, but not in the normal group (Contempre et al., 1992). The fall in T4 in the cretins can be attributed to an increase in the expression of hepatic IDI, which in turn increases conversion of plasma T4 to T3 (Vanderpas et al., 1993). Normal children, with adequate amounts of functional thyroid tissue, are able to cope with the increased IDI activity, but cretins, with small fibrosed thyroid glands with impaired iodine uptake, are unable to meet the requirement for increased thyroid hormone synthesis (Vanderpas et al., 1992). Since iodine supplementation has been found to improve thyroid function in cretins, it is probable that iodine availability is a limiting step in thyroid hormone production (Contempre et al., 1991). It is likely therefore that in cretins the increased requirement for thyroid hormone synthesis after selenium supplementation may lead to rapid depletion of iodine reserves (Arthur et al., 1999). Indeed, endemic cretins undergoing selenium supplementation can develop serious thyroid failure as a result of iodine loss by the kidney due to increased catabolism of both T4 and T3. It is for this reason that in cases where combined iodine and selenium deficiencies occur, caution must be exercised in using supplementation to correct the selenium deficiency before iodine deficiency has been attended to (Contempre et al., 1991).

References

Aaseth, J., Frey, H., Glattre, E., et al., 1990, Selenium concentrations in the human thyroid gland, *Biol. Trace Elem. Res.* **24**, 147–152.

Alfthan, G. and Nève, J., 1996, Reference values for serum selenium in various areas—evaluated according to the TRACY protocol, *J. Trace Elem. Med. Biol* **10**, 77–87.

Allander, E., 1994, Kashin-Beck disease: an analysis of research and public health activities based on a bibliography 1849–1992, *Scand. J. Rheumatol.* **S99**, 1–36.

Ankina, L.V., 1992, Selenium-deficient myocardiopathy (Keshan disease), in: *Fifth International Symposium on Selenium in Biology and Medicine. Abstracts*, Vanderbilt University, Nashville, TN, July 20–23, p. 122.

Aro, A., Kumpulainen, J., Alfthan, G., et al., 1994, Factors affecting the selenium intake of people in Transbaikalian Russia, *Biol. Trace Elem. Res.* **40**, 277–285.

Arthur, J.R., Beckett, G.J., and Mitchell, J.H., 1999, The interactions between selenium and iodine deficiencies in man and animals, *Nutr. Res. Rev.* **12**, 55–73.

Arthur, J.R., Bermano, G., Mitchell, J.H., and Hesketh, J.E., 1996, Regulation of selenoprotein gene expression and thyroid hormone metabolism, *Biochem. Soc. Trans.* **24**, 384–388.

Arthur, J.R., Nicol, F., and Beckett, G.J., 1990a, Hepatic iodothyronine deiodinase: the role of selenium, *Biochem. J.* **272**, 537–540.

Arthur, J.R., Nicol, F., Rae, P.W.H., and Beckett, C.J., 1990b, Effect of selenium deficiency on the thyroid gland and plasma and pituitary thyrotrophin and growth hormone concentrations in rats, *Clin. Chem. Enzymol. Commun.* **3**, 209–214.

Beck, M.A., Kolbeck, P.C., Shi, Q., et al., 1994, Increased virulence of a human enterovirus (coxsackievirus B3) in selenium deficient mice, *J. Infect. Dis.* **170**, 351–357.

Beck, M.A., Levander, O.A., and Handy, J., 2003, Selenium deficiency and viral infection, *J. Nutr.* **133**, 1463S–1467S.

Bergomi, M., Vinceti, M., Nacci, G., et al., 2002, Environment exposure to trace elements and risk of amyotrophic lateral sclerosis: a population-based case study, *Environ. Res.* **89**, 116–123.

Bratter, P., Negretti de Bratter, V.E., Jaffee, W.G., and Castellano, H.M., 1991, Selenium status of children living in a seleniferous areas of Venezuela, *J. Trace Elem. Electrolytes Health Dis.* **5**, 269–270.

Burk, R.F., Hill, K.E., Awad, J.A., et al., 1995, Pathogenesis of diquat-induced liver necrosis in selenium-deficient rats: assessment of roles of lipid peroxidation and selenoprotein P, *Hepathology* **21**, 561–569.

Chasseur, C., Suetens, C., Nolard, N., Bergaux, F., and Haubruge, E., 1997, Fungal contamination in barley and Kashin-Beck disease in Tibet, *Lancet* **350**, 1074.

Contempre, B., Duale, N.L., Dumont, J.E., et al., 1992, Effect of selenium supplementation on thyroid hormone metabolism in an iodine and selenium deficient population, *Clin. Endocrinol.* **36**, 579–583.

Contempre, B., Dumont, J.E., Ngo, B., et al., 1991, Effect of selenium supplementation in hypothyroid subjects of an iodine and selenium deficient area—the possible danger of indiscriminate supplementation of I-deficient subjects with selenium, *J. Clin. Endocrinol. Metabol.* **73**, 213–215.

Corvilan, B., Contempre, B., Longombe, A.O., et al., 1993, Selenium and the thyroid: how the relationship was established, *Am. J. Clin. Nutr. Suppl.* **57**, 244S–285S.

Croteau, W., Davey, J.C., Galton, V.A., and Germain, D.L., 1996, Cloning of the mammalian type II iodothyronine deiodinase—a selenoprotein differentially expressed and regulated in human and rat brain and other tissues, *J. Clin. Invest.* **98**, 405–417.

Delange, F. and Ermans, A.M., 1971, Role of cassava in the etiology of endemic goitre in Idjwi Island, *Am. J. Clin. Nutr.* **24**, 1354–1359.

Diplock, A.T., 1987, Trace elements in human health with special reference to selenium, *Am. J. Clin. Nutr.* **45**, 1313–1322.

Dongxu, M., 1987, Pathology and selenium deficiency in KBD, in: Combs, G.F. (ed.), *Selenium in Biology and Medicine*, Reinhold, New York, pp. 924–933.

Fang, W.X., Wu, P.W., and Hu, R.H., 2002, Environmental Se-Mo-B deficiency and its possible effects in Jiantou Keshan disease area in Shaanxi Province, China, *Environ. Geochem. Health* **24**, 349–358.

Finkleman, R.B., Belkin, H.E., and Zheng, B.S., 1999, Health impacts of domestic coal use in China, *Proc. Natl Acad. Sci. USA* **96**, 3427–3431.

Frost, D.V., 1972, The two faces of selenium—can selenophobia be cured? in: Hemphill, D. (ed.), *Critical Reviews In Toxicology*, CRC Press, Boca Raton, FL, pp. 467–514.

Frost, D.V. and Ingvoldstad, D., 1975, Ecological aspects of selenium and tellurium in human and animal health, *Chem. Scrip.* **8A**, 96–107.

Ge, K.Y. and Yang, G., 1993, The epidemiology of selenium deficiency in the etiology of endemic diseases in China, *Am. J. Clin. Nutr. Supp.* **57**, 259S–263S.

Ge, K.Y., Wang, S.Q., Bai, J., et al., 1987, The protective effect of selenium against viral myocarditis in mice, in: Combs, G.F., Spallholz, J., Levander, E., and Oldfield, J.E. (eds), *Selenium in Biology and Medicine*, Van Nostrand Reinhold, New York, pp. 761–768.

Glattre, E., Thomassen, Y., Thoresen, S., et al., 1989, Prediagnostic serum selenium in a case control study of thyroid cancer, *Int. J. Epidemiol.* **18**, 45–49.

Gnadinger, C.B., 1933, Selenium: insecticidal material for controlling red spider, *Indust. Eng. Chem.* **25**, 633.

Goyens, P., Goldstein, J., Nsombola, B., et al., 1987, Selenium deficiency as a possible factor in the pathogenesis of myxodematous cretinism, *Acta Endocrinol. (Copenhagen)* **114**, 497–502.

Gu, B., 1993, Pathology of Keshan disease: a comprehensive review, *Chinese Med. J.* **96**, 251–261.

Hadjimarkos, D.M., 1973, Selenium in relation to dental caries, *Food Cosmet. Toxicol.* **11**, 1083–1095.

Hadjimarkos, D.M., Storvick, C.A., and Remmert, L.F., 1952, Selenium and dental caries. An investigation among school children of Oregon, *J. Pediat.* **40**, 451–455.

Hensrud, D.D., Heimburger, D.C., Chen, J., and Parpia, B., 1994, Antioxidant status, erythrocyte fatty acids, and mortality from cardiovascular disease and Keshan disease in China, *Eur. J. Clin. Nutr.* **48**, 455–464.

Howie, A.F., Arthur, J.R., Nicol, F., et al., 1998, Identification of a 57-kilodalton selenoprotein in human thyrocytes as thioredoxin reductase and evidence that its expression is regulated through the calcium-phosphoinositol signalling pathway, *J. Clin. Endocrinol. Metabol.* **83**, 2052–2058.

Jaffe, W.G. and Velez, B.F., 1973, Selenium intake and congenital malformations in humans, *Archivos Latinoamericanos de Nutricion* **23**, 514–516.

Jaffe, W.G., Ruphael, M.D., Mondragon, M.C., and Cuevas, M.A., 1972, Clinical and biochemical studies on school children from a seleniferous zone, *Archivos Lationamericanos de Nutricion* **22**, 595–611.

Jiang, Y.F. and Xu, G.L., 1989, The relativity between some epidemiological characteristics of Kashin-Beck disease and selenium deficiency, in: Wendel, A. (ed.), *Selenium in Biology and Medicine*, Springer, Berlin, pp. 179–183.

Kerdel-Vegas, F., 1966, The depilatory and cytotoxic action of "Coco de Mono" (*Lecythis ollaria*) and its relationship to chronic selenosis, *Econ. Bot.* **20**, 187–195.

Keshan Disease Group of the Chinese Academy of Medicine, 1979, Epidemiological studies in the etiologic relationship of selenium and Keshan disease, *Chinese Med. J.* **92**, 477–482.

Kilness, A.W., 1973, Selenium and public health, *S. Dakota J. Med.* **26**, 17–19.

Kilness, A.W. and Hochberg, F.H., 1977, Amyotrophic lateral sclerosis in a high selenium environment, *JAMA* **238**, 2365.

Kurland, L.T., 1977, Amyotrophic lateral sclerosis and selenium, *JAMA* **238**, 2365–2366.

Larsen, P.R., 1996, Mammalian type 2 deiodinases sequences: finally, the end of the beginning, *J. Clin. Invest.* **98**, 242.

Lemley, R.E., 1943, Observations on selenium poisoning in South and North America, *Lancet* **63**, 257–258.

Levander, O.A., 1987, Etiological hypotheses concerning Kashin Beck disease, in: *Nutrition '87: American Institute of Nutrition Symposium Proceedings 1987*, American Institute of Nutrition, Bethesda, MD, pp. 67–71.

Li, Y., Peng, T., Yang, Y., et al., 2000, High prevalence of enteroviral genomic sequences in myocardium from cases of endemic cardiomyopathy (Keshan disease) in China, *Heart* **83**, 696–701.

Lin, N.F., Tang, J., and Bian, J.M., 2004, Geochemical environment and health problems in China, *Environ. Geochem. Health* **26**, 81–88.

Lin, Z.H., Liu, S.G., Shan, S., et al., 1992, The antagonistic effects of Se on the T-2 toxin-induced changes of ultrastructure and mitochondrial function of cultured chicken embryo chondriocytes, in: *Fifth International Symposium on Selenium in Biology and Medicine, Abstracts*, Vanderbilt University, Nashville, TN, July 20–23, 1992, p. 24.

Ma, T., Guo, J., and Wang, F., 1993, The epidemiology of iodine-deficiency diseases in China, *Am. J. Clin. Nutr.* **57**, 254S–266S.

Mahan, D.C. and Peters, J.C., 2004, Long-term effects of dietary organic and inorganic selenium sources and levels on reproducing sows and their progeny, *J. Anim. Sci.* **82**, 1343–1358.

Marjanen, H., 1969, Possible casual relationship between the easily soluble amounts of manganese on arable soil and susceptibility to cancer in Finland, *Ann. Agr. Fenn.* **8**, 326–333.

Mathieu, F., Begaux, F., Lan, Z.Y., et al., 1997, Clinical manifestations of Kashin-Beck disease in Nyemo valley, Tibet, *Int. Orthop.* **21**, 151–156.

Mitchell, J.H., Nicol, F., Beckett, G.J., and Arthur, J.R., 1997, Selenium and iodine deficiencies: effects on brain and brown adipose tissue selenoenzyme activity and expression, *J. Endocrinol.* **155**, 255–263.

Money, D.F.L., 1970, Vitamin E and selenium deficiencies and their possible aetiological role in sudden death in infants syndrome, *NZ Med. J.* **71**, 32–36.

Moreno-Reyes, R., Suetens, C., Mathieu, F., et al., 1998, Kashin-Beck osteoarthropathy in rural Tibet in relation to selenium and iodine status, *New Engl. J. Med.* **339**, 1112–1120.

Moriwako, F., 1993, Mercury and selenium contents in amyotrophic lateral sclerosis in Hokkaido, the northernmost island of Japan, *J. Neurol. Dis.* **118**, 38–42.

Nelson, A.A., Fitzhugh, O.G., and Calvery, H.O., 1943, Liver tumors following cirrhosis caused by selenium in rats, *Cancer Res.* **3**, 230–235.

Nève, J., 1992, Historical perspectives on the identification of type 1 iodothyronine deiodinase as the second mammalian selenoenzyme, *J. Trace Elem. Electrolytes Health Dis.* **6**, 57–61.

Nève, J., 1999, Combined selenium and iodine deficiency in Kashin-Beck osteoarthropathy, *Bull. Se-Te Dev. Assoc.* March 1999, pp. 1–3.

Nezelof, C., Bouvier, R., and Dijoud, F., 2002, Multifocal myocardial necrosis: a distinctive cardiac lesion in cystic fibrosis, lipomatous pancreatic atrophy, and Keshan disease, *Pediatr. Pathol. Mol. Biol.* **21**, 343–352.

Ngo, B., Dikassa, L., Okitolonda, W., et al., 1997, Selenium status of pregnant women of a rural population (Zaire) in relationship to iodine deficiency, *Trop. Med. Inte. Health* **2**, 572–585.

Norris, F.H. and Sang, K., 1978, Amyotrophic lateral sclerosis and low urinary selenium levels, *JAMA* **239**, 404.

Palace, V.P., Baron, C., Evans, R.E., et al., 2004, The assessment of the potential for selenium to impair reproduction in brown trout, *Environ. Biol. Fish.* **70**, 169–174.

Pamphlett, R., McQuilty, R., and Zarkos, K., 2001, Blood levels of toxic and essential metals in motor neuron disease, *Neurotoxology.* **22**, 401–410.

Peng, A., Wang, W.H., Wang, C.X., et al., 1999, The role of humic substances in drinking water in Kashin-Beck disease in China, *Environ. Health Perspect.* **107**, 293–296.

Porter, R., 1997, *The Greatest Benefit to Mankind: a Medical History of Mankind from Antiquity to the Present*, HarperCollins, London, p. 564.

Qing, Y. and Fan, W., 1991, Effect of sodium nitrite on myocardial glutathione peroxidase and protective action of vitamin E and selenium, *Biomed. Environ. Sci.* **4**, 373–375.

Research Group of Environment and Endemic Diseases, Institute of Geography, Beijing, 1990, Kashin-Beck disease in China: geographical epidemiology and its environmental pathogenicity, *J. Chin. Geog.* **1**, 71–83.

Robertson, D.S.F., 1970, Selenium, a possible teratogen? *Lancet*, **i**, 518–519.

Rosenfeld, I. and Beath, O.A., 1964, *Selenium, Geobotany, Biochemistry, Toxicity and Nutrition*, Academic Press, New York, p. 7.

Sector, C.L. and Lisk, D.J., 1989, Variations in the selenium content of individual Brazil nuts, *J. Food Safety* **9**, 279–281.

Shamberger, R.J. and Frost, D.V., 1969, Possible protective effect of selenium against human cancer, *Can. Med. Assoc. J.* **100**, 682–686.

Simón, P., 1953, Noticias historiales de las conquistas de tierra firme en las Indias Occidentales, año 1560, *Biblioteca Autores Colombianos* **4**, 222, cited in Kerdel-Vegas, 1966.

Smith, M.I. and Westfall, B.B., 1937, Further field studies on the selenium problem in relation to public health, *US Pub. Health Rep.* **52**, 1375–1384.

Smith, M.I., Franke, K.W., and Westfall, B.B., 1936, The selenium problem in relation to public health. A preliminary survey to determine the possibility of selenium intoxication in the rural population living on seleniferous soil, *US Pub. Health Rep.* **51**, 1496–1505.

Schwarz, K., 1977, Amyotrophic lateral sclerosis and selenium, *JAMA* **238**, 2365.

Tan, J.A., Zhu, W.Y., Wang, W.Y., et al., 2002, Selenium in soil and endemic diseases in China, *Sci. Total Environ.* **284**, 227–235.

Tank, G. and Storvick, C.A., 1960, Effect of naturally occurring selenium and vanadium in dental caries, *J. Dental Res.* **39**, 473–488.

Thompson, A.W.S. and Paul, A.H., 1971, Vitamin E deficiency and cot deaths, *Therapeutic Notes*, No.104, Government Printer, Wellington, New Zealand.

Vanderpas, J. and Nève, J., 1999, Kashin-Beck disease in China: osteochondrodysplasia related to nutrition and environment, *Bull. Mem. Acad. R. Med. Belg.* **154**, 177–184.

Vanderpas, J.B., Contempre, B., Duale, N.L., et al., 1993, Selenium deficiency mitigates hypothyroxinemia in I-deficient subjects, *Am. J. Clin. Nutr.* **57**, S271–S275.

Vanderpas, J.B., Dumont, J.E., Contempre, B., and Diplock, A.T., 1992, Iodine and selenium deficiency in northern Zaire, *Am. J. Clin. Nutr.* **56**, 957–958.

Vanderpas, J., Contempré, B., Duale, N.I., et al., 1990, Iodine and selenium deficiency associated with cretinism in northern Zaire, *Am. J. Clin. Nutr.* **52**, 1087–1093.

Voshchenko, A.V., Anikina, L.V., and Dimova, S.N., 1992, Towards the mechanism of selenium-deficient cardiopathy in sporadic cases, in: *Fifth International Symposium on Selenium in Biology and Medicine. Abstracts*, Vanderbilt University, Nashville, TN, July 20–23, p. 153.

Wang, G., Zhou, R., Sun, S., et al., 1979, Differences between blood selenium concentrations of residents of Keshan disease-affected and nonaffected areas – correlation between the selenium content of blood and hair, *Chinese J. Prevent. Med.* **13**, 204 (in Chinese), cited in Yang et al., 1984.

Wu, L., Xia, Y.M., Ha, P.C., and Chen, X.S., 1997, Changes in myocardial thyroid hormone metabolism and alpha-glycerophosphate dehydrogenase activity in rats deficient in iodine and selenium, *Br. J. Nutr.* **78**, 671–676.

Xia, Y., Hill, K.E., and Burk, R.E., 1990, Biochemical characterization of selenium deficiency in China, in: Trace Elements in Clinical Medicine. *Proceedings of the 2nd Meeting of the International Society for Trace Element Research in Humans (ISTERH),* August 28–September 1, 1989, Springer, Tokyo, pp. 349–352.

Xie, J.K., Yang, G., Ge, K., et al., 1964, Views on the etiology of Keshan disease and suggestions for future studies, in: *Selected Works on Keshan Disease*, Vol. 1, pp. 1–10 (in Chinese), cited in Keshan Disease Research Group of the Chinese Academy of Medical Science, 1979.

Yang, C., Niu, C.R., Bodo, M., et al., 1992, Selenium deficiency and fulvic acid supplementation disturb the posttranslational modification of collagen in the skeletal system of mice, in: *Fifth International Symposium on Selenium in Biology and Medicine, Abstracts*, July 20–23, 1992, Vanderbilt University, Nashville, TN, p. 117.

Yang, G., 1983, On the etiology of Keshan disease, *Adv. Physiol. Sci.* **14**, 313–317.
Yang, G., Chen, J., Wen, Z., et al., 1984, The role of selenium in Keshan disease, in: Draper, H.H. (ed.), *Advances in Nutritional Research*, Vol. 6, Plenum Press, New York, pp. 203–231.
Yang, G., Wang, S., Zhou, R., and Sun, S., 1983, Endemic selenium intoxication of humans in China, *Am. J. Clin. Nutr.* **37**, 872–881.
Yin, T., Sun, S., Wang, H., et al., 1979, Difference in the amount of selenium excreted in urine between children in Keshan disease-affected and nonaffected areas, *Chinese J. Prevent. Med.* **13**, 207 (in Chinese), cited in Yang et al., 1984.
Zheng, B.S., Ding, Z.H., Huang, R.G., et al., 1999, Issues of health and disease relating to coal use in southwestern China, *Int. J. Coal Geol.* **40**, 119–132.
Zhilun, W., Cai, B., Shemin, L., et al., 1993, Research on the relationship between selenium deficiency and KBD, *J. Xi'an Med. Uni.* **14**, 67–70.

6 Selenium in Health and Disease III: Nonendemic Selenium-Responsive Conditions, Cancer and Coronary Vascular Disease

6.1 Nonendemic Selenium Deficiency

Both KD and KBD are endemic diseases that occur in reasonably well-defined geographical regions of China and some neighboring countries. The diseases are associated with localized geological features in conjunction with geographical isolation and restricted food availability. Although there are well-recognized and extensive regions of selenium-deficient soils in some other countries, including New Zealand, neither KBD nor KD has been found to occur outside China and its northern neighbors. However, illnesses that show some of the features of KD and are related to selenium are not confined to the areas of endemic deficiency. These may be of iatrogenic origin or the consequences of other health conditions. Most cases reported in the medical literature are single and isolated instances of the effects of selenium deficiency. Although uncommon, such cases have important implications since they can be the result of accepted medical practices and therapies.

6.1.1 TPN-Induced Selenium Deficiency

Patients who require to be sustained for longer periods on total parenteral nutrition (TPN) can be at risk of developing selenium deficiency if there is little or no selenium in the infusion fluids (Gramm et al., 1995). This was not an uncommon situation until recently, because of lack of consensus about selenium requirements for such patients (Levander and Burk, 1986). In some early cases, selenium levels in TPN patients were found to be as little as one tenth of those in healthy adults, equivalent to those found in KD victims, though these low levels were not accompanied by symptoms of full-blown deficiency (AUSPEN, 1979). Selenium supplementation during TPN administration is now routine in practice (Abrams et al., 1992). Unfortunately, selenium deficiency can still be encountered in patients who are dependent on parenteral or enteral nutrition, particularly if they suffer from gastrointestinal disorders, which impair absorption (Rannem et al., 1998). There have been reports of selenium deficiency, e.g., in patients with Crohn's disease receiving long-term TPN (Inoue et al., 2003; Kuroki et al., 2003).

Skeletal problems, including myalgias and myopathies, have been reported in TPN patients. A New Zealand patient developed, within 1 month of the start of the therapy, muscular pain and tenderness, particularly in the lower limbs, and extreme difficulty in walking. Blood selenium levels and GPX activity were also very low. The condition cleared up rapidly when selenium was added to the infusion fluid (Van Rij et al., 1979). There have been reports of muscular weaknesses in children receiving parenteral nutrition, including home treatment, in the USA and the UK (Kelly et al., 1988; Kien and Ganther, 1983). The condition normally clears up rapidly once selenium is added to the infusion fluid (Chariot and Bignani, 2003).

6.1.1.1 TPN-Related KD-Like Cardiomyopathies

Muscular problems are not always associated with low selenium status resulting from TPN. Cardiomyopathies are also recognized as a potential problem in such circumstances. Among seven cases of cardiomyopathy due to nonendemic acquired selenium deficiency reported in the literature between 1980 and 1990, six were in patients undergoing TPN. Of these, three responded to treatment with selenium supplements, but the other three died. However, while selenium deficiency was the common factor in each of these patients, all were suffering from different underlying diseases, including cancer and Crohn's disease before they developed cardiomyopathy. Symptoms were similar to those observed in the victims of KD. Although it could not be proved that selenium deficiency was the cause of cardiomyopathy, the findings were strongly suggestive of this diagnosis (Lockitch et al., 1990).

6.1.1.2 Other Causes of Selenium Deficiency-Associated Cardiomyopathies

Several cases of cardiomyopathy linked to selenium deficiency caused by an inadequate diet, and not TPN, has been reported. A 2-year-old girl from a socially deprived background in New York was found to have congestive heart failure, with symptoms similar to those seen in Chinese KD victims. Her very low blood selenium level of 0.004 μmol/l (0.32 μg/l) was attributed to her poor diet, which contained almost no cereals or dairy products and just a little meat. Her daily intake of selenium was 10 μg. Her condition improved rapidly when selenium supplements were given, though 3 months later she still had cardiomegaly (Collip and Chen, 1981).

A more recent report was a case of cardiomyopathy in a patient at the Children's Hospital of Philadelphia. This was believed to be related to the use of a ketogenic diet (Bergqvist et al., 2003). The diet, which is very low in most of the vitamins and minerals, has been found to be an efficacious treatment with minimal side effects for intractable epilepsy. Selenium deficiency, determined by blood selenium determinations, was detected in nine young patients maintained on the diet, only one of whom developed cardiomyopathy. This patient was reported to have no detectable whole-blood selenium. Although cardiac physical examination did not reveal any abnormalities, cardiomyopathy was revealed by electrocardiogram. The selenium status of all the patients was improved by supplementation.

6.1.1.3 Low Selenium Intake and Muscular Problems in New Zealand

In the 1970s there were reports of muscular problems among people living in low soil selenium areas of the south island of New Zealand (Thomson and Robinson, 1980). Many of those who had these problems believed that they were related to a low dietary intake of selenium and were similar to WMD and other selenium deficiency conditions common in sheep in the area.

Symptoms reported included multiple muscular aches and pains and areas of tenderness. The condition was said to occur in nearly 50% of the population in some farming areas. It was reported most commonly in late winter and early spring. Intervention trials using sodium selenite and selenomethionine supplements up to 100 μg/day produced only inclusive results. In most cases it was found that use of a placebo was as effective as a supplement in treating the muscular conditions. In spite of the lack of medical evidence, many of the local people continued to use self-medication, usually with veterinary preparations, including selenium-containing sheep drenches. They claimed that this gave them relief from their muscular problems (Thomson et al., 1978).

6.2 Other Iatrogenic Selenium Deficiencies

Phenylketonuria (PKU) is an inherited defect of metabolism that interferes with the enzymatic pathway for converting the essential amino acid phenylalanine into tyrosine. Worldwide, approximately one child in 10,000 is born with the disease. In some countries and regions, such as Ireland, Queensland in Australia, and New England in the USA, where a high percentage of the population carry Celtic genes, incidence can be as high as 1 in 4,500 live births (Naughton et al., 1987). In affected children, phenylalanine, which enters the body as a normal component of proteins in the diet, and its metabolites accumulate in the blood. The consequences are serious, especially when these substances can cross the blood–brain barrier and cause permanent neurological damage (Scriver et al., 2001).

Since the 1950s PKU has been managed effectively by providing, as soon as possible after birth, a strictly controlled diet that restricts the intake of phenylalanine to the minimum required to meet essential needs, without any surplus for buildup in the blood (Bickel, 1954). This is achieved by excluding, or, where appropriate, severely restricting all natural protein foodstuffs, such as meat, dairy products, and certain cereals in the diet. In their place a mixture of purified amino acids containing a minimum of phenylalanine is provided. The diet must be followed strictly in infancy, with a gradual relaxation in later years. Although the vulnerability of the brain to damage from excessive phenylalanine decreases with maturity, lifelong use of the PKU diet is advocated in some circumstances, including pregnancy (Naughton et al., 1987).

Although effective in preventing the brain damage, the PKU diet, has, because of its restricted nature, continued to cause concern to nutritionists. A variety of micronutrient supplements had to be added to the diet as its deficiencies, such as iron and zinc, were recognized (Gropper et al., 1988). An Australian study (Reilly et al., 1990) found plasma levels of 0.38 ± 0.11 μmol/l in PKU children, a level considerably lower than that in normal children and equivalent to that found in KD children in China. The daily selenium intake of the PKU children was 8.4 ± 3.9 μg, comparable to that of Chinese KD children.

In spite of their very low selenium status the Australian children were not found to have any selenium-deficiency-related illness (Latham et al., 1989). Their growth rates were comparable to those of healthy children, their nails were undamaged, and they showed no symptoms of skeletal or cardiac myopathies. Similar absences of symptoms of selenium deficiency were reported in PKU children in Germany (Lombeck et al., 1984), and in the USA (Acosta et al., 1987). However, a subsequent study of German PKU children found that they had a significantly higher level of plasma thyroxine (T4) than did healthy controls (Terwolbeck et al., 1993). The significance of this finding was not clear at that time. In later studies, the same group again found that the increase in T4 levels in the PKU children was inversely correlated with plasma selenium values, and speculated that the increase was due to a decreased level of deiodination resulting from a decrease in IDI activity. They found no clinical signs of myopathy of the heart or skeletal muscles, or changes in the ECG or ultrasound measurements in the PKU children. However, there was a negative correlation between plasma selenium values and whole blood and plasma aspartate amino transferase (ASAT) activity, which might have indicated a subclinical stage of muscular damage (Reeve et al., 1989).

6.3 Selenium and Cancer

Although at one time selenium was officially listed as a carcinogen (Frost, 1972), its possible effectiveness in cancer therapy was considered as early as the second decade of the last century. The therapeutic use of selenium in cancer treatment was reported in a paper published in 1915 (Walker and Klein, 1915). Some 30 years later it was shown that addition of 5 mg/kg of sodium selenite to the diet reduced the incidence of tumors in rats exposed to dimethylaminobenzene (Clayton and Baumann, 1949). It is interesting that the investigation of azo dye-induced tumors began with the belief, as might have been expected at the time, that selenium was carcinogenic and its effect on the tumor could be expected to be additive to that of the dye. To the surprise of the investigators, the effects of the two substances were found to be opposite.

Following these early findings, much research was conducted on the possibly protective properties of selenium against several types of cancer. At the same time epidemiological studies on the relation between selenium intake in the diets of different populations and the incidence of a variety of cancers in different regions of the world were carried out by a number of investigators.

6.3.1 Epidemiological Studies of the Relation Between Selenium and Cancer

In the late 1960s Shamberger and Frost (1969) reported that there was evidence of an apparent inverse relationship between selenium levels in field crops and cancer mortality in different regions in the USA. Although their view was questioned by some commentators on the ground that they had overestimated the statistical significance of their findings (Schrauzer, 1979), several subsequent epidemiological studies produced supporting evidences for the hypothesis linking low selenium intake with an increased incidence of cancer (Ip, 1998).

Several of these later studies pointed towards epidemiological correlations of blood levels and dietary intakes of selenium with the occurrence of specific types of cancer. A major study by Schrauzer (1976) looked at published data from 27 countries and found evidence that dietary intake of selenium could be inversely correlated with total age-adjusted cancer mortality for both males and females. With regard to specific forms of the disease, he found evidence of a significant inverse correlation between selenium intake and mortality from cancer of the prostate, colon, rectum, and certain other tissues, while correlations in the case of cancer of the bladder, pancreas, and skin were weak and totally absent for cancer of the esophagus, stomach, and liver. Although there were criticisms of Schrauzer's findings, not least by the WHO Task Force on Selenium (1987), it was supported by several other epidemiologists (Jansson et al., 1978; Clark, 1985).

6.3.2 Case-Control Studies of Selenium and Cancer Associations

A number of studies in which blood and organ selenium levels in cancer patients were compared with those in subjects not suffering from the disease, but otherwise identical in origin and other parameters, have been carried out since the 1970s. The results of many of these studies indicated a significant inverse relationship between selenium levels and cancer incidence. Shamberger et al. (1973) were among the first to carry out this type of case-control study. They reported that blood selenium levels in patients with certain types of cancer were significantly lower than in healthy controls. However, the findings were not consistent within some groups with the same type of the disease. In a later study, which looked at age-specific death rates from cancer in relation to selenium levels in blood across the 50 US States, they found evidence that average cancer mortality was highest in the lower quintile of selenium values (Shamberger, 1985).

Doubts were expressed by some investigators about the significance of these findings. Diplock (1987) believed that much of the evidence was of little value since it is not possible to determine whether low blood and tissue selenium levels are a cause or a consequence of cancer. Robinson and Thomson (1981) carried out a similar exercise to that of Shamberger (Shamberger et al., 1973), using their own observations in New Zealand and data from ten other countries. At least in the case of colorectal and breast cancers, they failed to find any obvious relation between disease incidence rates and blood selenium levels.

Another study, which failed to show a clear relationship between selenium status and cancer, was the Nurse's Health Study (Garland et al., 1995). This was carried out in the USA in 1982 and involved over 60,000 nurses, none of whom has any previous history of cancer. Toenail clippings supplied by each of the participants were analyzed to determine selenium status. After three and a half years of data collection, selenium levels of nurses with and without cancer were compared. The investigators found that nurses with higher levels of selenium in their toenails did not have a reduced risk of cancer.

6.3.3 "Nested" Case-Control Studies

Several case-control studies which were "nested" within prospective studies, in which selenium levels in blood collected prospectively from subjects who did not have cancer at the time of collection but who developed the disease during the study, were compared at a later date with levels in those who remained cancer-free, have been carried out (Diplock, 1987). In general their findings lend support to the hypothesis of a link between low selenium status and an increased risk of cancer.

One of the earliest of these studies followed up some 10,000 US men and women over a period of 5 years, from 1973 to 1978 (Willett et al., 1983). Blood samples, which were analyzed for selenium, were taken from all participants at the beginning of the trial. During the 5 years, 111 new cases of cancer were detected. For each case, two controls as closely matching as possible, but without cancer, were selected. The initial selenium levels in controls were significantly higher than in the cancer patients. A significantly greater than expected cancer incidence was found in participants in the lower blood selenium groups, with an increased risk in the lower quintile of baseline selenium twice that in the highest quintile. The investigators concluded that although their findings supported the hypothesis that low selenium increases the risk of cancer, there was need for further investigation of the differences observed between cancer sites, as well as those related to age, sex, race, and smoking habits.

Several more recent prospective studies have strengthened the case for the view that a low selenium status is associated with a significantly increased risk of cancer incidence and mortality. A nested case–control study within a cohort of 9,000 Finns found that there was a significantly higher relative risk of lung cancer between the lowest and highest tertiles of serum selenium (Knekt et al., 1998). A study of more than 7,000 Taiwanese men with chronic hepatitis virus infection showed that there was a significant inverse relationship between selenium levels in stored plasma and later development of hepatocellular carcinoma (HCC) (Yu et al., 1999).

A large prospective study on the association between selenium intake and prostate cancer involved 34,000 men from the Harvard-based Health Professionals' Cohort Study (Yoshizawa et al., 1998). As in the Nurse's Health

Study (Garland et al., 1995), selenium status of participants was assessed by toenail selenium measurements. It was found that subjects in the lowest quintile of selenium status had three times the likelihood of developing advanced prostate cancer as those in the highest quintile.

While the results of these and several other prospective studies, apart from a few, such as the Nurse's Health Study, have provided evidence for the beneficial effect of higher selenium status in the prevention of certain forms of cancer, the most consistent association has been found in populations with low or moderate selenium intakes. It has been suggested, consequently, that selenium may only exert its protective effect against cancer, when the basic level is low in relation to oxidative stress (Knekt et al., 1990), or may provide protection only in certain circumstances, or in combination with other antioxidants (British Nutrition Foundation, 2001).

6.3.4 *Intervention Trials*

Several large-scale prospective studies, involving intervention with selenium alone or in combination with other micronutrient supplements, have been carried out in China. Their results, though not providing absolute evidence of the protective effects of selenium against cancer, do lend support to the hypothesis.

6.3.4.1 The Linxian Intervention Trials

One of the earliest of these intervention trials was carried out in Linxian, a remote rural county in north central China, whose inhabitants have one of the highest rates of esophageal cancer in the world. Incidence of gastric cancer is also very high (Anon, 1993). The trial involved nearly 30,000 adults, both male and female, and lasted for 5 years from 1985 to 1990. Subjects were randomly assigned to four groups, to receive one of four different combinations of different nutritional supplements or a placebo. The combinations were, vitamin A and zinc; riboflavin and niacin; vitamin C and molybdenum; and β-carotene, vitamin E, and selenium. At the end of the trial it was found that the combinations containing selenium and the two other antioxidants, had had a significant beneficial effect on mortality, especially from stomach, but not from other forms of cancer. None of the other combinations had a significant effect on cancer mortality. The investigators concluded that while their findings pointed towards a protective role of the combined antioxidant group of supplements, it was not possible to say whether this was due to selenium alone or to one of the other antioxidants, either on its own, or in combination with the others (Blot et al., 1993).

A subsequent survey of the nutritional intake of Linxian residents found evidence of a generally poor nutritional status, with intakes below RDAs for selenium, zinc and calcium, as well as for vitamins A, C, B2, and E. Protein intake was also low (Zou et al., 2003). These findings suggest that the observed fall in esophageal cancer following supplementation was unlikely to have been due to the additional intake of selenium alone but to a general improvement of the diet.

A 15-year follow-up study of 1,103 subjects randomly selected from the larger trial cohort, did find, however, a significant inverse association between baseline serum selenium concentrations and death from esophageal squamous cell carcinoma and gastric cardia cancer (Wei et al., 2004).

6.3.4.2 Qidong Intervention Trial

A second Chinese intervention trial was carried out between 1984 and 1990 in Qidong, Jiansu Province. This is a high-risk area for HCC, a disease which accounts for more than a quarter of a million deaths each year in China, with an incidence rate in some areas approaching 150 cases/100,000/year (Huang et al., 2003). More than 130,000 people living in five townships in Qidong were involved in the trial. The inhabitants of one township were provided with salt (sodium chloride) fortified with 15 mg/kg of sodium selenite. The other four townships had unfortified salt. After 6 years, the incidence of liver cancer in the fortified group had fallen from an initial 52.84/100,000 to 34.49/100,000, whereas in the control townships there was no decrease in incidence. It was concluded by the investigators at the Qidong Liver Cancer Institute, that fortification of domestic salt with selenium is a cheap, effective, and simple way of decreasing the risk of cancer in this high-risk area (Li et al., 1992). This may have been an overoptimistic conclusion. It has been shown that exposure to hepatitis B virus and aflatoxin B1 (AFB1) contributes to the development of hepatocarcinogenesis (Lunn et al., 1997; Hsia et al., 1992). It is believed that high levels of aflatoxin may be associated with a genetic mutation identified in several human cancers (Niu et al., 2002). This mutation of the p53 tumor suppressor gene in which there is a serine substitution at codon 249, which may be a SNP (Huang et al., 2003), has been detected in a high percentage of tumors from Qidong. Up to 15% of the residents of the area are chronically infected with the hepatitis B virus and more than 90% of them have serum aflatoxin-albumin adducts, indicating a very high exposure rate to the toxin (Huang et al., 2003). Thus, exposure to aflatoxins and the presence of the 249^{ser} p53 mutation in plasma appears to be strongly associated with HCC in Qidong patients. It has been suggested that further trials are required to examine the interrelationship between HCC, viral hepatitis infection, and selenium in order to understand better the etiological mechanisms involved and evaluate the true chemopreventive potential of selenium compounds for liver cancer (Sakoda et al., 2005).

6.3.4.3 The Nutritional Prevention of Cancer with Selenium Trial

The Nutritional Prevention of Cancer (NPC) Trial, carried out by Clark et al. (1996) in the USA, was the first double-blind, placebo-controlled intervention trial in a western population, designed to test the hypothesis that selenium supplementation could reduce the risk of cancer.

The primary purpose of the trial was to test the hypothesis that increased selenium status could reduce the risk of two forms of nonmelanoma carcinoma of the skin: basal (BCC) and squamous (SCC). Secondary end points included total and cancer mortality and incidents of lung, colorectal, prostate, and other forms of cancer.

The carefully designed and extensive trial was carried out in seven dermatological clinics in the eastern USA. It involved 1,312 adult patients with a history of BCC or SCC. Recruitment was sex neutral and the patients were randomized from 1983 to the end of 1991. They were given 200 μg of selenium, in the form of a high-selenium brewer's yeast tablet, or a placebo, daily for a mean of 4.5 years, with a follow-up of 6.4 years.

The results found that selenium supplementation did not significantly affect the incidence of either of the skin cancers. However, analysis of the secondary end points showed significant reductions in total cancer mortality, as well as incidents of lung (46% reduction), colorectal (58% reduction), and prostate (63% reduction) cancers. It was concluded by Clark and his colleagues that, while selenium treatment did not protect against development of nonmelanoma skin cancers, their results did support the hypothesis that supplemental selenium may reduce the incidence of, and mortality from, prostate and several other types of cancer.

Publication of the NPC trial findings caused considerable excitement among researchers in cancer research as well as in the popular media. Its importance was underlined by editorials, not only in the journal of the AMA, but also in several other major medical journals worldwide. However, while the report was generally received with considerable interest, it was also subject to criticism. It was pointed out that the results were not definitive (Fleshner and Klotz, 1999). Several commentators noted that reductions in prostate, lung, and colon cancers had not been a priori hypotheses of the study, and that interpretation of secondary end points required caution (Pocock and Hughes, 1990; Colditz, 1996; Fleet, 1997).

Clark and his colleagues were not unaware of the shortcomings of their trial. They did not claim that they had proved that selenium supplementation could prevent cancer, but only that selenium supplementation was found to be associated with significant reductions in secondary end points of total cancer incidence, lung, colorectal, and prostate cancer incidents, and lung cancer mortality. They were careful to conclude their report with a statement that these apparent beneficial effects of selenium supplementation require confirmation in independent trials of appropriate design before health recommendations regarding selenium supplementation could be made (Clark et al., 1996). The numerous follow-up and other trials, including those by Clark's own group, that have been planned and undertaken since that time, show that their advice that further, independent and appropriately designed investigations should be undertaken, has been widely accepted in the scientific community. Unfortunately, that has not been the case in some areas of the pharmaceutical and health food industries, nor by some journalists who have raised unrealistic expectations of a cure for cancer by selenium supplementation in their readers (Anon, 1998).

One of the first of the additional studies was that by Clark et al. (1998) which found further evidence of a decreased incidence of prostate cancer with selenium supplementation. It was a follow-up, over 10 years, of participants who had taken part in the original NPC trial. Interestingly, while the results showed a significant treatment effect in participants in the lowest and middle tertiles of baseline plasma selenium, there was only a nonsignificant reduction in risk in the highest third.

6.3.4.4 The PRECISE Intervention Trial

Shortly before his untimely death in 2000 from prostate cancer, Clark with colleagues from the USA and several other countries, designed a large-scale, international trial as a definitive test for the hypothesis that selenium supplementation can prevent several different types of cancers in humans. The Prevention of Cancer with Selenium in Europe and America (PRECISE) trial was to be a 5-year, double-blind randomized, placebo-controlled cancer study, involving as many as 50,000 subjects in the USA and several European countries, including the UK, Denmark, the Netherlands, and Scandinavia. It was designed to replicate and extend the design of the NPC study by including participants in other countries and by using supplementation doses of 100, 200, and 300 μg/day (Rayman and Clark, 1999). Two pilot studies following the PRECISE protocol, using selenium supplements up to 300 μg/day, but with relatively small numbers of subjects, are currently underway in the UK and in Denmark (Rayman, 2004). Trials, using daily selenium doses of up to 800 μg and even higher, have been carried out at the University of Arizona Cancer Center, as a follow-up to the NPC trial. They were designed to look at the effects of long-term selenium supplementation in men who are either at high risk of prostate cancer or are already diagnosed as having it (Stratton et al., 2003a). In one of the trials, known as the "Watchful Waiting Trial," it involved men with localized prostate cancer and life expectancy of <10 years. The majority of the participants were given 200 or 800 μg of selenium (as selenium-enriched yeast), daily for up to 3 years (Stratton et al., 2003b). No side effects of selenosis were observed in any of the subjects on this regime. In a small subgroup, eight subjects were given a daily selenium dose of 1,600 μg, and 16 others 3,200 μg for up to a year. Mean plasma selenium levels increased to 492 ± 188 and 640 ± 491 μg/l, respectively. Side effects, such as garlic breath, nail and hair damage, dizziness, and stomach upsets were experienced, especially by those taking the higher selenium dose. However, it was reported that blood chemistry and hematology results were within normal ranges and no severe or serious selenium-related toxicity was observed. However, because of the lack of safety information about such high doses in the literature, the trial was discontinued for the high intake subgroup at the end of its first year (Reid et al., 2004).

6.3.4.5 The SELECT Intervention Trial

The Selenium and Vitamin E Cancer Prevention Trial (SELECT) is another ongoing trial at the present time in the USA (Klein et al., 2003). It is a randomized, prospective, double-blind study designed to determine whether selenium and vitamin E, alone and in combination, can reduce the risk of prostate cancer among healthy men, with a PSA not greater than 4 ng/ml. The daily supplement dose is 200 μg of selenium in the form of selenomethionine and/or 400 mg of racemic α-tocopherol or matched placebo. The primary end point is the clinical incidence of prostate cancer. Enrolment began in 2001 with the aim of recruiting more than 30,000 men. Results are expected in 2013.

6.3.4.6 The SU.VI.MAX Trial

A French study, Supplementation en Vitamines et Mineraux AntioXydants (SU.VI.MAX), designed to assess the effect of vitamin and mineral supplements on chronic disease risk, including prostate and other forms of cancer, begun in 1994, has followed more than 12,000 adult men and women over a period of 8 years (Hercberg et al., 1998a). Participants were given 100 μg selenium daily, and in addition, one to three times the RDA of vitamins E and C, as well as β-carotene and zinc (Hercberg et al., 1998b).

At the end of the 8 years of intervention, there was, overall, a moderate non significant reduction in prostate cancer rate in the men who were given the vitamin and mineral supplements. However, the rate differed significantly between men with normal baseline prostate-specific antigen (PSA) levels (<3 μg/l), and those with an elevated PSA. Those with a normal PSA showed a significant reduction in the rate of prostate cancer, while in those with a higher PSA, the supplement was associated with an increased incidence of prostate cancer of borderline statistical significance. The results were interpreted as supporting the hypothesis that chemoprevention of prostate cancer can be achieved with nutritional doses of antioxidant vitamins and minerals (Meyer et al., 2005).

6.3.5 Evidence for an Association Between Cancer-Prevention and Selenium

Although evidence has been accumulating in support of the hypothesis of an association between cancer and selenium, it is still not fully established, nor is it likely that such large-scale intervention trials will finally provide the definitive proof that is still lacking. Indeed, it has been suggested that what is needed is smaller supplementation trials within the larger population so that the effect of the micronutrient can be separated from any other dietary and medical interventions taking place and, moreover, take account of the full range of biochemistry and functions of selenium and their individual variations in humans (Arthur, 2003). Until that is done, doubts that have been expressed, e.g., by the UK's Department of Health (1998), as to whether there are adequate grounds to support the view that there are specific links for selenium in the causation or prevention of cancer, will continue to held by many. There may, indeed, be need for further investigations, even after the results of current intervention trials become available, to answer other questions regarding selenium's role in disease prevention. Not least of these relates to the problem of assessment of selenium status, especially the absence of absolutely reliable biochemical and functional markers. Possibly even more important is the need for a better understanding of individual variation in ability to utilize selenium and the role of genetic polymorphisms in this process.

It is of some interest that the negative views of the UK's Department of Health on the possibility of the role of selenium in relation to cancer prevention do not appear to be followed by the US FDA. The Bureau, in considering the possible use of a claim for a connection between selenium and health on food labels, has concluded that there is sufficient evidence to permit a qualified health claim for selenium and cancer (Trumbo, 2005).

6.3.5.1 Baseline Selenium Levels and Dose Size in Cancer Prevention Trials

Rayman (2000) made a significant observation when she drew attention to differences in baseline blood selenium levels in participants in the NPC trial in the USA and in potential participants in European trials. She noted that the NPC trial was carried out in a region of the USA in which daily dietary intake of selenium is 90 μg. This intake is low by US standards, but well above the level needed to optimize selenoenzyme activity (Thomson et al., 1993). Rayman suggests that while these observations do not preclude a role for selenoenzymes in cancer prevention, they do suggest the operation of additional important mechanisms. These possible mechanisms include the ability of selenium to enhance the immune response or the ability to produce antitumorigenic metabolites that can interfere with tumor cell metabolism, inhibit angiogenesis, and induce apoptosis of cancer cells and also activate stress kinase pathways (Fleming et al., 2001). This view is supported by the fact that antitumorigenic effects in experimental carcinogenic models have been consistently associated with supranutritional intakes of selenium, at least ten times the levels required to prevent clinical signs of selenium deficiency (Combs, 2001). It is noteworthy that supranutritional levels of selenium have been used in the intervention trials, such as Clark's NPC (Clark et al., 1996) and its successors, that have reported a positive relation between selenium intake and a reduction in cancer incidence.

6.4 The Carcinostatic Properties of Selenium Compounds

The first known report of the use of a selenium compound to treat a preexisting cancer was that of Walker and Klein et al. (1915), which described the successful treatment of a patient with a lingual cancer by directly injecting sodium selenite into the tumor. Subsequently, several different selenium compounds were shown to be able to affect the development of a range of tumors, though in animal models, not in humans. The results of a number of these experiments have been summarized by Medina (1986). Rats and mice were the animals most commonly used, and hamsters in a few cases. Carcinogens tested included 1,2-dimethylbenzanthracene (DMBA), benzo[*a*]pyrene (BP), dimethylnitrosamine (DMN), AFB1, and mouse mammary tumor virus (MMTV). Tumors investigated were in the liver, colon, mammary gland, skin, stomach, esophagus, pancreas, kidney, lung, and some other organs. The cytotoxic effects of selenium compounds were also investigated using cultured tumor cell lines, with results similar to those obtained with experimental animals (Poirer and Milner, 1979). The selenium compounds investigated were both inorganic and organic, including selenite, selenate, and selenium dioxide, as well as the selenoamino acids, selenomethione, and selenocysteine and several other organic forms. It was shown that most but not all selenium compounds have anticarcinogenic activity that will arrest cancer growth and prevent or reduce induced carcinogenesis in a variety of cell culture and animal experiments (Combs and Gray, 1998). Carcinostatic activity of selenium was not observed in animals when dietary supplemental levels were <1 to 1.5 mg/kg. Diets needed to be supplemented to considerably higher dose of selenium of 20 to 30 mg/kg of diet, 10 to 150 times the nutritional requirement of 0.10 to –0.30 mg/kg, to bring about cancer preventing activity (Spallholz, 2001).

6.4.1 How Selenium Compounds May Prevent Cancer

A number of hypotheses have been postulated to account for the experimental data, which indicates that selenium compounds have carcinostatic properties. Five of these are discussed by Spallholz (2001): (1) selenium's antioxidant role; (2) its ability to enhance immunity; (3) its effect on the metabolism of carcinogens; (4) its role in protein synthesis and cell division; and (5) the formation of anticancer selenium metabolites.

6.4.1.1 Hypotheses of Cancer Prevention by Dietary Selenium

Although GPX and other antioxidant selenoprotein enzymes are capable of protecting cells against reactive oxygen species, and thus against genetic damage and possibly cancer, it has been pointed out by Beckett et al. (2003) that it is unlikely that selenium exerts its anticancer activity through a mechanism related to recognized selenoproteins. In the NPC trial (Clark et al., 1996), those found to benefit from supplementation already had an intake sufficient to saturate selenoprotein activities. Moreover, it has been found that supplementation at supranutritional levels is required to bring about the chemopreventive effects, in humans and experimental animals. Thus, it is likely that the carcinostatic effects of selenium are brought about in a manner unrelated to the saturated levels of selenoproteins that can normally be provided by an adequate dietary intake of the element.

Lipinski (2005) has drawn attention to a paradox relating to the possible role of antioxidant selenoenzymes in inhibiting cancer. Because there appears to be a relationship between free radical generation and carcinogenesis, there are good grounds for believing that antioxidants should be beneficial in inhibiting cancer tumor growth. However, since tumor growth is associated with tissue hypoxia accompanied by the formation of reductive rather than oxidative free radicals, this antioxidant role is open to question. Nevertheless, an oxidizing role of selenium in the inhibition of cancer can still be postulated. Under the reducing conditions of hypoxic tumor tissue, tumor cells can become surrounded by a fibrin-like polymer coat, which is formed by a disulfide reaction between polythiols which are associated with the tumor and plasma proteins, mainly fibrinogen. This coat is protease-resistant and can mask specific tumor antigens, thus allowing the cancer cells to escape immune recognition and elimination by natural killer (NK) cells. Selenite is capable of oxidizing cell membrane thiols and can prevent the formation of the tumor coat, thus making the tumor vulnerable to immune surveillance and destruction.

Immune system enhancement by selenium is a more satisfactory explanation for the carcinostatic properties of selenium. Selenium is essential for optimal immune function, and stimulation of the immune system can be brought about by selenium supplementation. Experiments using mice have shown that selenium supplementation enhances the cellular immune response of the T-cell and the NK cell systems. In humans, stimulation with both vitamin E and selenium is believed to enhance all aspects of the immune system, through stimulation of interleukines and other associated T-cell genes (Kiremidjian-Schumacher and Roy, 1998). How this comes about is not yet fully understood, and the relation of immune system enhancement by selenium supplementation to cancer prevention remains a subject of considerable current investigation (Jackson et al., 2005).

The third hypothesis discussed by Spallholz (2001) is that selenium interferes with the metabolism of carcinogens, derived both externally and internally from normal metabolism. It may do this by reacting directly with carcinogens to prevent their binding to DNA, or by the formation of reactive selenium metabolites, which could make the carcinogens noncarcinogenic. Selenium has been shown in experimental animals to be able to raise the levels of xenobiotic enzymes in liver, such as cytochrome P450 and mixed-function oxidases responsible for the detoxification of carcinogens (Ip and Lisk, 1997).

Selenium may prevent cancer by its effects on the cell cycle and protein synthesis. Many selenium compounds have been shown in cell culture to affect cell viability and DNA integrity (Spallholz, 1994). Selenite, for instance, arrests the cell cycle of cancer cells at low concentration by inhibiting cell division and protein synthesis (Combs and Grey, 1998). It can also cause DNA damage and cell death (Batist et al., 1986). Other selenium compounds have been shown to have similar effects in cell culture. The most effective of these are selenodiglutathione and methylseleninic acid; less effective are organic compounds such as selenomethionine and methylselenocysteine. How these selenium compounds initiate cellular change is not clear (Spallholz, 2001).

The last, and probably the best supported, of the hypotheses discussed by Spallholz explains the carcinostatic activity of selenium supplementation by the formation of selenium metabolites that are toxic to cancer cells, such as hydrogen selenide, selenodiglutathione, and a number of methylated selenium compounds. The findings of Ip's group, which has extensively investigated the chemopreventive properties of natural and man-made selenium compounds (Ip and Ganther, 1994), indicate that methylselenol (CH_3SeH) is the most likely of these metabolites to be responsible for selenium chemoprevention. The methylselenide anion is formed in the body from dietary selenide and selenomethionine and from other less common naturally occurring selenium compounds, such as L-Se-methylselenocysteine, as well as from the synthetic methylseleninic acid (Ip et al., 2000; Whanger, 2004). Evidence from cell culture experiments suggests that selenium compounds that form methylselenides are able not only to arrest growth of cancer cells, but also to induce apoptosis (Zou et al., 2000). This is a highly significant observation. Apoptosis, or, as it is often called, programmed cell death, is a normal event at the end of the life cycle of most cells, except brain, cardiac, and cancer cells. Cancer cells are normal cells that have been "immortalized" and continue to divide, because they have lost the restraints imposed by the cell's normal life cycle. The controlling factor for the induction of cellular apoptosis is the mitochondrion. Certain drugs, proteins, and event signals outside the cell that produce changes in the integrity of the cellular mitochondria, induce apoptosis (Lemasters et al., 1998). Selenium compounds are known to cause mitochondrial swelling, a precursor event to apoptosis (Wakabayashi and Spodnik, 2000). It is believed that they do this by generating oxidative stress within the cells by reacting with glutathione to produce a selenide, the selenopersulfide anion. This in turn generates a free radical, superoxide, and other reactive oxygen species (Spallholz, 1997). The induction of apoptosis in human cancer cells by this free radical mechanism has been shown to occur in the case of selenite by Shen et al. (1999).

Spallholz (2001) concluded with a statement that all the research data he has reviewed leads to a single conclusion that catalytic redox selenium metabolites are the cancer-preventing agents formed by selenium metabolism in vivo. Such metabolites may even account, he believes, for all the hypotheses he has presented to explain selenium's chemopreventive activity. More recent findings add support to his conclusion, not least in relation to the role of selenium compounds in modulating the mitochondrial redox equilibrium and the induction of apoptosis (Fleming et al., 2001).

6.5 Selenium and Cardiovascular Disease

There is evidence of an association between low antioxidant status and an increased risk of developing coronary vascular disease (CVD). It is from this context that a possible role of low selenium status in the pathogenesis of CVD has been suggested (Coppinger and Diamond, 2001).

It is believed that oxidative stress from free radicals plays a major part in the development of heart disease (Ozer et al., 1995). Oxidation of low-density lipoprotein (LDH) promotes the build up of plaques in coronary arteries. The selenoenzyme GPX4 reduces hydroperoxides of phospholipids and cholesteryl esters associated with lipoproteins and thus could reduce the accumulation of oxidized LDHs in the artery wall and the formation of atherosclerotic lesions (Lapenna et al., 1998). Hydroperoxides produced in eicosanoid synthesis by the lipoxygenase and cyclo-oxygenase pathways, can inhibit both the enzyme prostacyclin synthetase and thus production of vasodilatory prostacyclin, and at the same time stimulate production of thromboxane which is associated with vasoconstriction and platelet aggregation (Nève, 1996). GPX is able to prevent a buildup of these hydroperoxides and thus prevent the development of blood clots.

6.5.1 Epidemiological Studies of CVD Incidence

Evidence in support of an association between CVD and a low intake of dietary selenium has been provided by several, though not all, epidemiological studies. A 1967 Swedish investigation, which looked at trace elements in drinking water and rates of CVD in different parts of the country, found evidence of a possible inverse relationship between selenium intake and heart disease (Bostrom and Wester, 1967). Shamberger (1978), using the same descriptive epidemiological approach as he was to do later in his investigations of cancer (Shamberger, 1985), found, in a study of data from 25 different countries, evidence of a higher rate of CVD mortality in those with a low selenium intake, compared to those with a higher selenium status. Evidence from other related studies was less supportive of a connection between selenium status and CVD. Westermark et al. (1977) failed to find a difference between selenium levels in heart and lung tissue from CVD victims and those dying from other diseases in Finland. Thomson and Robinson (1980) in a report on their observations in New Zealand, noted that their findings did not support the suggestion that hypertension and vascular disease could be due to selenium deficiency "unless the whole population of New Zealand is at increased risk."

In a survey of data on regional differences in mortality rates from CVD in Britain, Brown (1993) noted that Scotland and Northern Ireland, which ranked among the highest regions for death from heart disease in the world, showed a 25% higher rate than did England and Wales. He argued that the high mortality rate was due to consumption of a poor diet, lacking in fruits and vegetables, and hence of antioxidants, including selenium. Although another study (MacPherson et al., 1993) found that the average dietary intake of selenium in Scotland was indeed low, at 30 μg/day, it failed to find any differences in plasma selenium levels between heart disease patients and controls.

6.5.2 Prospective Epidemiological Studies of Selenium and CVD Associations

Several prospective epidemiological studies have found supportive evidences for an association between low selenium status and CVD, though others have failed to do so. A large study by Salonen et al. (1982) in Finland, which involved some 11,000 subjects over a 7-year period, found a 3.6-fold increase in coronary mortality and a 2.7-fold increase in myocardial infarction among men with serum selenium below 45 μg/l, compared to 51.8 μg/l in controls. In a subsequent study by the same group (Virtamo et al., 1985) in which 1,710 men were followed up over 5 years, it was found that serum selenium levels <45 μg/l were related to total mortality risk, with a possible relationship between selenium levels and stroke, but not significantly to CVD.

Both these Finnish studies had been carried out before selenium supplementation of fertilizers was introduced into the country and selenium intakes were very low. Studies carried out with other groups, and in other countries with a higher dietary intake of selenium, have not produced supporting evidence for an association between selenium status and CVD. An investigation carried out in Tromso in Norway, where selenium intakes are high, and also has high CVD mortality rates, failed to find any differences in tissue selenium levels in patients who died from heart disease or other conditions, nor were their serum selenium levels different from controls (Ringstead et al., 1987). Another extensive prospective study by Kok et al. (1987) in the Netherlands, failed to find an association between selenium and CVD mortality. These and similar findings by other investigators (Salvini et al., 1995; Nève, 1996) may be interpreted as indicating that, perhaps, cardiovascular risk may be influenced only by very low selenium status. This conclusion is supported by the findings of the ten-center European Antioxidant Myocardial Infarction and Breast Cancer (EURAMIC) study (Kardinaal et al., 1997) where a significant inverse association between selenium status (as measured by toenail selenium) and the risk of a nonfatal heart attack was shown only for Germany, the country with the lowest selenium status.

Toenail selenium was also used in an investigation of a possible association between selenium status and coronary heart disease (CHD) in a case-control study nested within the Health Professionals Follow-up Study between 1987 and 1992 (Yoshizawa et al., 2003). No association was found between toenail selenium levels and total risk of CHD. However, selenium levels were inversely associated with risk of nonfatal myocardial infarction for extreme quintiles. It was concluded that while the findings suggested no overall relation between selenium status and CHD, a specific protective role for myocardial infarction could not be ruled out.

The disparity between the results of these studies may also to some extent be due to another factor, namely differences in the levels of intake of other antioxidants, such as vitamin E. Selenium is only one of a group of antioxidants that may help to limit the oxidation of LDL cholesterol and thereby help to prevent CVD.

References

Abrams, C.K., Siram, S.M., Galsim, C., et al., 1992, Selenium deficiency in long-term parenteral nutrition, *Nutr. Clin. Pract.* **7**, 175–178.

Acosta, P.B., Gropper, S.S., Clarke-Sheehan, N., et al., 1987, Trace element intake of PKU children ingesting an elemental diet, *J. Parent. Ent. Nutr.* **11**, 287–292.

Anon, 1993, Antioxidants and cancer: the Linxian general population study, *Antiox. Vit. Newsletter*, Hoffman-La Roche, New York, November 1993, pp. 5–8.

Anon, 1998, An element of hope, *The Times* (Lond.), 21 May, p. 12.

Arthur, J.R., 2003, Selenium supplementation: does soil supplementation help and why? *Proc. Nutr. Soc.* **62**, 1–5.

AUSPEN (Australian Society for Parenteral and Enteral Nutrition), 1979, *Vitamin and Mineral Supplements for Total Parenteral Nutrition*, Report 3/78, Therapeutic Advisory Committee, AUSPEN, Sydney.

Batist, G., Katki, A.G., Klecker, R.W.J., et al., 1986, Selenium-induced cytotoxicity of human leukemia cells: interaction with reduced glutathione, *Cancer Res.* **46**, 5482–5485.

Beckett, G.J., Arthur, J.R., Miller, S.M., and McKenzie, R.C., 2003, Selenium, in: Hughes, D.A., Darlington, G., and Bendich, A. (eds), *Dietary Enhancement of Human Immune Function*, Humana Press, Totowa, NJ, pp. 217–240.

Bergqvist, A.G.C., Chee, C.M., Lutchka, L., et al., 2003, Selenium deficiency associated with cardiomyopathy: a complication of the ketogenic diet, *Epilepsia* **44**, 618–620.

Bickel, H., 1954, The effect of phenylalanine-free and phenylalanine-poor diet in phenylpyruvic oligophrenia, *Exp. Med. Surg.* **12**, 114–118.

Blot, W.J., Li, B., Taylor, W., et al., 1993, Nutrition intervention trials in Linxian, China: multiple vitamin/mineral supplementation, cancer incidence, and disease-specific mortality in the general population, *J. Natl Cancer Inst.* **85**, 1483–1492.

Bostrom, H.J. and Wester, P.O., 1967, Trace elements in drinking water and death rates of cardiovascular disease, *Acta Med. Scand.* **181**, 465–470.

British Nutrition Foundation, 2001, *Briefing Paper: Selenium and Health*, British Nutrition Foundation, London, p. 22.

Brown, A.J., 1993, Regional differences in coronary heart disease in Britain: do antioxidant nutrients provide the key? *Asia Pacific J. Clin. Nutr.* **2**, Suppl. 1, 33–36.

Chariot, P. and Bignani, O., 2003, Skeletal muscle disorders associated with selenium deficiency in humans, *Muscle Nerve* **27**, 662–668.

Clark, L.C., 1985, The epidemiology of selenium and cancer, *Fed. Proc.* **44**, 2584–2589.

Clark, L.C., Combs, G.F., Jr., Turnbill, W., et al., 1996, Effects of selenium supplementation for cancer prevention in patients with carcinomas of the skin; a randomized controlled trial, *J. Am. Med. Assoc.* **276**, 1957–1963.

Clayton, C.C. and Baumann, C.A., 1949, Diet and azo dye tumors: dimethylaminobenzene, *Cancer Res.* **9**, 575–582.

Colditz, G.A., 1996, Selenium and cancer prevention. Promising results indicate further trials required [editorial], *J. Am. Med. Assoc.* **81**, 1984–1985.

Collip, P.J. and Chen, S.Y., 1981, Cardiomyopathy and selenium deficiency in a two year old girl, *New Eng. J. Med.* **304**, 1304–1305.

Combs, G.F., Jr., 2001, Selenium in global food systems, *Br. J. Nutr.* **85**, 517–547.

Combs, G.F., Jr. and Gray, W.P., 1998, Chemopreventive agents: selenium, *Pharmacol. Therapeut.* **79**, 179–192.

Coppinger, R.J. and Diamond, A.M., 2001, Selenium deficiency and human disease, in: Hatfield, D.L. (ed.), *Selenium: its Molecular Biology and Role in Health*, Kluwer Academic, Boston, MA, pp. 219–233.

Department of Health, 1998, Nutritional Aspects of the Development of Cancer, HMSO, London.

Diplock, A.T., 1987, Trace elements in human health with special reference to selenium, *Am. J. Clin. Nutr.* **45**, 1313–1322.

Fleet, J.C., 1997, Dietary selenium repletion may reduce cancer incidence in people at high risk who live in areas with low soil selenium, *Nutr. Rev.* **55**, 277–286.

Fleming, J., Ghose, A., and Harrison, P.R., 2001, Molecular mechanisms of cancer prevention by selenium compounds, *Nutr. Cancer* **40**, 42–49.

Fleshner, N.E. and Klotz, L.H., 1999, Diet, androgens, oxidative stress and prostate cancer susceptibility, *Cancer Metast. Rev.* **17**, 325–330.

Frost, D.V., 1972, The two faces of selenium—can selenophobia be cured? in: Hemphill, D. (ed.), *Critical Reviews in Toxicology*, CRC Press, Boca Raton, FL, pp. 467–512.

Garland, M., Morris, J.S., Stampfere, M.J., et al., 1995, Prospective study of toenail selenium levels and cancer among women, *J. Natl Cancer Inst.* **87**, 497–505.

Gramm, H.J., Kopf, A., and Bratter, P., 1995, The necessity of selenium substitution in total parenteral nutrition and artificial alimentation, *J. Trace Elem. Med. Biol.* **9**, 1–12.

Gropper, S.S., Acosta, P.B., Clarke-Sheehan, N., et al., 1988, Trace element status of children with PKU and normal children, *J. Am. Diet. Assoc.* **88**, 459–465.

Hercberg, S., Galan, P., Preziosi, P., et al., 1998a, Background and rationale behind the SU.VI.MAX Study, *Int. J. Vitam. Res.* **68**, 3–20.

Hercberg, S., Preziosi, P., Briancon, S., et al., 1998b, A primary prevention trial using nutritional doses of antioxidant vitamins and minerals in cardiovascular diseases and cancers in a general population: the SU.VI.MAX study, *Control Clin. Trials* **19**, 336–351.

Hsia, C.C., Kleiner, D.E., Jr., Axiotis, C.A., et al., 1992, Mutations of p53 gene in hepatocellular carcinoma: roles of hepatitis B virus and aflatoxin contamination in the diet, *J. Natl Cancer Inst.* **84**, 1638–1641.

Huang, X.H., Sun, L.H., Lu, D.D., et al., 2003, Codon 249 mutation in exon 7 of p53 gene in plasma DNA: maybe a new early diagnostic marker of hepatocellular carcinoma in Qidong risk area, China, *World J. Gastroenterol.* **9**, 692–695.

Innoue, M., Wakisaka, O., Tabuki, T., et al., 2003, Selenium deficiency in a patient with Crohn's disease receiving long-term total parenteral nutrition, *Intern. Med.* 424–157.

Ip, C., 1998, Lessons from basic research in selenium and cancer research, *J. Nutr.* **28**, 1845–1854.

Ip, C. and Ganther, H.E., 1994, Novel strategies in selenium cancer chemoprevention research, in: Burk, R.F. (ed.), *Selenium in Biology and Human Health*, Springer, New York, pp. 171–180.

Ip, C. and Lisk, D.J., 1997, Modulation of Phase I and Phase II xenobiotic-metabolizing enzymes by selenium-enriched garlic in rats, *Nutr. Cancer* **28**, 184–188.

Ip, C., Thomson, H.J., Zhu, Z., and Ganther, H.E., 2000, In vitro and in vivo studies of methylseleninic acid: evidence that a monomethylated selenium metabolite is critical for cancer chemoprevention, *Cancer Res.* **60**, 2882–2886.

Jackson, M.J., Dillon, S.A., Broome, C.S., et al., 2005, Are there functional consequences of a reduction in selenium status in the UK? *Proc. Nutr. Soc.* **63**, 513–517.

Jansson, B., Jacobs, M.M., and Griffin, A.C., 1978, Gastrointestinal cancer: epidemiological and experimental studies, in: Schrauzer, G.N. (ed.), *Inorganic and Nutritional Aspects of Cancer*, Plenum, New York, pp. 305–322.

Kardinaal, A.F., Kok, F.J., Kohlmeier, L., et al., 1997, Association between toenail selenium and risk of acute myocardial infarction in European men. The EURAMIC Study, *Am. J. Epidemiol.* **145**, 373–379.

Kelly, D.A., Coe, A.W., Shenkin, A., et al., 1988, Symptomatic selenium deficiency in a child on home parenteral nutrition, *J. Pediat. Gastroent. Nutr.* **7**, 783–786.

Kien, C.L. and Ganther, H.E., 1983, Manifestation of chronic selenium deficiency in a child receiving total parenteral nutrition, *Am. J. Clin. Nutr.* **33**, 2076–2085.

Kiremidjian-Schumacher, L. and Roy, M., 1998, Selenium and immune responses, *Z. Ernahrungswiss.* **37**, 50–56.

Klein, E.A., Lippman, S.M., Thompson, I.M., et al., 2003, The selenium and vitamin E cancer prevention trial, *World J. Urol.* **21**, 21–27.

Knekt, P., Aromaa, A., Maatela, J., et al., 1990, Serum selenium and subsequent risk of cancer among Finnish men and women, *J. Natl Cancer Inst.* **82**, 864–868.

Knekt, P., Marniemi, J., Teppo, L., et al., 1998, Is low selenium status a risk factor for lung cancer? *Am. J. Epidemiol.* **14**, 975–982.

Kok, F.J., de Bruijn, A.M., Vermeeren, R., et al., 1987, Serum selenium, vitamin antioxidants, and cardiovascular mortality: a 9-year follow-up study in the Netherlands, *Am. J. Clin. Nutr.* **45**, 462–468.

Kuroki, F., Matsumoto, T., and Lida, M., 2003, Selenium is depleted in Crohn's disease on enteral nutrition, *Digest. Dis.* **21**, 266–270.

Lapenna, D., de Gioia, S., Ciofani, G., et al., 1998, Glutathione-related antioxidant defences in human atherosclerotic plaques, *Circulation* **97**, 1930–1934.

Latham, S.C., Reilly, C., Tinggi, U., et al., 1989, Do children with phenylketonuria have a clinically balanced diet? [Abstract], *Australian Coll. Pediat. Meeting* Adelaide, South Australia, May 25–26, 1989, p. 38.

Lemasters, J.J., Nieminen, A.L., Quian, T., et al., 1998, The mitochondrial permeability transition in cell death: a common mechanism in necrosis, apoptosis and authophagy, *Biochim. Biophys. Acta.* **1366**, 177–196.

Levander, O.A. and Burk, R.F., 1986, Report on the 1986 ASPEN research workshop on selenium in clinical nutrition, *J. Parent. Ent. Nutr.* **10**, 545–549.

Li, W.G., Yu, S.Y., Zhu, Y.J., et al., 1992, Six year prospective observation of ingesting selenium-salt to prevent primary liver cancer, in: *Fifth Intern. Symp. Sel. Biol. Med. Abs.*, July 20–23, 1992, Vanderbilt University, Nashville, TN, p. 140.

Lipinski, B., 2005, Rationale for the treatment of cancer with sodium selenite, *Med. Hypoth.* **64**, 806–810.

Lockitch, G., Taylor, G.P., Wong, L.T.K., et al., 1990, Cardiomyopathy associated with nonendemic selenium deficiency in a Caucasian adolescent, *Am. J. Clin. Nutr.* **52**, 572–577.

Lombeck, I., Ebert, K.H., Kasperek, K., et al., 1984, Selenium intake of infants and young children, healthy children and dietetically treated patients with phenylketonuria, *Eur. J. Pediatr.* **143**, 99–102.

Lunn, R.M., Zhang, Y.J., Wang, L.Y., et al., 1997, p53 mutations, chronic hepatitis B virus infection, and aflatoxin exposure in hepatocellular carcinoma in Taiwan, *Cancer Res.* **57**, 3471–3477.

MacPherson, A., Barclay, M.N.I., Dixon, J., et al., 1993, Decline in dietary selenium intake in Scotland and effect on plasma concentrations, in: Anke, A., Meissner, D., and Mills, C.F. (eds), *Trace Elements in Man and Animals – TEMA 8*, Verlag Media Touristik, Gersdorf, Germany, pp. 269–270.

Medina, D., 1986, Selenium and murine mammary tumorigenesis, in: Shamberger, R.J. (ed.), *Diet, Nutrition and Cancer: a Critical Evaluation*, Vol. 11, CRC Press, Boca Raton, FL, pp. 23–42.

Meyer, F., Galan, P., Douville, P., et al., 2005, Antioxidant vitamin and mineral supplementation and prostate cancer prevention in the SU.VI.MAX trial, *Int. J. Cancer* **116**, 182–186.

Naughton, E.R., Kiely, B., Saul, I., and Murphy, D., 1987, Phenylketonuria: outcome and problems in a "diet-for-life" clinic, *Eur. J. Clin. Pediatr.* **146**, Suppl. 1, A23–A24.

Nève, J., 1996, Selenium as a risk factor for cardiovascular disease, *J. Cardiovasc. Dis.* **3**, 42–47.

Niu, Z.S., Li, B.K., and Wang, M., 2002, Expression of p53 and C-myc genes and its clinical relevance in the hepatocellular carcinomatous and pericarcinomatous tissues, *World J. Gastroenterol.* **8**, 822–826.

Ozer, N.K., Boscoboinik, D., and Azzi, A., 1995, New roles of low density lipoproteins and vitamin E in the pathogenesis of atherosclerosis, *Biochem. Mol. Biol. Int.* **35**, 117–124.

Pocock, S. and Hughes, M, 1990, Estimation issues in clinical trials and overviews, *Stat. Med.* **9**, 657–671.

Poirer, K.A. and Milner, J.A., 1979, The effects of various seleno-compounds on Ehrlich Ascites tumor cells, *Biol. Trace Elem. Res.* **1**, 25–34.

Rannem, T., Ladefoged, K, Hylander, E., et al., 1998, Selenium depletion in patients with gastrointestinal disease: are there predictive factors? *Scand. J. Gastroenterol.* **33**, 1057–1061.

Rayman, M.P., 2000, The importance of selenium to human health, *Lancet* **356**, 233–241.

Rayman, M.P., 2004, The use of high-selenium yeast to raise selenium status: how does it measure up? *Br. J. Nutr.* **92**, 557–573.

Rayman, M.P. and Clark, L.C., 1999, Selenium in cancer prevention, in: Roussel, A.M., Anderson, R.A., and Favier, A.E. (eds), *Trace Elements in Man and Animals* 10, Kluwer/Plenum, New York, pp. 575–580.

Reeves, W.C., Marcuard, S.P., Willis, S.E., and Movahed, A., 1989, Reversible cardiomyopathy due to selenium deficiency, *JPEN* **13**, 663–665.

Reid, M.E., Stratton, M.S., Lillico, A.J., et al., 2004, A report of high-dose selenium supplementation: response and toxicities, *J. Trace Elem. Med. Biol.* **18**, 69–74.

Reilly, C., Barrett, J.E., Patterson, C.M., et al., 1990, Trace element status and dietary intake of children with phenylketonuria, *Am. J. Clin. Nutr.* **52**, 159–162.

Ringstead, J., Jacobsen, B.K., Thomassen, Y., and Thelle, D.S., 1987, The Tromso heart study: serum selenium and risk of myocardial infarction: a nested case control study, *J. Epidemiol. Comm. Health* **41**, 329–332.

Robinson, M.F. and Thomson, C.D., 1981, Selenium and cancer, in: Spallholz, J.E., Martin, J.L., and Ganther, H.E. (eds), *Selenium in Biology and Medicine*, Avi, Westport, CT, pp. 283–302.

Salonen, J.T., Alfthan, G., Huttenen, J.K., et al., 1982, Association between cardiovascular death and myocardial infarction and serum selenium in a matched pair longitudinal study, *Lancet* **ii**, 175–179.

Salvini, S., Hennekens, C.H., Morris, J.S., et al., 1995, Plasma levels of the antioxidant selenium and risk of myocardial infarctions among US physicians, *Am. J. Cardiol.* **76**, 1218–1221.

Schrauzer, G.N., 1976, Cancer mortality correlation studies II. Regional associations of mortalities with the consumption of foods and other commodities, *Med. Hypoth.* **2**, 39–49.

Schrauzer, G.N., 1979, Trace elements in carcinogenesis, in: Draper, H.H. (ed.), *Advances in Nutritional Research*, Vol. 2, Plenum, New York, pp. 219–244.

Scriver, C.R., Kaufman, C., Eisensmith, R.C., and Woo, S.L.C., 2001, The hyperphenylalaninemias, in: Scriver, C.R., Beaudet, A.L., Sly, W.S., and Valle, D. (eds), *The Metabolic and Molecular Basis of Inherited Disease*, 8th edn., McGraw-Hill, New York, pp. 1667–1724.

Shamberger, R.J., 1978, Selenium and heart disease II: selenium and other trace element intakes and heart disease in 25 countries, in: Hemphill, D.D. (ed.), *Trace Substances in Environmental Health*, University of Missouri Press, Columbia, MO, pp. 48–50.

Shamberger, R.J., 1985, Selenium and cancer, in: Bostrom, H. and Ljungstedt, N. (eds), *Trace Elements in Health and Disease*, Almqvist & Wiksell, Stockholm, pp. 283–302.

Shamberger, R.J. and Frost, D.V., 1969, Possible protective effect of selenium against human cancer, *Can. Med. Assoc. J.* **100**, 682–686.

Shamberger, R.J., Rukovena, E., Longfield, A.K., et al., 1973, Antioxidants and cancer I: Selenium in blood of normal and cancer patients, *J. Natl Cancer Inst.* **50**, 863–70.

Shen, H.M., Yang, D.F., and Ong, D.N., 1999, Induction of oxidative stress and apoptosis in sodium selenite treated human hepatoma cells ($HepG_2$), *Int. J. Cancer* **81**, 820–828.

Sakoda, L.C., Graubard, B.I., Evans, A.A., et al., 2005, Toenail selenium and the risk of hepatocellular carcinoma mortality in Hainen City, China, *Int. J. Cancer* **115**, 618–624.

Spallholz, J.E., 1994, On the nature of selenium toxicity and carcinostatis activity, *Free Rad. Biol. Med.* **17**, 45–64.

Spallholz, J.E., 1997, Free radical generation by selenium compounds and their pro-oxidant toxicity, *Biomed. Environ. Sci.* **10**, 260–270.

Spallholz, J.E., 2001, Selenium and the prevention of cancer, Part II: mechanisms for the carcinostatic activity of Se compounds, *Bull. STDA*, October 2001, pp. 1–12.

Stratton, M.S., Reid, M.E., Schwartzberg, G., et al., 2003a, Selenium and prevention of prostate cancer in high-risk men: the Negative Biopsy Study, *Anticancer Drugs* **14**, 589–594.

Stratton, M.S., Reid, M.E., Schwartzberg, G., et al., 2003b, Selenium and inhibition of disease progression in men diagnosed with prostate carcinoma: study design and basic characteristic of the "Watchful Waiting" Study, *Anticancer Drugs* **14**, 595–600.

Terwolbeck, K., Behne, D., Meinhold, H., et al., 1993, Low selenium status, thyroid hormones, and other parameters in children with phenylketonuria, in: Anke, M., Meissner, D., and Mills, C.F. (eds), *Trace Elements in Man and Animals—TEMA8*, Verlag Media Touristik, Gersdorf, Germany, pp. 535–538.

Thomson, C.D. and Robinson, M.F., 1980, Selenium in human health and disease with emphasis on those aspects peculiar to New Zealand, *Am. J. Clin. Nutr.* **33**, 303–323.

Thomson, C.D., Burton, C.E., and Robinson, M.F. 1978, On supplementing the selenium intake of New Zealanders. 1. Short experiments with large doses of selenite or selenomethionine, *Br. J. Nutr.* **39**, 579–587.

Thomson, C.D., Robinson, M.F., Butler, J.A., and Whanger, P.D., 1993, Long-term supplementation with selenate and selenomethionine: selenium and glutathione peroxidase (EC 1.11 1.9) in blood components of New Zealand women, *Br. J. Nutr.* **69**, 577–588.

Thorn, J., Robertson, J., Buss, D.H., and Bunton, N.G., 1978, Trace nutrients: selenium in British foods, *Br. J. Nutr.* **39**, 391–396.

Trumbo, P.R., 2005, The levels of evidence for permitting a qualified health claim: FDA's review of the evidence for selenium and cancer and vitamin E and heart disease, *J. Nutr.* **135**, 354–356.

Van Rij, A.M., Thomson, C.D., McKenzie, J.M., et al., 1979, Selenium deficiency in total parenteral nutrition, *Am. J. Clin. Nutr.* **32**, 2076–2085.

Virtamo, J., Valkeila, E., Alfthan, G., et al., 1985, Serum selenium levels and the risk of coronary heart disease and stroke in elderly Finnish men, *Am. J. Epidemiol.* **122**, 276–282.

Wakabayashi, T. and Spodnik, J.H., 2000, Structural changes of mitochondria during free radical-induced apoptosis, *Folia. Morphol.* **59**, 61–75.

Walker, C.H. and Klein, F., 1915, Selenium—its therapeutic value, especially in cancer, *American Med.* **628**, as cited by Schrauzer, C.H., 1979, Trace elements in carcinogenesis, in: Draper, H.H. (ed.), *Advances in Nutritional Research*, Vol. 2, Plenum, New York, pp. 219–244.

Wei, W.Q., Abnet, C.C., Qiao, Y.L., et al., 2004, Prospective study of serum selenium concentrations and esophageal and gastric cardia cancer, heart disease, stroke, and total death, *Am. J. Clin. Nutr.* **79**, 80–85.

Westermark, T., Raunn, P., Kirjarinta, M. and Lappalainen, M., 1977, Selenium content of the whole blood and serum in adults and children of different ages from different parts of Finland, *Acta Pharmacol. Toxicol.* **40**, 465–475.

Whanger, P.D., 2004, Selenium and its relation to cancer: an update, *Br. J. Nutr.* **91**, 11–28.

Willett, W.C., Polk, B.F., Morris, J.S., et al., 1983, Prediagnostic serum selenium and risk of cancer, *Lancet* **ii**, 130–134.

World Health Organization, 1987, *Environmental Health Criteria 58: Selenium*, WHO, Geneva.

Yoshizawa, K., Willett, W.C., Morris, S.J., et al., 1998, Study of prediagnostic selenium level in toenails and the risk of advanced prostate cancer, *J. Natl Cancer Inst.* **90**, 1219–1224.

Yoshizawa, K., Ascherio, A., Morris, J.S., et al., 2003, Prospective study of selenium levels in toenails and risk of coronary heart disease in men, *Am. J. Epidemiol.* **158**, 852–860.

Yu, M.W., Hornig, I.S., Chiang, Y.C., et al., 1999, Plasma selenium levels and the risk of hepatocellular carcinoma among men with chronic hepatitis virus infection, *Am. J. Epidemiol.* **150**, 367–374.

Zou, Z., Jiang, W., Ganther, H.E., et al., 2000, Activity of Se-allylselenocysteine in the presence of methionine gamma-lyase on cell growth, DNA integrity, apoptosis, and cell-cycle regulatory molecules, *Mol. Carcinogen.* **29**, 191–197.

Zou, X.N., Taylor, P.R., Mark, S.D., et al., 2003, Seasonal variation of food consumption and selected nutrient intake, in Linxian, a high risk area for esophageal cancer in China, *Int. J. Vitam.. Res.* **72**, 375–382.

7 Selenium in Health and Disease IV: The Immune Response and Other Selenium-Related Conditions

7.1 The Immune System

The immune system is a collection of tissues, cells, and molecules whose prime physiological function is protection of the body against harmful influences, both external and internal, that can damage health. It is also involved in other functions, such as wound healing and removal of cells that have died through natural processes. In a restricted sense, immunity refers to mechanisms established by a host to resist disease after exposure to a foreign infectious agent. In a broader sense, it can also include hypersensitive biological phenomena of altered tissue reactivity such as allergies, acquired tolerance to—and rejection of—foreign tissues, and autoimmune diseases (Maurer, 1961).

There is evidence that selenium plays a part in many of the mechanisms of immunity. How it does so is still only partially understood and, because of the complexity of the processes involved, final answers to many, as yet unresolved, questions are unlikely to be found for some time. For some readers the language of immunity is largely unfamiliar and highly specialized, yet an understanding of it is useful for those who want to appreciate the role of selenium in human health. It is for this reason that the following brief overview of some of the principal elements in the body's immune system is given. It is hoped that it will help to clarify the picture for those who might otherwise be deterred from looking into what is, in fact, a very important and fascinating role of selenium. This introduction is largely based on the text by Staines et al. (1993).

7.1.1 Components of the Immune System

The mechanisms of immunity, like the language used to describe them, are complex. The body's immune system must always be in a state of alert, ready to defend it against infection. It is designed to give protection against several different classes of infective organisms, including viruses, bacteria, fungi, protozoa, and helminths. Although its processes are, to a large extent, dependent on lymphoid organs, such as thymus, spleen, and lymph nodes, the immune system does not operate in isolation in just one type of organ or tissue. It interacts dynamically with the endocrine, gastrointestinal, respiratory, and other tissues, and its cells are distributed throughout every part of the body.

The system operates at several levels. A first line of defense is its *innate* or *natural immunity*, which provides physical and chemical protection against infection. This is a function of skin and other epithelial and mucous membrane barriers in the gastrointestinal, respiratory, and urogenital tracts. The defensive processes include phagocytosis and killing of invading organisms, as well as secretion of enzymes, such as lysozymes and other compounds to form a chemical barrier against invasion. This level of immunity is nonspecific and is not always effective.

Organisms that manage to get through the first barrier are tackled by a variety of other agents. These include *acute phase proteins*, a mixed group of molecules that can attach themselves to invading materials and prepare them for phagocytosis. *C-reactive proteins* and *lactoferrin* are two of these proteins that are synthesized in the liver in response to inflammation at other sites. Another group of the acute phase proteins are the *interferons*, which increase the resistance of cells against viral attack. They function as *cytokines* or intercellular signaling molecules.

Two groups of phagocytotic cells ingest and destroy foreign materials that enter the cell. The first comprises *polymorphonuclear neutrophil leucocytes* (PMNs), or white blood cells (*neutrophils*). The second is the *reticulo-endothelial system* composed of monocytes found in the blood and macrophages found especially in the liver, kidney, spleen, and lymph nodes.

Phagocytosis is comparable to the mechanism whereby amebae eat food particles. Macrophages, for instance, recognize a foreign material, bind it to their cell membrane, and engulf it in a vacuole. Oxygen free radicals are generated within the vacuole and kill the entrapped microorganism, which is then digested by lysosomes. This is the final act of the body's first line of defense, the natural immune system. The foreign material is bound to the macrophages or neutrophils usually with the help of what is known as *opsonization*. This is a process in which the foreign particle is coated with specific antibodies and components of the *complement system*. This system is composed of a complex group of protein molecules working as a molecular cascade. They are involved in the control of inflammation and in the activation of phagocytes and lysis of cell membranes.

Phagocytes can also destroy invading organisms and other unwanted cells, including some types of tumor cells, directly without phagocytosis. This is done by a special type of lymphocyte, the *large granular lymphocytes*. These cytotoxic cells are known as *natural killer* (NK) cells.

Acquired or adaptive immunity is the body's *secondary immune response*. Unlike natural immunity, it is characterized by specific immunological memory. Acquired immunity takes place in a number of different cells and tissues. They include the *lymphocytes*, which are found in blood and lymph fluids and in organized lymphoid tissue. These cells recognize and react to antigens, proteins foreign to the organism that are capable of triggering formation of antibodies. Lymphocytes originate in bone marrow as lymphoid stem cells. They can develop into two different forms, *T cells* and *B cells*, depending on which developmental pathway they follow.

Those that pass through the blood to the thymus gland before moving on to the lymph nodes and spleen are the T cells. In the thymus they mature and acquire antigen reactivity. This gives them the ability to recognize foreign antigens by means of the *major histocompatibility complex* (MCH) molecules, known as *T cell receptors* (TCRs), which react with antigens on their surface. TCRs are not specific for any one antigen, though they have considerable diversity in immunocompetence. T cells provide what is known as *cell-mediated immunity*.

The second type of lymphocyte, B cells, which are responsible for what is known as *humoral immunity*, do not pass through the thymus but settle directly in the lymph nodes and spleen. They acquire their name from the *bursa of Fabricius*, the tissue in which they are produced in chicks. B cells also have antibody protein receptor molecules on their surface, but unlike TCRs, these are specific for one antibody only. However, though they differ from each other in their development and response to antigens, both T and B cells cooperate closely with each other and form a combined defense against invading organisms.

B cell activation occurs when an antigen comes into contact with the cell and combines with an antibody receptor molecule on its surface. This generates signals within the cell that switch on antibody production and converts it into an antibody-secreting *plasma cell*. The cell then multiplies, differentiates into a clone of daughter cells, and starts a chain reaction, leading to the destruction of the invader.

The life of most of these daughter cells is short and ends when their work of secreting antibodies is done. A few, however, which do not take part in secreting antibodies, survive for up to several years. These are *memory cells* that can recognize the antigen responsible for their original formation if exposed to it once more. The same antibody is produced, but now at a faster rate, because in the meantime clonal expansion has resulted in the production of additional antigen-reactive cells. This secondary immune response provides a highly efficient rapid response to antigen invasion, since it does not require the initial presence of large numbers of each specific leucocyte.

The antibodies secreted by B cells in response to antigens are immunoglobulins, one of several different groups of proteins that occur in blood. Between about a quarter and a half of the protein in human plasma is composed of a mixture of globulins. These can be separated by electrophoresis into six different categories, which includes the *alpha-globulins* (α-globulins) and the *gamma-globulins* (γ-globulins). These latter are the immunoglobulins or antibodies.

Immunoglobulins consist of different types or classes of closely related molecules. The commonly used abbreviation for immunoglobulin is Ig, followed by a letter signifying the subclass, such as IgG and IgA. The most abundant of them in human plasma is IgG, making up about 80% of the total, with IgA next (13%), followed by IgM, IgD, and IgE in lesser amounts.

The five principal classes of Ig are heterogeneous, and each class in its turn is made up of possibly thousands of individual immunoglobulins. Their molecular structure, comprising two small and two large polypeptide chains, accounts for their overall similarities and also their specific individuality. The sequence of amino acids at the site where the antigen binds to the N-terminal end of each pair of polypeptide chains is variable and accounts for the unique specificity of each antibody. The C-terminal ends have a constant amino acid sequence and provide the basic framework that all Ig molecules require to carry out their functions (Montgomery et al., 1977).

Each antibody is manufactured by the body in response to a specific antigen. The Ig has the ability to recognize this antigen and combines with it tightly through specific bonds. The antigen–antibody reaction is analogous to the specificity and bonding of an enzyme to its substrate. Once the body has manufactured antibodies against a particular antigen, the procedure is recorded in the molecular memory of its cells and may never be forgotten in most cases.

The activation of T cells differs considerably from the process in B cells. Unlike B cells, they do not make antibodies or secrete special forms of their antigen receptor molecules when they react with antigen. However, like B cells, they do respond to activation by growth and differentiation. In addition, they secrete a number of different types of cytokines. These mediators are very important for regulating the function of other lymphocytes. Among these other cells are a number of different types of T cells that have special accessory molecules on their surfaces that allow them to perform a number of different functions. These cells include *T-helper cells*, which help B cells to make antibodies; *T-suppressor cells*, whose function is to suppress immune response and thus moderate it when necessary; and *T-cytotoxic cells*, which can destroy other cells that have been invaded by a virus. Another type of cell resulting from antigen reaction of T cells is the *delayed-type hypersensitivity cell* (Tdth, or THI), which can be involved in cell-mediated immune response, such as destruction of intracellular bacteria, autoimmune diseases, and rejection of tissue implants.

Other cells, in addition to B and T cells, are also involved in immune responses. *Mast cells*, which occur in large numbers in mucosal tissue, contain granules of pharmacologically active compounds. These have IgE antibodies on their surface and when, during an infection of the body, these bind to specific antigens, the cells are triggered to degranulate and release their contents. This causes local inflammation, which in turn calls neutrophils, monocytes, and lymphocytes to the site to oppose the infection. *Basophils* (basophilic polymorphonuclear leucocytes), which are related to neutrophils, contain similar granules and function in a similar manner to the mast cells. *Eosinophils*, also related to neutrophils, are particularly concerned with defense against parasites that are too large to be phagocytosed. They function by coating the parasite with IgG and IgE antibodies and destroy it outside the cell. These, and certain other cells with similar functions, are known as *killer cells* (K cells).

7.1.2 The Role of Selenium in the Immune Response

Adequate dietary selenium is known to be essential for optimum activity of virtually all arms of the immune system, though mechanisms of this requirement are not yet fully understood (Arthur et al., 2003). Selenium deficiency affects the efficiency of both the innate nonadaptive and the acquired adaptive immune systems

(Spallholz, 1990; Turner and Finch, 1991; Kiremidjian-Schumacher and Roy, 1998; Brown and Arthur, 2001).

Selenium, however, is not the only nutrient required for the optimum function of the body's immune response to attack. A study of the development of the acquired immune system in chickens has shown that while deficiency of selenium on its own can impair bursal growth, stunting of the thymus occurs only when both selenium and vitamin E are inadequate (Marsh et al., 1986). Thus, it appears that while deficiency of both vitamin E and selenium blocks the normal flow of inductive signals from epithelial cells to the developing lymphocytes, B cells are more vulnerable than T cells to selenium deficiency. The effect of selenium deficiency on antibody production appears to be age-dependent. When the mitogen sheep red blood cell (SRBC) was used to assess immune response in vitro, 2-week-old chicks maintained on a selenium-deficient diet had reduced antibody titres, whereas 3-week-old chicks only showed a reduction when they were both selenium- and vitamin E–deficient (Marsh et al., 1986).

Studies on a number of different animal species, both ruminants and nonruminants, have shown that not all classes of antibodies are affected to the same extent by selenium deficiency (Larsen, 1993). It has been found to impair the proliferation of both T and B cell lymphocytes in response to mitogens as well as the activity of NK cells and lymphokine-activated killer cells (Kiremidjian-Schumacher et al., 1994). The humoral system is also adversely affected, with decreased production of, for example, IgG and IgM titre in humans. Supplementation with selenium results in improvements in these processes. Mice given a low-selenium diet, with adequate vitamin E, had reduced IgG, but had normal IgM responses to SRBC mitogen. However, when the deficient diet was continued into the second generation, IgM-producing cells also became affected (Mulhern et al., 1985).

Differences in animal species, age, sex, and antigen have also been found to affect the degree to which antibody production responds to selenium supplementation. Early experiments appeared to indicate that high concentrations of selenium are necessary to boost IgG and IgM antibody response (Spallholz et al., 1975). However, it has been shown that supplementation at the supranutritional level may not be necessary to do this. Levels required appear to depend on species and antigen. In the case of lambs, for example, selenium at a level of 0.1 μg/g in the diet gave a better antibody response to parainfluenza-3 virus than did a dose of 1.0 μg/g in response to tetanus toxin (Larsen et al., 1988). A difference in antibody response to toxins has been shown between lambs and certain other animals. Supplementation with both vitamin E and selenium was found to be necessary in cattle and horses to increase their antibody response to *Pasteurella haemolytica* and certain other toxins, but no such additive effect of the two micronutrients was observed in lambs (Larsen, 1993).

Tests using phytolectin mitogens of different types to investigate the effect of selenium on the proliferative response of T and B cells have confirmed that selenium deficiency affects the immune systems of different animal species in different ways. While, for example, the antibody response of T cells to Concanavalin

A (Con A) was increased in selenium-deficient chickens and pigs (Larsen and Tollersrud, 1981; Marsh et al., 1987), as well as in marginally deficient humans (Arvilommi et al., 1983), it was depressed in sheep (Larsen et al., 1988). Deficiency of both selenium and vitamin E depressed T-cell response to mitogens more severely than did selenium deficiency alone in chicks and rats (Eskew et al., 1985; Marsh et al., 1987).

Adult ruminants appear to be more resistant than their young to the effects of selenium deficiency on lymphocyte response to mitogens (Turner and Finch, 1991). Ewes with combined vitamin E and selenium deficiencies responded well to phytohemoglutinin (PHA), but their lambs did not and their T cell reactivity ultimately failed (Turner and Finch, 1990). It may be that this difference is due to the high levels of selenium that can be concentrated in the rumens of adult sheep, almost 50 times higher than levels in their dry diet (Whanger et al., 1978) and, consequently, to the difference in availability of microbial selenium to lymphocytes in lambs and ewes.

Failure of lymphocyte response to mitogens in selenium-deficient lambs is easily reversed by the provision of supplementary selenium. However, the amount of the element used can affect the outcome significantly. While in vitro studies have shown that doses even less than 1 ng/ml are sufficient to enhance the response in selenium-deficient lambs to PHA, when the dose was increased to 10 ng/ml, the response plateaued out and above 1 μg/ml toxic effects were observed (Turner and Finch, 1990). A similar concentration-related effect has been found to occur in human lymphocytes stimulated with PHA. When the selenium concentration in the culture medium was increased, the risk of chromosomal aberrations was found to be increased significantly (Khalil, 1989).

7.1.2.1 Selenium and the Immune Response to Infection

It is well established that selenium plays a role in the defense systems of animals against bacteria and other infectious agents (Boyne et al., 1984). Selenium deficiency has been shown to impair in vitro the ability of neutrophils and macrophages to kill ingested cells of the yeast *Candida albicans* (Boyne and Arthur, 1986). This impairment is associated with changes in enzymes and structures in the cells (Serfass and Ganther, 1975).

As has been noted by Arthur et al. (2003), one of the most widely investigated associations between selenium and the immune system is the effect of the element on neutrophil function. Reactive oxygen species produced by neutrophils play a major role in the destruction of invading microorganisms. However, these free radicals, if not scavenged by GPX once their primary role has been completed, can destroy the very neutrophils that produce them.

A balance must be maintained between production of sufficient radicals to kill invaders and the enzyme systems that protect the neutrophils from the same radicals. This balance can be upset by selenium deficiency. This does not actually affect production of neutrophils in a number of different animal species, but it can interfere with their function (Turner and Finch, 1991). Neutrophils from selenium-deficient mice, rats, and cattle, for instance, have been shown to be able to ingest pathogens in vitro, but are unable to kill them as efficiently as neutrophils from selenium-sufficient animals can (Boyne and Arthur, 1986). Evidence from in vitro experiments that investigated production of superoxide by neutrophils from selenium-deficient mice stimulated with phorbal myristate acetate supports the view that the inability to destroy pathogens is related to decreased activity of GPX1 in the neutrophils. This allows the free radicals produced in the respiratory burst to kill the neutrophils themselves.

The effect of selenium on GPX activity is not the only selenium-related function involved in neutrophil activity. In vitro studies that investigated the response of selenium-deficient mice to *C. albicans* found evidence that neutrophil candidacidal activity has a biphasic pattern (Boyne and Arthur, 1986). When very low doses of selenium were given to deficient mice, candidacidal activity increased from approximately 9 to 14%. Additional supplementation did not increase this activity until much higher doses were given, which also correlated with changes in GPXI activity. These findings suggest that, in addition to GPX1, candidacidal activity of neutrophils is dependent on other selenium-dependent factors, including possibly phospholipid hydroperoxide GPX and cytosolic or mitochondrial TR.

It has been pointed out by Arthur et al. (2003) that the evidence for the foregoing views concerning neutrophil function in immunity relies on findings using in vitro cultures, and that it is highly likely that, in vivo, several other factors are involved. Thyroid hormone metabolism, for example, has been shown to play an important part in immune function. Hypothyroidism generally reduces the ability of neutrophils to respond to a challenge. Moreover, depression of thyroid function, by selenium deficiency, leading to a decrease in IDII, could lead to suboptimal development and function of thymic cells (Molinero et al., 1995).

Selenium is known to be essential for other aspects of cell-mediated immunity besides the destruction of pathogenic viruses and fungi, such as destruction of neoplastic cells. While GPX, in its role as protector against peroxides, must play a major part in such activities, it is unlikely that this is the only mediator of these functions of selenium. The anti-inflammatory role of selenium is also of importance. Both GPX and, possibly, the thioredoxin reductases also play a part by influencing eicosanoid metabolism to modulate inflammation. Fatty acids of the (n–3) and (n–6) series act as substrates for the lipoxygenase pathway that gives rise to the leukotrienes, which are proinflammatory, and also for the cyclooxygenase pathway to the inflammatory prostaglandins and thromboxanes (McKenzie et al., 2000).

7.1.2.2 Selenium and Inflammatory Diseases in Humans

There is a limited amount of evidence from human studies which indicates that conditions associated with increased oxidative stress or inflammation may be related to dietary selenium intake. Low blood selenium levels occur in a number of inflammatory diseases, suggesting that selenium supplementation could be effective in their treatment. In rheumatoid arthritis, for instance, there is progressive erosion of joint cartilage that appears to be exacerbated by free radicals. Selenium supplementation has the potential to prevent this occurring by reducing the production and concentration of these reactive oxygen species. It was reported by Peretz et al. (1992) that short-term (3 months) supplementation with 200 μg/day of selenium significantly reduced pain and joint involvement in a group of rheumatoid arthritis patients. In a large case-control study of Finnish subjects who had no arthritis at baseline, those in the highest tertile of serum selenium were found to have a lower risk of rheumatoid factor–negative arthritis than those in the lower tertile (Knekt, 2000). However, selenium supplementation has not been found to alleviate arthritic symptoms in some forms of arthritis.

Asthma is another condition in which oxidative stress and selenium deficiency have been identified as risk factors (Shaheen et al., 1999). The evidence for this, however, is not clear. While asthmatic adults have been shown to be protected against asthmatic wheeze, and clinical symptoms of children with intrinsic asthma improved on supplementation with selenium, some studies have found higher levels of GPX activity in blood of younger patients with asthma than in controls (Ward et al., 1984).

A UK study has shown that supplementation with selenium, and other antioxidants, can benefit patients suffering from pancreatitis by reducing pain and frequency of attacks (McCloy, 1998). It has also been reported that lethality from acute pancreatitis has been reduced by intravenous administration of selenite (Kuklinsky and Schweder, 1996). It is believed that the effect of the supplementation is to reduce the high level of oxidative stress associated with the disease.

7.2 Selenium and Viral Infections

It has been demonstrated by Beck and her colleagues that the association between viral disease and nutrition is due not only to the effects on the host's immune system but also to the fact that the host's nutritional status can have a direct effect on the viral pathogen itself (Beck, 1999). The group's interest in the relationship between infectious disease and host nutritional status began with their study of KD. They noted that, though KD was found only in regions of China with selenium-poor soils, many of the features of the endemic cardiomyopathy, such as its seasonal and annual incidence, and the fact that not all selenium-deficient individuals developed KD, could not be explained entirely on the basis of an inadequate intake of selenium. An infectious cofactor, possibly cocksackievirus, an enterovirus known to cause myocarditis, that had been isolated from the blood of KD victims was believed to be involved (Bai et al., 1979; Su et al., 1979). Beck and her colleagues used a mouse model to investigate the relationship between cocksackie infection and myocarditis (Beck et al., 1994). The mice were fed a diet deficient or adequate in selenium for 4 weeks and were then infected with either a benign strain of cocksackie B virus (CVB3/0), which was not known to cause cardiomyopathy, or with another strain (CVB3/20), which is myocarditic in mice. Both the selenium-deficient and the nondeficient mice injected with CVB3/20 developed myocarditis, as might have been expected, though symptoms were much more severe in the selenium-deficient than in the nondeficient animals, showing that the pathogenicity of the virus was increased by the deficiency. The results of infection with the benign strain CVB3/0 were unexpected. The selenium-adequate mice did not develop any myocarditis, as had been anticipated, while the selenium-deficient mice developed moderate myocarditis. Thus, the virulence of the normally benign virus was altered in the selenium-deficient animals—deficiency of selenium was seen to increase the pathogenicity of CVB3 virus, raising the severity of myocarditis caused by a virulent strain, and changing a normally benign strain into a virulent one (Beck, 1997). The same effects occurred in vitamin E-deficient mice and in GPX-knockout mice, which suggests that oxidative stress was involved in the mechanisms that caused the mutations in the virus (Beckett et al., 2003). It was also found that the change in virulence was due to specific mutations in the virus itself, such that once the mutation had occurred, even mice with normal nutrition became vulnerable to the virus (Beck et al., 1995).

The significance of these findings is considerable in relation to the occurrence, virulence, and disease progression of viral infections in general (Beck, 2001). The possibility that other viruses, such as poliovirus, hepatitis, influenza, or HIV, can also become more virulent by passing through a selenium-deficient host would have considerable public health implications. These, like coxsackievirus, are RNA viruses, and are prone to mutation in an oxidative environment (Beck, 1997) and in GPX-knockout mice (Beck et al., 1998). This is because RNA viruses, unlike DNA viruses, do not have proofreading enzymes, and thus genomic mistakes that occur in them cannot be repaired during replication (Steinhauer et al., 1992). It has been suggested that the emergence of new strains of influenza that has been reported in recent decades in China, a country with extensive regions of selenium-deficient soils, may be due to mutation of formerly less-virulent strains of the virus by passage through a low-selenium status population (Beckett et al., 2003). Beck et al. (2004) have stressed the urgent need to take particular account of the nutritional status of the host when investigating the emergence of new infectious diseases and of old diseases with new pathogenic properties, such as severe acute respiratory syndrome (SARS).

7.2.1 Selenium, Human Immunodeficiency Virus, and Acquired Immunodeficiency Syndrome

Selenium is believed to play a multifactorial role in human immunodeficiency virus (HIV) and acquired immunodeficiency syndrome (AIDS). A decline in blood selenium levels and GPX activity occurs in individuals with HIV and AIDS (Mantero-Atienza et al., 1991; Altavena et al., 1995). This decline begins in the early stages of HIV infection, when malnutrition and malabsorption are unlikely to be involved.

Selenium deficiency is a recognized feature of advanced HIV disease, and may be due either to malnutrition and/or the presence of opportunistic infections (OI) (Look et al., 1997a). A low selenium status has been implicated in accelerated disease progression and poorer survival of HIV victims, especially pregnant women (Kupka et al., 2004). Plasma selenium levels are believed to be a strong predictor of the outcome of HIV infection (Baum et al., 1997). The fall in blood selenium is paralleled by a reduction in $CD4^{+}$ T-helper cells. These are cells that recognize viral antigen on the surface of infected cells and release chemotactic factors and cytokines that activate the cells to become resistant to the infection (Look et al., 1997b).

HIV, like certain other viruses, has the ability to acquire, through transduction, GPX-like genes that are believed to protect the virus from respiratory burst products of host neutrophils and macrophages. The use of GPX-like selenoproteins by the virus has been described as "hijacking" the selenium supply of the host by incorporating selenium into viral selenoproteins. The result is that the ability of the host to mount an effective immune response is reduced (Rayman, 2000). Several types of virus, including cocksackievirus B3 and measles, as well as HIV-1, are known to have the ability to make viral, GPX-like, selenoproteins (Zhang et al., 1999).

The mechanisms that underlie the relationship between selenium status and HIV progression are not yet clear (Baum et al., 2001), and several studies of the mechanisms involved, as well as clinical trials to investigate the effect of supplementation on HIV, are currently being carried out. As has been noted by Semba and Tang (1999) in a report on the pathogenesis of human HIV, since 90% of those infected with HIV are in developing countries, it is especially important that micronutrient deficiencies be identified and trials be carried out to determine whether micronutrient supplementation will improve clinical outcomes.

7.3 Selenium and Human Fertility

Selenium is known to play a part in both males and females in reproduction. This has been long recognized in animal husbandry (Underwood, 1977; Hidiroglou, 1979). Low selenium blood levels have been associated with abortions in cattle and pigs (Stuart and Oehme, 1982). There are conflicting views on whether low selenium status is also implicated in infertility or miscarriages in humans. Evidence of significantly lower serum selenium in women who had either first-trimester or recurrent miscarriages has been reported by one group (Barrington et al., 1997). However, a subsequent study failed to confirm this finding (Nicoll et al., 1999).

The evidence for a requirement of selenium for fertility is stronger for males than for females. Selenium has been shown, in animal experiments, to be an essential requirement for the synthesis of testosterone and normal development of spermatozoa (Behne et al., 1996). In the absence of adequate selenium, structural abnormalities occur in sperm and their motility is affected (Wu et al., 1973). It is believed that this is a result of a deficiency of GPX4, which in healthy animals accounts for about 50% of the sperm capsule material and confers the structural integrity necessary for sperm stability and motility (Ursini et al., 1999). Selenoprotein P has been shown to be required for the development of functional sperm in mice (Olson et al., 2005).

Investigations of the relation between selenium and fertility in humans also indicate the essential role of the element in spermatogenesis. In a group of subfertile Norwegian men, selenium levels in seminal plasma were found to be positively correlated with concentration of spermatozoa (Oldereid et al., 1998). However, while such results appear to support the view that selenium supplementation could improve fertility in subfertile men, this has not always been found to be the case. A Scottish study of subfertile men did find that supplementation with 100 μg of selenium daily for 3 months resulted in significantly increased sperm motility and was followed by the fathering of a child in 11% of the group, compared to none in an unsupplemented control group (Scott et al., 1998). In contrast, a Polish study in which subfertile men were given a supplement of 200 μg/day found that though there was an increase in selenium levels in seminal fluid, there was no increase in sperm fertility (Iwanier and Zachara, 1995).

7.4 Selenium and Preeclampsia

Preeclampsia, though not directly a problem of infertility, is another condition related to fertility, believed to be associated with low selenium status. The disease is a major problem of pregnancy, with a high maternal and perinatal morbidity and mortality (Rayman et al., 2003). Placental ischemia and oxidative stress, resulting from poor placentation (Redman and Sargent, 2000), are believed to produce bloodborne agents that cause a maternal systemic inflammatory response and generalized endothelial dysfunction. This gives rise to the characteristic symptoms of hypertension, protinurea, and sudden edema (Roberts et al., 1989). The bloodborne agents are believed to be the products of oxidative stress (Redman et al., 1999). A recent study has found evidence indicating that elevated lipid peroxide levels, impaired antioxidant defense mechanisms, and lower trace element status may be related at least partly to the pathogenesis of preeclampsia (Atamer et al., 2005).

There is evidence that the peroxynitrite may play a major role in the endothelial dysfunction and the resulting oxidative stress of preeclampsia. Peroxynitrite is a potent inflammatory mediator, and causes vasoconstriction, platelet aggregation, and thrombus formation (Arteel et al., 1999). It occurs in the placenta of all women, but is produced to a significantly greater extent in those with preeclampsia (Myatt et al., 1996).

It has been shown that supplementation with the antioxidants vitamins C and E can reduce the incidence of preeclampsia in women with a high risk of the disease (Chappell et al., 1999). Another study looked at the possibility that selenoproteins, which are known to be able to limit adverse endothelial effects, with selenoprotein P having a unique capacity for scavenging peroxynitrite at the endothelial surface (Anteel et al., 1999), could have similar effect. When the selenium status of a group of preeclampsic (assessed by toenail clippings) patients was compared with that of a matched group of nonpreeclampsic women, it was shown that the former had a significantly lower selenium status than had the controls. Being in the lower tertile of toenail selenium was associated with a 4.4-fold greater incidence of the disease, and within the preeclampsic group, lower selenium status was significantly associated with more severe expression of the disease (Rayman et al., 2003).

These findings have not provided clear evidence that selenium deficiency is a cause of preeclampsia, though they do indicate that there is a connection between low selenium status and the condition. This conclusion is given some support by the results of a small-scale Chinese study in which selenium supplementation (at 100 μg/day) was shown to prevent pregnancy-induced hypertension and gestational edema in women at risk of developing hypertension (Han and Zhou, 1991). A further trial, to test the hypothesis that an adequate selenium status is important for antioxidant defense and peroxynitrite scavenging in pregnant women at risk of preeclampsia, is planned in the UK (Rayman et al., 2003).

References

Altavena, C., Dousset, B., May, T., et al., 1995, Relationship of trace element, immunological markeres, and HIV1 infection progression, *Biol. Trace Elem. Res.* **47**, 133–138.

Arteel, G.E., Briviba, K., and Sies, H., 1999, Protection against peroxynitrite, *FEBS Lett.* **115**, 226–230.

Arthur, J.R., McKenzie, R.C., and Beckett, G.J., 2003, Selenium in the immune system, *J. Nutr.* **133**, 1457S–1459S.

Arvilommi, H., Poikonen, K., Jokinen, I., et al., 1983, Selenium and immune functions in humans, *Infect. Immun.* **41**,185–189.

Atamer, Y., Kocyigit, Y., Yokus, B., et al., 2005, Lipid peroxidation, antioxidant defense, status of trace metals and leptin levels in preeclampsia, *Eur. J. Obstet. Gynecol. Reprod. Biol.* **119**, 60–66.

Bai, J., Wu, S., Ge, K., et al., 1979, Preliminary results of viral etiology of Keshan disease, *Chin. Med. J.* **59**, 466–472.

Barrington, J.W., Taylor, M., Smith, S., and Bowen-Simpkins, P., 1997, Selenium and recurrent miscarriage, *J. Obstet. Gynaecol.* **17**, 199–200.

Baum, M.K., Shor-Posner, G., Lai, S., et al., 1997, High risk of HIV-related mortality is associated with selenium deficiency, *J. Acquir. Immune Defic. Syndr.* **15**, 370–374.

Baum, M.K., Campa, A., Miguez-Burbano, M.J., et al., 2001, Role of selenium in HIV/AIDS, in: Hatfield, D.L. (ed.), *Selenium: Its Molecular Biology and Role in Health*, Kluwer Academic, Boston, MA, pp. 232–235.

Beck, M., 2001, Selenium as an antiviral agent, in: Hatfield, D.L. (ed.), *Selenium: Its Molecular Biology and Role in Health*, Kluwer Academic, Boston, MA, pp. 235–245.

Beck, M.A., 1997, Rapid genomic evolution of a non-virulent coxsackievirus B3 in selenium-deficient mice, *Biomed. Environ. Sci.* **10**, 307–315.

Beck, M.A., 1999, Selenium and host defense towards viruses, *Proc. Nutr. Soc.* **58**, 707–711.

Beck, M.A., Shi, Q., Morris, V.C., and Levander, O.A., 1995, Rapid genomic evolution of nonvirulent cocksackievirus B3 in selenium deficient mice results in selection of identical virulent isolates, *Nat. Med.* **1**, 433–436.

Beck, M.A., Esworthy, R.S., Ho, Y.S., and Chu, F.F., 1998, Glutathione peroxidase protects mice from viral-induced myocarditis, *FASEB J.* **12**, 1143–1149.

Beck, M.A., Handy, J., and Levander, O.A., 2004, Host nutritional status: the neglected virulence factor, *Trends Microbiol.* **12**, 417–423.

Beckett, G.J., Arthur, J.R., Miller, S.M., and McKenzie, R.C., 2003, Selenium, in: Hughes, D.A., Darlington, G., and Bendich, A. (eds), *Dietary Enhancement and Human Immune Function*, Humana Press, Totowa, NJ, pp. 217–240.

Behne, D., Weiler, H., and Kyriamopoulos, A., 1996, Effects of selenium deficiency on testicular morphology and function in rats, *J. Reprod. Fertil.* **106**, 291–297.

Boyne, R. and Arthur, J.R., 1986, The response of selenium deficient mice to *Candida albicans* infection, *J. Nutr.* **116**, 816–822.

Boyne, R., Mann, S.O., and Arthur, J.R., 1984, Effects of *Salmonella typhimurium* infection on selenium deficient rats, *Microbios Lett.* **27**, 83–87.

Brown, K.M. and Arthur, J.R., 2001, Selenium, selenoproteins and human health: a review, *Public Health Nutr.* **4**, 593–599.

Chappell, I.C., Seed, P.T., Briely, A.I., et al., 1999, Effect of antioxidants on the occurrence of preeclampsia in women at increased risk: a randomised trial, *Lancet* **351**, 810–816.

Eskew, M.L., Scholz, R.W., Reddy, C.C., et al., 1985, Effects of vitamin E and selenium deficiencies on rat immune function, *Immunology* **54**, 173–180.

Han, I. and Zhou, S., 1991, Selenium supplementation in the prevention of pregnancy induced hypertension, *Chin. Med. J.* **107**, 870–871.

Hidiroglou, M., 1979, Trace element deficiencies and fertility in ruminants: a review, *J. Dairy Sci.* **62**, 1195–1206.

Iwanier, K. and Zachara, B., 1995, Selenium supplementation enhances the element concentration in blood and seminal fluid but does not change the spermatozoal quality characteristics in subfertile men, *J. Androl.* **16**, 441–447.

Khalil, A.M., 1989, The induction of chromosome aberrations in human purified peripheral blood lymphocytes following in vivo exposure to selenium, *Mutat. Res.* **224**, 503–506.

Kiremidjian-Schumacher, L. and Roy, M., 1998, Selenium and immune function, *Z. Ernahrungswiss.* **37**, 50–56.

Kiremidjian-Schumacher, L., Roy, M., Wishe, H., et al., 1994, Supplementation with selenium and human immune cell functions. II. Effect on cytotoxic lymphocytes and natural killer cells, *Biol. Trace Elem. Res.* **41**, 115–127.

Knekt, P., Heliövaara, M., Aho, K., et al., 2000, Serum selenium, serum alpha-tocopherol and the risk of rheumatoid arthritis, *Epidemiol*ogy **11**, 402–405.

Kuklinsky, B. and Schweder, R., 1996, Acute pancreatitis, a free radical disease: reducing the lethality with sodium selenite and other antioxidants, *J. Nat. Environ. Med.* **6**, 393–394.

Kupka, R., Msamanga, G.I., Spiegelman, D., et al., 2004, Selenium status is associated with accelerated HIV disease progression among HIV-1-infected pregnant women in Tanzania, *J. Nutr.* **134**, 2556–2560.

Larsen, H.J. and Tollersrud, S., 1981, Effect of dietary vitamin E and selenium on the phytohemoglutinin response of pig lymphocytes, *Res. Vet. Sci.* **31**, 301–305.

Larsen, H.J., Moksnes, K., and Overnes, G., 1988, Influence of selenium on antibody production in sheep, *Res. Vet. Sci.* **45**, 4–10.

Larsen, H.J.S., 1993, Relations between selenium and immunity, *Norwegian J. Agric. Sci. Suppl.* **11**, 195–119.

Look, M.P., Rocstroh, J.K., Rao, G.S., et al., 1997a, Serum selenium, plasma glutathione (GSH) and eryhtrocyte glutathione peroxidase (GSH-Px)-levels in asymptomatic versus symptomatic human immunodeficiency virus-1 (HIV-1)-infection, *Eur. J. Clin. Nutr.* **51**, 266–272.

Look, M.P., Rockstroh, J.K., Rao, G.S., et al., 1997b, Serum selenium versus lymphocyte subsets and markers of disease progression and inflammatory response in human immunodeficiency virus-infection, *Biol. Trace Elem. Res.* **56**, 31–41.

Mantero-Atienza, E., Beach, R.S., Gavancho, M.C., et al., 1991, Selenium status of HIV-1 infected individuals, *J. Parent. Ent. Nutr.* **15**, 693–694.

Marsh, J.A., Combs, G.F., Whiteacre, M.E., and Dietert, R.R., 1986, Effect of selenium and vitamin E deficiencies on chick lymphoid organ developments, *Proc. Soc. Exp. Biol. Med.* **182**, 425–436.

Marsh, J.A., Dietert, R.R., and Combs, G.F., 1987, Effect of dietary selenium and vitamin E deficiencies in the chicken on Con A-induced splenocyte prolifereation, *Prog. Clin. Biol. Res.* **238**, 333–345.

Maurer, P.H., 1961, Immunology, in: Gray, P. (ed.), *Encyclopedia of the Biological Sciences*, Reinhold, New York, pp. 503–505.

McCloy, R., 1998, Chronic pancreatitis in Manchester, UK: focus on antioxidant therapy, *Digestion* **59** (Suppl. 4), 36–48.

McKenzie, R.C., Arthur, J.R., Miller, S.M., et al., 2000, Selenium and the immune system, in: Calder, P.C., Field, C.J., and Gill, N.S. (eds), *Nutrition and Immune Function*, CAB International, Oxford, pp. 229–250.

Molinero, P., Osuna, C., and Guerrero, J.M., 1995, Type I thyroxine 5′-deiodinase in the rat thymus, *J. Endocrinol.* **146**, 816–822.

Montgomery, R., Dryer, R.L., Conway, T.W., and Spector, A.A., 1977, *Biochemistry, a Case-Orientated Approach*, 2nd edn., Mosby, St Louis, MO, pp. 65–67.

Mulhern, S.A., Taylor, G.L., Magruder, L.E., and Vessey, A.R., 1985, Deficient levels of dietary selenium suppress the antibody response in first and second-generation mice, *Nutr. Res.* **5**, 201–210.

Myatt, I., Rosenfield, R.B., Eis, A.I., et al., 1996, Nitrotyrosine residues in placenta. Evidence for peroxynitite formation and action, *Hypertension* **28**, 188–193.

Nicoll, A.E., Norman, J., McPherson, A., and Acharya, U., 1999, Association of reduced selenium status in the aetiology of recurrent miscarriage, *Br. J. Obstet. Gynaecol.* **106**, 1188–1191.

Oldereid, N.B., Thomassen, Y., and Purvis, K., 1998, Selenium in human males reproductive organs, *Hum. Reprod.* **13**, 2172–2176.

Olson, G.E., Winfey, V.P., NadDas, N.K., Hill, K.E., and Burk, R.F., 2005, Selenoprotein P is required for mouse sperm development, *Biol. Reproduct.* **73**, 201–211.

Peretz, A., Nève, J., Duchataeu, J.P., and Famaey, J.P., 1992, Adjuvant treatment of recent onset rheumatoid arthritis by selenium supplementation: preliminary observations, *Br. J. Rheumatol.* **31**, 281–286.

Rayman, M.P., 2000, The importance of selenium to human health, *Lancet*, **356**, 233–241.

Rayman, M.P., Bode, P., and Redman, C.W.G., 2003, Low selenium status is associated with the occurrence of the pregnancy disease preeclampsia in women from the United Kingdom, *Am. J. Obstet. Gynecol.* **189**, 1343–1349.

Redman, C.W.G. and Sargent, H., 2000, Placental debris, oxidative stress and preeclampsia, *Placenta* **21**, 597–602.

Roberts, J.M., Taylor, R.N., Musci, T.J., et al., 1989, Preeclampsia: an endothelial cell disorder, *Am. J. Obstet. Gynecol.* **161**, 1200–1201.

Scott, R. and McPherson, A., 1998, Selenium supplementation in sub-fertile human males, *Br. J. Urol.* **82**, 625–629.

Semba, R.D. and Tang, A.M., 1999, Micronutrients and the pathogenesis of human immunodeficiency virus infection, *Br. J. Nutr.* **81**, 181–189.

Serfass, R.E. and Ganther, H.E., 1975, Defective microbiocidal activity in glutathione peroxidase deficient neutrophils of Se deficient rats, *Nature (Lond.)*, **225**, 640–641.

Shaheen, S.O., Sterne, J.A.C., Thompson, R.L., et al., 1999, Dietary antioxidants and asthma in adults, *Eur. Respir. J.* **14** (Suppl. 30), 141–150.

Spallholz, J.E., 1990, Selenium and glutathione peroxidase: essential nutrient and antioxidant component of the immune system, *Adv. Exp. Med. Biol.* **262**, 145–158.

Spallholz, J.E., Martin, J.L., Gerlach, M.L., and Heizerling, R.H., 1975, Injectable selenium: effect on the primary immune response of mice, *Proc. Soc. Exp. Biol. Med.* **148**, 37–40.

Staines, N.A., Brostoff, J., and James, K., 1993, *Introducing Immunology*, 2nd edn., Mosby, St Louis, MO.

Steinhauer, D., Domingo, E., and Holland, J.J., 1992, Lack of evidence for proofreading mechanisms associated with an RNA virus polymerase *Gene* **122**, 281–288.

Stuart, L.D. and Oehme, F.W., 1982, Environmental factors in bovine and porcine abortion, *Vet. Hum. Toxicol.* **24**, 435–441.

Su, C., Gong, C., Li, J., et al., 1979, Preliminary results of viral etiology study of Keshan disease, *Chinese Med. J.* **59**, 466–472, cited in Ge, K. and Yang, G., 1993, The epidemiology of selenium deficiency in the etiology of endemic diseases in China, *Am. J. Clin. Nutr. Suppl.* **57**, 259S–263S.

Turner, R.J. and Finch, J.E., 1990, Immunological malfunctions associated with low selenium-vitamin E diets in lambs, *J. Compar. Pathol.* **102**, 99–109.

Turner, R.J. and Finch, J.M., 1991, Selenium and the immune response, *Proc. Nutr. Soc.* **50**, 275–285.

Underwood, E.J., 1977, *Trace Elements in Human and Animal Nutrition*, 4th edn., Academic Press, New York, pp. 303–345.

Ursini, F., Heim, S., Kiess, M., et al., 1999, Dual function of the selenoprotein PHGPx during sperm maturation, *Science* **285**, 1393–1396.

Ward, K.P., Arthur, J.R., Russell, G., and Aggett, P.J., 1984, Blood selenium content and glutathione peroxidase activity in children with cystic fibrosis, coeliac disease, asthma and epilepsy, *Eur. J. Paediatr.* **142**, 21–24.

Whanger, P.D., Weswig, P.H., and Oldfield, J.E., 1978, Selenium, sulfur and nitrogen levels in ovine rumen microorganisms, *J. Anim. Sci.* **46**, 515–519.

Wu, S.H., Oldfield, J.E., Whanger, P.D., and Weswig, P.H., 1973, Selenium and reproduction in sheep, *Biol. Reprod.* **8**, 625–629.

Zhang, W., Ramanathan, C.S., Nadimpalli, R.G., et al., 1999, Selenium-dependent glutathione peroxidase modules encoded by RNA viruses, *Biol. Trace Elem. Res.* **70**, 97–116.

8 Selenium in Health and Disease V: Selenium Deficiency in Search of a Disease?

8.1 Selenium and other Health Conditions

There have been numerous reports and claims, both in the scientific papers and in the popular media, that selenium deficiency is implicated in a considerable number of other human diseases, in addition to those discussed above. Casey (1988), writing in a UK scientific journal, listed a dozen such conditions, for which the taking of selenium was advocated by supplement suppliers and popular writers. A few years later a newsletter produced by an international pharmaceutical company claimed that there were more than 50 diseases against which selenium could have a protective role (Anon, 1993). Evidence for the involvement of selenium in these and other diseases is not in every case apodictic. Nevertheless, among them are several health conditions in which selenium appears to play a part and for which there is support from the results of some clinical and other trials. Few would now subscribe to the somewhat cynical comment made nearly 20 years ago by Burke (1988), in a paper with the provocative title *Selenium deficiency in search of a disease*, that there was little agreement on pathological conditions in human beings related to lack of selenium and that, as a consequence, a vacuum in knowledge had been filled by speculation.

8.2 Selenium and Ageing

Ageing is not, of course, an illness, though the process of growing old is often accompanied by deterioration in health and the development of certain age-related and other diseases. It is believed that oxidative damage to cells, mostly caused by free radicals, increases with age (Beckman and Ames, 1998). Damage is caused to both mitochondrial and nuclear DNA by reactive oxygen species (ROS), which also lead to an accumulation of carbonyl moieties on proteins and thiobarbituric reactive substances (TBARS) from lipid peroxidation. ROS appear to be able to activate a senescence program, leading to cessation of cell growth (Chen and Ames, 1994). A decrease in selenium status in the elderly could result in an inability to "mop up" ROS, with consequent cellular damage leading to cellular ageing (Beckett et al., 2003).

Another feature of old age is a decline in immune function and a consequent decrease in the ability to fight off infection. There is a lessening of lymphocyte proliferation, especially in those who have a low selenium status (Peretz et al., 1991). There is also a decrease in the body's ability to detect and destroy cancerous tumors, possibly because of a decrease in effectiveness of NK cells (Ravaglia et al., 2000).

A number of studies have looked at the effects of micronutrient supplementation on the health of elderly persons, both institutionalized and independently living. Although selenium was contained in the supplements, none of the reported trials used the element on its own. In one study of institutionalized persons, with an average age of 84 ± 8 years (range 65 to 102 years), supplementation with a combined dose of zinc and selenium was followed by a significant decrease in the number of respiratory and urogenital infections (Girdon et al., 1997). A study using a multinutrient supplement of vitamins and minerals, again including selenium, found that independently living elderly subjects given the supplement over a 1-year period, had fewer days of illness owing to infections, and fewer days in which antibiotics were used than did a control group (Chandra, 1992). However, another study of independently living elderly subjects, also using a multimicronutrient supplement, though for only 4 months, reported no reduction in incidence of infections (Chavance et al., 1993).

8.3 Selenium and Age-Related Degenerative Disorders of the Eye

There is evidence that selenium, as well as other antioxidant micronutrients, may play a part in the prevention of a number of degenerative eye disorders. These disorders include age-related cataract and macular degeneration. These are major causes of visual impairment and blindness among elderly people in western countries. Both are believed to be associated with progressive damage caused by accumulation in the eye of ROS. There are a number of reports indicating that supplementation with antioxidants, including selenium, can be beneficial in their prevention and treatment (Sperduto et al., 1990).

8.3.1 Age-Related Macular Degeneration

Age-related macular degeneration (AMD) occurs in almost 35% of people over 65 years of age in the USA (Eye Disease Control Study Group, 1993). It is characterized by features that include the presence of drusen or retinal pigment epithelial changes, and choroidal neovascularization and scarring. It has been shown in animals that the retinal pigment can be damaged by light-induced free radical formation. It has been postulated that GPX plays a protective role against oxidation (Weiter et al., 1985).

Findings from a number of human clinical trials have been contradictory. A US study (Eye Disease Control Study Group, 1993) of 400 AMD patients found that the risk of developing the most severe form of the disease was inversely related to levels in blood of antioxidant micronutrients (including selenium). A British study, however, failed to find any connection between the levels of antioxidant micronutrients and the development of maculopathy (Sanders, 1993).

8.3.2 Cataract

The situation appears to be much the same in the case of age-related cataract, with some support in theory, but contradictory evidence from clinical trials. An association between the development of cataract and nutrition has been claimed by a number of investigators (Taylor, 1989). However, evidence from clinical trials has not been clear-cut. A Finnish study found that, while low serum levels of antioxidant vitamins could be used to predict development of the condition, there appeared to be no association between risk of cataract and selenium status (Knect et al., 1992). A much larger trial in China, which took advantage of the extensive Linxian esophageal dysplasia study, found a statistically significant reduction in the risk of nuclear cataract in subjects given the antioxidant multivitamin/mineral supplement, which contained selenium. However, the supplement had no significant effect on prevalence of another common form of the condition, cortical cataract (Sperduto, 1993).

8.4 Sudden Infant Death Syndrome

Among other possible selenium-related conditions that have been suggested by some investigators, is sudden infant death syndrome (SIDS), also known as cot or crib death. In the late 1960s, Money, a New Zealand veterinary surgeon, noted similarities between the sudden deaths that occur in selenium-deficient piglets and SIDS in humans (Money, 1970). This was a significant observation in a country where selenium deficiency-related conditions in farm animals are common and, in addition, a high level of incidence of crib death occurs in human infants.

Money proceeded to investigate selenium levels in the diet of infants and correlated the results of his findings with the incidence of SIDS in New Zealand. He found that the syndrome occurred more frequently in cow's milk-based formula-fed infants than in those who were breast-fed, and that the latter received twice as much dietary selenium as did the former. His conclusion was that the underlying cause of SIDS was an inadequate intake of selenium. However, in a later study he failed to find a significant difference between dietary levels of selenium in SIDS cases and controls. What he did find was that the SIDS victims had significantly higher iron levels in their blood than did other infants. He now concluded that rather than a deficiency of selenium, an imbalance of antioxidants and iron might be important in the etiology of the disease (Money, 1978). In 1992 Money once more entered the debate, with a review in which he again proposed a hypothesis of a dietary link between SIDS, deficiency of both vitamin E and selenium, and an excess of iron, as the etiological factor for what he described as a largely unexplained and avoidable factor in infant mortality (Money, 1992).

Money's reports attracted a great deal of attention, not only from pediatricians and other medical professionals, but also in the general media and, not least, in certain commercial circles. His claims that inadequate levels of selenium in infant formula might be responsible for SIDS caused much concern to certain infant food manufacturers in New Zealand whose reputation, and profitability, according to one of the experts they consulted, depended greatly on the use of their baby foods (Cuthbertson, W.F.J., 2001, personal communication). No less concerned was the dairy industry at the possible damage to New Zealand's image as a producer of high-quality food and a shipper of "very large quantities of dried milk, much of it to developing countries where infant malnutrition is rife" (Editorial, 1971).

Money's theory of a connection between selenium status and SIDS received support from some, but by no means all, of those who looked into the problem. Another New Zealand group found evidence which suggested that heat stress in sleeping infants can cause a decrease in vitamin E and an increase in GPX activity, which, they concluded, pointed to a protective role for selenium against the syndrome (Dolamore et al., 1990). A finding by a Canadian group of an apparent correlation between SIDS incidence and iodine intake has been interpreted as indicating a possible connection with selenium, since iodine deficiency and selenium deficiency often overlap (Oldfield, 1991). More recently the hypothesis of a connection between the syndrome and selenium has received some support from Reid (2000), who has drawn attention to the possibility that nitric oxide (NO) overload plays a part in SIDS. He believes that the findings in autopsies of victims of SIDS show that it leaves "footprints" analogous to those that follow a flood of NO, including elevated hepatic iron, bone marrow hyperplasia, and cerebral hypoperfusion resembling lesions caused by chronic hypoxemia. The hypoxia, he believes, stimulates the immune response and this in turn triggers a flood of NO, which results in respiratory failure. Since selenium is known to be important in combating the effect of NO, this could account for its proposed role in SIDS prevention.

Several other studies failed to find a link between selenium intake and SIDS (McGlashan and Cook, 1996; Rhead et al., 1972). Today, the debate about a possible role for selenium continues to rumble on, resurfacing every now and again, at least in the popular press. SIDS is, in fact, most likely to be multifactorial in origin and, like other conditions of a similar nature, many different theories have been put forward to account for it, and a variety of preventive measures proposed. Rather than concentrating on nutrition alone, these include modification of the physical condition of the sleeping infant.

8.5 Selenium and Brain Function

One of the most striking aspects of selenium metabolism is that, during times of deficiency, the element is retained in the brain to a greater extent than in other organs. This priority of supply indicates how important the element is to the brain

(Benton, 2002). There is increasing evidence of a close connection between selenium supply and brain function. Selenium deficiency has been shown to change the turnover rate of dopamine and other neurotransmitters in the brain (Castano et al., 1997). A low selenium status has been associated with senility and cognitive decline in the elderly, and low brain selenium levels have been detected in Alzheimer patients (Berr et al., 2004). Selenium deficiency has been linked with intractable epilileptic seizures in children (Ramaekeres et al., 1994).

One of the clearer examples, supported by a number of experimental and clinical findings, of an aspect of psychological functioning that is modified by selenium intake is mood. In several studies selenium status has been shown to be associated with mood changes, with deficiency resulting in poorer mood and hostile activity (Hawkes and Hornbostel, 1996; Benton, 2002). Improvements in mood, with decreased anxiety, depression, and tiredness, have been reported in subjects given selenium supplements (Benton and Cook, 1991; Finley and Penland, 1998). The improvements were greatest in those whose diets were the lowest in selenium. The mechanism underlying these effects is unclear. Although there are suggestions that oxidative damage is involved in some forms of brain malfunction, the finding that a higher intake of selenium than is necessary for maximal GPX activity is required to bring about mood improvement (Benton, 2002) suggests that other functions of selenoproteins, besides that of an antioxidant, are involved. It is possible that thyroid hormones and the deiodinase selenoenzymes play a role in these brain activities. Hypothyroidism, even at a subclinical level, is known to result in depression and lethargy (Sher, 2002a).

Selenium supplementation has been recommended for patients with mood and behavior problems caused by a number of different conditions. Depression and behavioral problems are common in patients undergoing dialysis, which also results in low serum selenium levels. It has been suggested that such dialysis-related selenium loss plays a role in the biological mechanisms of psychiatric disorders in these patients and that selenium supplementation could be used in their treatment (Sher, 2002b). A micronutrient supplement, containing a range of trace elements, including selenium, has been used with good effect in the treatment of mood lability and explosive rage in two boys. The conditions of the two—one an 8-year-old with a typical obsessive-compulsive disorder; the other, a 12-year-old with pervasive developmental delay—were stabilized by the supplementation over a 2-year period. While these results may be interpreted as indicating the benefits of dietary supplemetation with trace elements and other micronutrients, they leave open the question of whether selenium, on its own, will have a similar effect (Kaplan, 2002).

8.6 Other Possible Selenium-Related Conditions

Protein-energy malnutrition (PEM) is a common feature of pediatric health and one of the most serious health problems in countries affected by poverty, famine, periodic food shortages, and unbalanced diet. It is not a single condition but covers a range of clinical disorders. At one end is marasmus, caused by restriction of dietary energy and protein, as well as other nutrients; at the other end is kwashiorkor, caused by quantitative and qualitative protein deficiency, but in which energy may be sufficient. Between these two extremes are clinical conditions with a range of features related to various combinations of deficiencies of energy, protein, vitamins, and minerals.

Kwashiorkor has been extensively studied for some 70 years since its name was first introduced into medical literature by Cicely D. Williams in her reports on her pioneering investigations in West Africa (Williams, 1935). The pathophysiology of kwashiorkor, however, is still unclear (Krawinkel, 2003). A feature of the disease is loss of ability to resist microbial attacks, resulting in almost ubiquitous infection, with an overgrowth of bacteria in the small intestine (Golden and Ramdath, 1987).

Several different theories have been proposed to account for the loss of immunocompetence and progression of the syndrome, including dysadaptation to protein-deficient stress (Gopalan, 1968) and aflatoxin intoxication (Hendrickse, 1984). Golden (1985) believed that kwashiorkor results from an imbalance between the production of free radicals and their safe disposal by the body. This imbalance is caused by low concentrations of antioxidant nutrients, with selenium prominent among them. This view is supported by the finding of low selenium levels in children with kwashiorkor (Burk et al., 1967). Reduced GPX activity is a significant feature of the disease (Sive et al., 1991). According to Golden (1985), provision of supplementary selenium and other antioxidant micronutrients must be made in any rehabilitation regime for kwashiorkor victims to allow for an essential improvement in their immunocompetence. However, a recent study of Malawian children found that daily consumption of a mixed supplement containing riboflavin, vitamin E, selenium, and N-acetylcysteine, all at about three times their recommended dietary intakes, did not prevent the onset of the disease. This finding has been interpreted as evidence that neither selenium nor any of the other components of the supplement has a role to play in the development of kwashiorkor (Ciliberto et al., 2005). It is possible, however, that an increase in the length of the trial and/or the size of the dose might have produced a different result.

Low selenium levels are commonly found in children suffering from marasmus and other forms of PEM. Both marasmus and kwashiorkor are common in severely malnourished urban and rural children living in Andean regions of Ecuador, where the soil is low in selenium. A study of a group of such children found that serum selenium concentrations were lower in those with marasmus than in normally nourished controls. Levels in children with kwashiorkor were significantly lower than in the marasmic children (Sempertegui et al., 2003).

Congestive heart failure (CHF) is a common feature of kwashiorkor, as it is of selenium deficiency in people living in low-selenium regions. In a study of a group of children with kwashiorkor, including marasmic kwashiorkor, all the children were found to have low serum selenium levels, but these were significantly lower in those who developed CHF than in those who did not (Manary et al., 2001).

8.7 Other Health Conditions and Selenium

There are several other health conditions for which a connection with selenium deficiency has been suggested. These include Crohn's disease, ulcerative colitis, diabetes, hemophilia, multiple sclerosis, arsenic toxicity, bronchopulmonary displasia in preterm infants, and several others. Evidence in support of these views is seldom convincing. They often depend on findings of low blood selenium levels in victims of the disease, but whether these low levels are a cause or a consequence of the condition is difficult to determine. Moreover, many diseases are multifactorial in origin and it is unlikely that if there is a connection with selenium, the element will be more than one of several factors involved. There is still, in spite of the considerable amount of investigation being undertaken at present, a great deal of uncertainty in our understanding of selenium in relation to human health. It is probably premature to look for a final answer to all our questions about the role of the element in human lives. Fresh information continues to appear in every issue of the scientific journals, and new hypotheses are still being proposed. While hope and enthusiasm are legitimate, there is still a place for some degree of caution, and perhaps even scepticism, about several of the claims.

References

Anon, 1993, Oxidative stress and human disease: a broad spectrum of effects, *Antioxidant Vitamins Newsletter*, No. 7, Hoffman-La Roche, New York, p. 12.

Beckett, G.J., Arthur, J.R., Miller, S.M., and McKenzie, R.C., 2003, Selenium, in: Hughes, D.A., Darlington, G., and Bendich, A. (eds), *Dietary Enhancement of Human Immune Function*, Humana Press, Totowa, NJ, pp. 217–240.

Beckman, K.B. and Ames, B.N., 1998, The free radical theory of aging matures, *Physiol. Rev.* **78**, 547–581.

Benton, D., 2002, Selenium intake, mood and other aspects of psychological functioning, *Nutr.. Neurosci.* **5**, 363–374.

Benton, D. and Cook, R., 1991, Selenium supplementation improves mood in a double-blind crossover trial, *Biol. Psychiatry* **29**, 1092–1098.

Berr, C., Richard, M.J., Gourlet, V., et al., 2004, Enzymatic antioxidant balance and cognitive decline in aging—the EVA study, *Eur. J. Epidemiol.* **19**, 133–138.

Burk, R.F., 1988, Selenium deficiency in search of a disease, *Hepatology* **8**, 421–423.

Burk, R.F., Pearson, W.N., Wood, R.P., and Viteri, F., 1967, Blood selenium levels and in vitro red blood cell uptake of ^{75}Se in kwashiorkor, *Am. J. Clin. Nutr.* **20**, 723–730.

Casey, C.E., 1988, Selenophilia, *Proc. Nutr. Soc.* **47**, 55–62.

Castano, A., Ayala, A., Rodriguez-Gomes, J.A., et al., 1997, Low selenium diet increases the dopamine-turnover in prefrontal cortex of the rat, *Neurochem. Int.* **30**, 549–555.

Chandra, R.K., 1992, Effect of vitamin and trace-element supplementation on immune responses and infection in elderly subjects, *Lancet* **340**, 1124–1127.

Chavance, M., Herbeth, B., Lemoine, A., and Bao-Piong, Z. 1993, Does multivitamin supplementation prevent infections in healthy elderly subjects? A controlled trial, *Int. J. Vitam. Nutr. Res.* **63**, 11–16.

Chen, Q. and Ames, B.N., 1994, Senescence-like growth arrest induced by hydrogen peroxide in human diploid fibroblast F65 cells, *Proc. Natl Acad. Sci. USA* **91**, 4130–4134.

Ciliberto, H., Ciliberto, M., Briend, A., et al., 2005, Antioxidant supplementation for the prevention of kwashiorkor in Malawian children: randomised, double blind, placebo controlled trial, *BMJ* **330**, 1109–1111.

Dolamore, B.A., Sluis, K.B., McGrouter, J.C., et al., 1990, Low selenium and infant death in Christchurch, *Proc. Nutr. Soc. NZ.* **15**, 181–186.

Editorial, 1971, Selenium and vitamin E in cow's milk in relation to infant health, *NZ Agric.* **19**, 2.

Eye Disease Control Study Group, 1993, Antioxidant status and neovascular age-related macular degeneration, *Arch. Ophthalmol.* **111**, 104–109.

Finley, J.W. and Pentland, J.G., 1998, Adequacy or deprivation of dietary selenium in healthy men: clinical and psychological findings, *J. Trace Elem. Exp. Med.* **11**, 11–27.

Girdon, F., Lombard, M., Galan, P., et al., 1997, Effect of micronutrient supplementation on infection in institutionalized elderly subjects: a controlled study, *Ann. Nutr. Metab.* **41**, 98–107.

Golden, M.H.N., 1985, The consequences of protein deficiency in man and its relationship to the features of kwashiorkor, in: Blaxter, K. and Waterlow, J.C. (eds), *Nutritional Adaptations in Man*, Applied Science, London, pp. 169–187.

Golden, H.M.N. and Ramdath, D., 1987, Free radicals in the pathogenesis of kwashiorkor, *Proc. Nutr. Soc.* **46**, 53–68.

Gopalan, G., 1968, Kwashiorkor, in: McCance, R.A. and Widdowson, E.M. (eds), *Calorie Deficiencies and Protein Deficiency*, Churchill, London, pp. 48–58.

Hawkes, W.C. and Hornbostel, L., 1996, Effects of dietary selenium on mood in healthy men living in a metabolic research unit, *Biol. Psychiatry* **39**, 121–128.

Hendrickse, R.G., 1984, Aflatoxin intoxication and kwashiorkor, *Trans. Roy. Soc. Trop. Med. Hyg.* **78**, 427–435.

Kaplan, B.J., Crawford, S.G., Gardner, B., and Farrelly, G., 2002, Treatment of mood lability and explosive rage with minerals and vitamins: two case studies in children, *J. Child Adolesc. Psychopharmacol.* **12**, 205–209.

Knect, P., Heliövaara, M., Rissanen, A., et al., 1992, Serum antioxidant vitamins and risk of cataract, *Br. Med. J.* **305**, 1392–1394.

Krawinkel, M., 2003, Kwashiorkor is still not fully understood, *Bull. World Health Organ.* **81/12**, 1–4.

McGlashan, N.D., Cook, S., Melrose, W., et al., 1996, Maternal selenium and Sudden Infant Death Syndrome (SIDS), *Aust. NZJ. Med.* **26**, 677–682.

Manary, M.J., MacPherson, G.D., McArdie, F., Jackson, M.J., and Hart, C., 2001, Selenium status, kwashiorkor and congestive heart failure, *Acta Paediatr.* **90**, 950–952.

Money, D.F.L., 1970, Vitamin E and selenium deficiencies and their possible aetiological role in the sudden death in infants syndrome, *NZ Med. J.* **71**, 32–34.

Money, D.F.L., 1978, Vitamin E, selenium, iron and vitamin A content of livers from sudden infant death syndrome cases and control children: interrelationships and possible significance, *NZJ. Sci.* **21**, 41–44.

Money, D.F.L., 1992, The Sudden-Infant-Death Syndrome—the vitamin E-selenium-iron hypothesis (dietary anti/pro-oxidant imbalance), *Med. Hypoth.* **39**, 286–290.

Oldfield, J., 1991, Some implications of selenium for human health, *Nutr. Today* **26**, 6–11.

Peretz, A., Nève, J., Desmedt, J., et al., 1991, Lymphocyte-response is enhanced by supplementation of elderly subjects with selenium-enhanced yeast, *Am. J. Clin. Nutr.* **53**, 1323–1328.

Ramaekeres, V.T., Calomme, M., Vanden Berghe, D., et al., 1944, Selenium deficiency triggering intractable seizures, *Neuropediatrics* **25**, 217–223.

Ravaglia, G., Forti, P., Maioli, F., et al., 2000, Effect of micronutrient status on natural killer cell immune function in healthy free-living subjects aged ≥90 y. *Am. J. Clin. Nutr.* **53**, 1323–1328.

Reid, G., 2000, Association of sudden infant death syndrome with grossly deranged iron metabolism and nitric oxide overload, *Med. Hypoth.* **54**, 137–139.

Rhead, W.J., Cary, E.E., Allaway, W.H., et al., 1972, The vitamin E and selenium status of infants and the sudden infant death syndrome, *Bioinorg. Chem.* **1**, 289–295.

Sanders, T.A.B., 1993, Plasma cholesterol, and fat-soluble vitamins in subjects with age-related maculopathy and matched control subjects, *Am. J. Clin. Nutr.* **57**, 428–433.

Sempertegui, F., Estrella, B., Vallejo, W., et al., 2003, Selenium serum concentrations in malnourished Ecuadorian children: a case-control study, *Int. J. Vit. Nutr. Res.* **73**, 181–186.

Sher, L., 2002a, Selenium, thyroid hormones, mood, and behaviour, *Can. J. Psychiatry*, **47**, 284–285.

Sher, L., 2002b, Role of selenium depletion in the effects of dialysis on mood and behaviour, *Med. Hypoth.* **59**, 89–91.

Sive, A.A., Hesse, H.de V., Demster, W.S., et al., 1991, Protein energy malnutrition: selenium, glutathione peroxidase and glutathione in children with acute kwashiorkor and during refeeding, in: Momčilović;, B. (ed.), *Trace Elements in Man and Animals—TEMA 7*, Institute for Medical Research and Occupational Health, University of Zagreb, Croatia, pp. 19.15–19.16.

Sperduto, R.D., 1993, The Linxian cataract studies, two nutrition intervention trials, *Arch. Ophthalmol.* **111**, 1246–1253.

Sperduto, R.D., Ferris, F.L., and Kurinij, N, 1990, Do we have a nutritional treatment for age-related cataract and macular degeneration? *Arch. Ophthalmol.* **108**, 1403–1405.

Taylor, A., 1989, Associations between nutrition and cataract, *Nutr. Revs* **47**, 225–234.

Weiter, J., Dratz, E., Fitch, K., and Handelman, G., 1985, Role of selenium nutrition in senile macular degeneration [Abstract], *Invest. Ophthalmol. Vis. Sci.* **26** (Suppl.), 58.

Williams, C.D., 1935, Kwashiorkor: a nutritional disease of children associated with a maize diet, *Lancet* **229**, 1151–1152.

9
Selenium in Foods

9.1 Selenium in Food

Only a decade ago it was possible to write in the first edition of this book (Reilly, 1996) that, compared with several other inorganic components of food, selenium has received relatively little attention in the technical literature. That is no longer the case. In spite of being a relative newcomer in the nutrition and food science fields, long dominated by metals such as iron, zinc, mercury, and lead, selenium is one of the most widely investigated and written-about of all the nutritionally significant inorganic food components.

9.1.1 Selenium in Foods: National and International Databases

Reliable data on selenium concentrations in foods are now readily available, following the development of rapid and accurate procedures for its determination. This was not the case as recently as the end of the 1980s when, as noted by Versieck and Cornelis (1989), accurate determination of selenium concentrations in biological samples was beyond the capabilities of not a few analysts. Today well-equipped and highly professional analytical laboratories, government, university and industrially funded have been established in many countries and food composition databases, which include selenium, are available.

The availability of data on selenium levels in foods in a wide range of countries has helped to correct a misconception, or rather a distortion in the perception of not a few nutritionists that was not uncommon some decades ago, probably due to the paucity of information then available. Among the earliest and most widely referred to surveys of selenium levels in foods and diets were those carried out either in selenium-rich regions of the USA or in countries where deficiencies of soil selenium occurred, such as Finland and New Zealand. Subsequent reports from China were also usually concerned with extreme conditions of either excess or deficiency. These reports gave an impression that selenium was only of real nutritional interest in countries where it either posed a danger of toxicity through excess, or of deficiency leading to locally endemic illnesses such as Keshan disease. However, as data on selenium concentrations in foods and diets in countries and regions with intermediate levels of soil selenium became available, balance began to be introduced into the picture. The importance of even moderate levels of deficiency and the implications for health of living in areas with lower levels of soil selenium than in the USA midwest, are now well recognized.

9.1.2 Selenium in Food Composition Databases

Although information on selenium levels in foods in different countries began to be published in the last decades of the 20th century, it usually appeared in reports and reviews in specialist journals and was not incorporated into national food composition databases. However, as the importance of selenium as an essential component of the diet became clear, the situation changed. In the UK, the pioneering text by McCance and Widdowson, *The Composition of Foods*, first published in 1940 and then several new editions over the next more than half a century, did not include selenium among the inorganic food constituents until the 5th edition in 1991 (Holland et al., 1991). Now food composition tables that include data on selenium are available in many countries, both in printed form and on readily accessible websites. In addition to official published tables, data on levels of selenium in foods in a great number of countries, both developed and developing, appear in the scientific literature (McNaughton and Marks, 2002). Table 9.1, based on a sample selected from several sources, summarizes some of the data on selenium in a range of basic foodstuffs consumed in different countries. As the table shows, levels in majority of foods are less than 1 mg/kg, or as sometimes reported in food technology and popular literature, 1 ppm (parts per million).

TABLE 9.1 Selenium levels (μg/kg) in foods from different countries

Food	UK	USA	Australia	Ireland	Thailand	New Zealand
Bread	43–92	282–366	92.6–125	15–158	–	31.6–59.4
Rice	4–13	75	25	10–17	29–65	0
Beef	30–76	134–190	72–121	61–105	72–226	22.3–83
Pork	140	144–450	94–205	82–129	142–250	19.3–150
Chicken	60–70	190–276	116–280	86–147	156–271	137–145
Eggs	90–120	225–308	190–414	56–282	145–420	157–161
Fish	200–500	126–502	20–632	268–298	196–1137	195–512
Milk	10–15	20–21	2.5–25.9	14–22	19–36	1.0–14
Cheese	7.4–12	13.9	70–78.9	9.5–11.5	–	23
Vegetables	3–22	2–19	0.5–32	10–38	1–127	0–2.5
Mushrooms	90	88	255	25–38	8–15	76.6
Peanuts	30	75	140	–	32–186	46–105

Source: Adapted from McNaughton, S.A. and Marks, G.C., 2002, Selenium content of Australian foods: a review of literature values, *J. Food Comp. Anal.* **15**, 169–182, with additional data from Murphy, J. and Cashman, K.D., 2001, Selenium content of a range of Irish foods, *Food Chem.* **74**, 493–498, and, Sirichakwal, P.P., Puwastien, P., Polngam, J., and Kongkachuichai, R., 2005, Selenium content of Thai foods, *J. Food Comp. Anal.* **18**, 47–59.

9.1.2.1 Selenium in Total Diet Studies

Many countries conduct ongoing programmes to monitor, on a regular basis, levels of nutrients in the national diet. These *market basket*, or equivalent, surveys analyze foods (either as individual items or as composites), purchased on the domestic market in different geographical regions of the country, as part of a programme designed to represent the national or regional diet. In USA the *core food model*, in which some 300 foods considered to be the major contributors of energy, nutrients, and other food components, are analyzed in the Total Diet Study (TDS), has been developed by the FDA to assess dietary intakes nationally as well as of regions and individual groups. The selection of core foods is regularly updated to reflect changes in food consumption patterns (Pennington, 1983, 1992, 2001).

A similar approach to that of the FDA, though with a shorter list of representative foods, is used in the UK to monitor constituents of the nation's food supply. This is done via a series of dietary surveys, including an ongoing National Food Survey and a National Diet and Nutrition Programme (Peattie et al., 1983). Similar TDS procedures are used in many other countries.

9.1.3 Variations in Levels of Selenium in Foods

In a report published in 1987, the World Health Organization (WHO) summarized worldwide data on selenium levels in different food groups as follows:

> organ meats and seafood: 0.4 to 1.5 µg/g; muscle meats: 0.1 to 0.4 µg/g; cereals and grains: <0.1 to >0.8 µg/g; dairy products: <0.1 to 0.3 µg/g; fruits and vegetables: <0.1 µg/g (World Health Organization, 1987).

The report drew particular attention to the wide range of concentrations of selenium in different types of food and commented that the variations were due to differences in the availability of selenium in the soils on which an animal is raised or a plant is grown. As a result, selenium levels in foods can vary manyfold, not only between countries but also between regions in a country. A food may have more than a 10-fold difference in selenium content, depending on where it was produced. Does this mean, however, as has been stated in a key document published by the US Institute of Medicine (IOM) that "food tables that reflect average selenium contents [of food] are unreliable" (Institute of Medicine, 2000)? It may, but only if the tables are misused and an assumption is made that they can be employed for the determination of the nutrient intake of individuals, rather than of population groups. It is true that food composition tables cannot be relied on to give accurate information on the precise intakes by an individual of a particular nutrient, especially one such as selenium, levels of which can be so variable in foods. However, it is highly unlikely that the IOM comment was intended to imply that food tables published in such reputable works as the UK's *McCance and Widdowson's The Composition of Foods* (Food Standards Agency, 2002) and intended to reflect average nutrient contents of foods should be abandoned as misleading.

9.1.4 Selenium Levels in Individual Foodstuffs

The overall coefficient of variation (CV) for selenium in some 234 foods surveyed in the US TDS had a range of 19 to 47%, with a mean of 32% for selenium (Pennington and Young, 1990). This is four times greater than for any of the other trace elements investigated in the survey. The high CV in meat products was attributed to variable amounts of the element consumed by the animals, and this in turn was related to variations in soil levels in the areas of production. The wide range of CVs for selenium that has also been reported in other countries has been attributed to similar causes (Molnar, 1995).

9.1.4.1 Selenium Levels in Cow's Milk

An example of the levels of variation of selenium concentrations in a widely, if not universally consumed food, is seen in cow's milk. A worldwide range of 2 to 140 μg/l has been estimated on the basis of published data on milk composition (Alejos and Romero, 1995). A range of 10 to 260 μg/kg has been reported in milks from different parts of the USA (Combs, 2001). There can be significant differences between selenium levels in milk produced not only in different countries or regions but also in adjacent farms. An Australian study (Tinggi et al., 2001) found that raw milk from one farm contained 38.5 μg/l, while milk from a neighboring dairy had only 21.0 μg/l. Pasteurized and homogenized milk produced across Australia over a 2-year period had concentrations ranging from 38.34 ± 6.01 to 15.87 ± 4.49 μg/l. The same study found that there were significant differences between selenium levels in milks produced in different seasons of the year, with, on one farm in Queensland, a summer (wet season) high of 38.5 μg/l in raw milk, compared to a low of 19.0 μg/l in winter (dry season). The Australian Market Basket Survey of 1994 reported a mean level of 27.0 μg/g (range 90—not detected), in milk purchased nationwide (Marro, 1996).

9.1.4.2 Selenium Levels in Human Milk

Although, of course, consumed at any one time by only a small section of the population, human breast milk is a very important food, recognized as the optimal source of nutrients throughout at least the first year of life (Institute of Medicine, 1991). As such breast milk must meet all the nutritional requirements, including that of selenium. Like cow's milk, human milk, depending on various circumstances, can fail to meet those requirements, leading to malnutrition in the infant who depends on it. However, selenium levels in human milk do not vary as greatly as do those in cow's milk, and appear to reflect mainly dietary intake rather than environmental conditions. There can still be a considerable spread of concentrations in reported ranges in different countries. Assessing these reports can be made difficult in the absence of information about the times and other conditions of sample collection. There can also be difficulties with some of the earlier studies that suffered from analytical problems before reliable methods became generally available for the determination of selenium at the low concentrations normally encountered in breast milk. Consequently, as was noted in the report on trace elements in breast milk published jointly by the WHO and the International Atomic Agency in 1989, "the scientific literature is full of inconsistent data and it is generally impossible to decide a priori whether the differences are real (representing biological or geographical variability) or whether they are simply the result of analytical error" (World Health Organization/International Atomic Energy Agency, 1989).

There is evidence that concentrations of selenium in breast milk change over the period of lactation. A US study found higher selenium levels in colostrum (41 μg/l) than in mature milk (16 μg/l), and a reduction from 20 μg/l one month postpartum to 15 μg/l at 3 and 6 months postpartum (Levander et al., 1987). Cumming and her colleagues in Australia (Cumming et al., 1992) reported that levels were significantly higher in hind milk, at the end of suckling, than in fore milk at the beginning of feeding.

Although there can also be wide interindividual, as well as regional variations (Higashi et al., 1983; Dorea, 2002), the average selenium content of mature human milk sampled between 2 and 6 months lactation appears to be relatively constant within a population group (Debski et al., 1989). Levels are related to the maternal dietary intake. Levels of 15 to 20 μg/l have been recorded in women across the USA and Canada (Levander et al., 1987). Another study found that in milk of women living in US states with high soil selenium levels the mean level was 28 μg/l, compared to 13 μg/l in those in areas with a low soil selenium level (Smith et al., 1982). A range of 6 to –39 μg/l in mature breast milk has been reported in studies carried out in a range of different countries (Smith et al., 1982; Levander et al., 1987; Cumming et al., 1992). An interesting finding that points to a possible effect of climate, and, as a consequence of changes in dietary intakes, are the results of a study of rural women in Africa (Funk et al., 1990). This found a mean level of selenium in breast milk of 15.5 μg/l in the rainy season, compared to 21.3 μg/l in the dry season. An effect of differences in diet on selenium levels in breast milk is indicated by the finding of levels of 22.2 ± 0.8 μg/l in vegetarian women, compared to 16.8 ± 1.3 μg/l in nonvegetarians (Debski et al., 1989). These data fall within the international reference range of selenium in breast milk of 10 to 62 μg/l (median 18.5 μg/l) proposed by Iyengar and Wooittiez (1988) on the basis of a survey of world literature.

9.1.4.3 Selenium in Infant Formula

Not all mothers can, for a variety of reasons, breast-feed their infants. Consequently if their infants are to survive and develop properly, they must be supplied with a substitute food. Ideally this should contain all the nutrients, including selenium, found in breast milk. Most of these infant formulae are based on cow's milk and are normally modified by manufacturers so that they match nutritional qualities of human milk. Cow's milk alone is an inadequate food for infants and fails to meet their daily dietary requirements for selenium, as well as for some other nutrients (Cumming et al., 1992). Even specially manufactured infant formulae may also be an inadequate feed. This was commonly the situation as recently as 2 decades ago. A 1982 study of cow's milk-based infant formulae in the USA found a mean selenium concentration of 6.7 μg/l (range 5.1 to 9.2), which would provide a 3-month-old infant with approximately 7.2 μg/day, nearly 3 μg less than the 10 μg/day which was considered at the time to be the RDA for an infant of that age (Smith et al., 1982). An earlier German study (Lombeck et al., 1975) found that the average selenium concentration in 10 different commercially available fluid and powdered cow's milk formulae was only about one third that of mature human milk. A 2-month-old infant consuming one of the formula feeds would receive approximately 7.8 μg of selenium each day, compared with about 22.4 μg if it had been human breast milk.

Several other studies confirmed the low levels of selenium in formula-based infant feeds and their inability to meet nutritional requirements for selenium. One of the reasons for the low levels of selenium in infant foods was that manufacturers relied on the protein naturally present in cow's milk to provide the required level of selenium in the formulae. In the 1980s they began gradually to reduce the protein content of infant formulae by, for example, replacing casein with higher levels of whey, to reflect more closely the protein level and amino acid profile of human breast milk (Räihä, 1989). As a consequence, the selenium content of formulae was also reduced (Labbé, 1996).

It was to overcome this problem that manufacturers began to supplement their products with selenium to meet the recommended intakes of the infants. This is a normal practice today. A recent survey of commercial formulae and manufactured infant foods on sale in the UK found that their selenium mean concentration was 0.055 mg/kg with a range of 0.0027 to 0.14 mg/kg (Ministry of Agriculture, Fisheries and Food, 1999). These figures are not dissimilar to the range of 0.019 to 0.091 found in Spanish infant formulae (Rodríguez et al., 1998).

9.1.4.4 Selenium in Bread and Flour

Selenium levels in bread are of major importance for nutrition, though the actual concentration in this food may be relatively low. Because of the quantities in which bread is consumed, it a significant source of selenium in the diet of many people, especially in western societies. However, whether this will continue to be the case in the future is uncertain, especially in the UK and several other European countries. There are two reasons for this. Changes in dietary patterns in recent years have resulted in a fall in bread consumption in many countries and, possibly of even more importance, there has been a significant reduction in selenium concentrations in the bread-making flour used in Europe. In the late 1980s it was estimated that bread supplied 47% of selenium in the UK diet. Some 10 years later the contribution had fallen to approximately 20% of the dietary intake (Barclay et al., 1995). This decrease reflected a fall in bread consumption by the UK population from 1,080 g/person/week in 1970 to 775 g/person/week in 1995 (Ministry of Agriculture, Fisheries and Food, 1996). A more recent survey found that the contribution to selenium intake made by wheat-based products in the

UK was 6.4 μg, about one-tenth of the UK's RNI, significantly less than the approximately 30 μg estimated to have been provided by bread in the 1980s (Adams et al., 2002).

Some 20 years ago bread was the second most important dietary source of selenium in the USA (Schubert et al., 1987). However, as a consequence of changes in eating patterns, this is no longer the case.

Not all types of bread, even of the same brand and quality and produced in the same geographical area, contain similar amounts of selenium. This has been shown by results of a survey that looked at 90 samples of white bread representing major brands available in supermarkets and other stores in large cities in nine different geographical regions of the USA (Holden et al., 1991). Mean selenium concentrations in white bread ranged from 0.46 μg/g in an east coast (Boston) to 0.17 μg/g on the west coast (Los Angeles), with an overall range for all cities of 0.06 to 0.74 μg/g (CV 49%). A single national brand, manufactured in one city (Boston) had a mean selenium content of 0.60 μg/g (range 0.24 to 0.92; CV 41%).

There can be differences in selenium levels between white, brown, and other types of bread. A study by Murphy and Cashman (2001) found that selenium levels in Irish brown bread had a range of 0.094 to 0.146 μg/g, while in white bread it was 0.053 to 0.095, compared to 0.039 to 0.048 μg/g in English brown/wholemeal bread and 0.043 to 0.044 μg/g in English white bread. These figures probably reflect some differences between bread manufacturing procedures in the two neighboring countries as well as differences in the amounts of North American high selenium flour mixed with the locally produced flour used by the bakers. The significance of this factor can be seen by comparing the selenium contents of the Irish and UK breads with those found in American products. US brown, for instance, has been reported to contain 0.41 to 0.676 μg/g, and Canadian brown 0.06 to 0.71 μg/g of selenium (Murphy and Cashman, 2001), all considerably higher than the European breads.

The Irish study has highlighted a problem faced by sufferers from celiac disease who, because of their gluten intolerance, have to use gluten-free bread. Coeliacs have been reported to have lower blood selenium levels than do healthy individuals (Hinks et al., 1984), a condition that must be related to the fact that gluten-free bread has extremely low selenium levels (0.013 to 0.018 μg/g).

9.1.4.5 Selenium Levels in Other Cereals

In many countries, rice, not wheat, is the most commonly consumed cereal. It is a staple of the diet for a high proportion of the world's population, especially in Asian countries. Although selenium concentrations in rice are normally low, because of the total amount of the cereal consumed in such countries, rice supplies substantial amounts of the nutrient in the diet. In Thailand where average rice consumption is 250g/peron/day each day, as much as 12.5 μg of selenium comes from rice (Sirichakwal et al., 2005). Selenium levels in rice, as in other food plants, depend on the availability of the element in the soil on which it is produced. This can vary and thus there can be, overall, a wide variability in selenium levels in the grain.

A Japanese study of rice grown in different regions of the country found that its selenium content ranged from 0.011 to 0.182 μg/g and that levels were related to soil selenium content, not to differences between cultivars (Yoshida and Yasumoto, 1987). A wide range of selenium levels has also been reported in rice sold for domestic consumption in several countries worldwide. Mean levels that have been reported, as μg/g, are 0.05 in Thailand (Sirichakwal et al., 2005), 0.02 in China (Wang et al., 1997), 0.073 in New Zealand (Thomson and Robinson, 1980), 0.319 in the USA (Morris and Levander, 1970), and 0.10 in the UK (Barclay et al., 1995).

9.1.4.6 Selenium in Meat and Meat Products

For many people meat is the main source of dietary intake of selenium, especially in Northern Europe and America (Koutnik and Ingr, 1998). In Ireland meat and meat products contribute 30% of total selenium intake of adults, compared to 24% contributed by bread (Murphy et al., 2002). Liver, kidney, and other offal meat are particularly rich sources, with, e.g., a mean level of 1.45 μg/g in pork kidney, compared to 0.14 μg/g in pork carcass meat (British Nutrition Foundation, 2001). There are differences in selenium levels in different kinds of muscle meat, with higher levels in pork than in beef, lamb, and chicken. Levels reflect the nutrient intakes of the animals and thus differences in animal husbandry practices, as well as in selenium content of feeds, of different countries.

9.1.4.7 Selenium in Fish and Other Seafoods

Fish and other seafoods constitute a major source of selenium in the diet of many different people, especially communities, such as the Inuits of Greenland who traditionally rely on the ocean to supply the bulk of their food (Hansen et al., 1984). Even in populations whose intake of seafoods is relatively low, fish consumption can make an appreciable contribution towards meeting selenium requirements. In the UK, for example, where average fish consumption per person per day was, in 1997, 14 g, seafoods were estimated to contribute 5 μg, or 12.7% of total daily selenium intake (Ministry of Agriculture, Fisheries and Food, 1999).

However, not all types of seafoods are equally good sources of selenium. An Australian study found that five different types of ocean fish sold at commercial outlets had selenium contents ranging from 0.30 to 0.70 μg/g (Tinggi et al., 1992). A larger New Zealand study of more than 80 species of marine and freshwater fish and crustaceans, reported a range of 0.11 to 0.97 μg selenium/g in edible portions of these foods (Vlieg, 1990), as shown in Table 9.2. Similar findings have been reported in other countries. An Irish study found a mean of 0.282 (range 0.268 to 0.298) μg/g in plaice and 0.265 (range 0.299 to 0.233) μg/g in cod. Interestingly, the same study found higher selenium levels in tinned sea foods, compared to fresh products, with, tuna canned in brine containing 0.70 (range 0.637 to 0.789) μg/g, and in crab, also canned in brine, 0.390 (range 0.347 to 0.437) μg/g (Murphy and Cashman, 2001). Similar figures have been reported for the UK, though with the exception of a high of 1.30 μg selenium/g in crab

TABLE 9.2 Selenium levels in New Zealand marine and freshwater fish, crustaceans and molluscs

Sample type (mean and range)	Selenium content (μg/g, fresh weight, edible part)
Marine finfish	0.42 (0.11–0.97)
Freshwater finfish	0.34 (0.18–0.68)
Molluscs	0.36 (0.19–0.77)
Crustaceans	0.30 (0.19–0.41)

Source: Adapted from Vlieg, P., 1990, Selenium concentration of the edible part of 74 New Zealand fish species, *J. Food Comp. Anal.* **3**, 67–72.

(Barclay et al., 1995). The UK study also found that at least one form of popular fish, much promoted in the diet of children, cod fish fingers, had a relatively low mean selenium content of 0.11 μg/g.

Very high levels of selenium in certain marine foods traditionally used by Inuit people in Greenland and the Canadian Arctic have been reported. Levels up to 18 μg/g have been found in the liver of ringed seals, with an even higher level of 34.4 μg/g in bearded seal liver (AMAP, 1998). Levels in whales were also high, at 24.2 μg/g in liver of Belugas and 1.78 μg/g in Baleen whales. Levels in muscle were about one tenth of those in livers. Whale skin, which is known as muktuk and is eaten as a delicacy, has been reported to contain as much as 47.9 μg selenium/g. Interestingly, similar foods consumed by Inuit communities in Arctic Canada have been reported to have lower levels of selenium. Canadian muktuk contained 2.0 μg/g, Bearded seal meat 0.2 μg/g, and Ringed seal liver 1.0 μg/g (Kuhnlein et al., 2002).

9.1.4.8 The Relation Between Selenium and Mercury in Seafoods

Although fish is an important source of selenium in the diets of many people, it can also contribute significantly to their intake of mercury. Accumulation of this toxic metal, especially in its organic form, is a well-recognized problem for populations whose diet includes a high intake of fish (Turner et al., 1980). However, there is evidence that fish that accumulate mercury also accumulate selenium in equivalent amounts and the simultaneous presence of the selenium is believed to be able to counteract the toxic effects of the mercury.

A study of a population of Inuit sealers in East Greenland whose daily intake of marine foods was made up of 200 g of fish and 180 g of seal meat, found that blood mercury levels often exceeded 200 μg/l, a level regarded as the lowest concentrations observed in clinical methyl mercury intoxication (Margolin, 1980). In spite of these high levels of mercury, there were no signs of toxicity. This was attributed to the presence of high levels of selenium in the fish and seal meat consumed by the sealers and their families (Hansen et al., 1984).

This view is supported by a study of residents of the Faroe Islands (Grandjean et al., 1992). The Faroes are a group of islands in the North Atlantic, with a population of about 45,000 whose main occupation is fishing. Their consumption of marine foods is very high by world standards, with a daily intake by adults of 72 g of fish, 12 g of whale meat, and 7 g of seal blubber. Levels of mercury, much of which is methylated, and of selenium in these foods are high. These are reflected in blood levels of the islanders. A median level of 24.2 μg/l (range 13 to 40 μg/l) of mercury and 110 μg/l (range 100 to 122 μg/l) of selenium were found in umbilical cord blood of more than 1,000 neonates. Mercury and selenium levels were significantly correlated, with selenium generally being in excess on a molar basis. No symptoms of mercury toxicity were detected, either in mothers or infants. It was surmised that this was due to the formation of a bis(methyl–mercury)–selenide complex that is less toxic than methyl mercury. It is possible that a high selenium intake may also be responsible for modifying the toxic action of methyl mercury in the Seychelles, another fish-eating island population with a high intake of mercury-rich fish (Clarkson and Strain, 2003).

9.1.4.9 Selenium in Vegetables and Fruits

Selenium levels in plant foods are generally low, usually at <0.1 μg/g (World Health Organization, 1987). This is because plants do not require selenium for growth and, unless the soil is selenium-rich, do not normally accumulate it, except in a few particular instances. Members of the *Allium* family, which includes garlic (*A. sativum*) and onion (*A. cepa*), and contain a variety of sulfur compounds which are responsible for their distinctive odors and flavors, are also able to accumulate significant amounts of selenium, especially if grown on selenium-rich soil. While levels of 0.03 to 0.25 μg selenium/g have been reported in garlic grown on normal soil, this was increased to 68 μg/g when the soil was enriched in selenium. Similarly onion, with about 0.002 to 0.01 μg/g under normal growing conditions, has had its selenium content increased up to 96 μg/g when grown on selenium-enriched soil. In both garlic and onion the increased levels of selenium attributed to the production of organoselenium compounds, including Se-methyl selenocysteine (Block, 1998).

In a similar manner, though to a lesser extent, leafy members of the *Brassica* family, such as broccoli (*B. oleracea*), which also contain organic compounds of selenium, can accumulate relatively high levels of selenium. When grown on enriched soil they have been shown to accumulate up to 1.5 μg/g of selenium (Finley et al., 2004).

Mushrooms have also been shown to be able to provide a not insignificant amount of selenium to the diet, even without being grown on enriched soil or compost. Levels of 0.08 to 0.1 μg/g (wet wt.) have been reported in the UK (Thorn et al., 1978), and 0.13 μg/g (wet wt.) in ordinary store-bought mushrooms (*Agaricus spp.*) in the USA (Morris and Levander, 1970). A Finnish study of several different species of wild mushroom used for human consumption, found considerable differences in selenium levels between species, with 17 μg/g (dry wt.) in *Boletus edulis*, compared to 2.1 μg/g (dry wt.) in *Agaricus spp.* (Piepponen et al., 1983). Mushrooms grown on enriched growing medium can contain more than 100 μg/g (dry wt.) of selenium (Lázló and Csaba, 2004).

9.1.4.10 Selenium in Brazil and Other Nuts

Certain types of tree nut, especially those of tropical origin, can contain relatively high levels of selenium. A UK study found levels of 0.17 to 0.39 µg/g in cashew nuts, 0.049 to 0.08 in coconut, and 0.034 to 0.087 in macademia nuts, all three imported, compared to 0.008 to 0.036 in locally grown hazelnut (Barclay et al., 1995). None of these nuts approached the levels of 0.85 to 6.86, with a mean of 2.54 µg/g found in the same study in Brazil nuts. Brazil nuts have been reported to be the richest natural source of dietary selenium. In the US nuts purchased in supermarkets averaged 36 ± 50 µg/g, with the extraordinarily high level of 512 µg in an individual nut. However, not all Brazil nuts contain such high levels, and concentrations, even in batches of nuts from the same source, can be highly variable. The nuts are produced by *Bertholletia excelsa*, a large tree that grows in the tropical rainforest of the Amazon basin in South America. Concentrations of selenium in the nuts depend on how effectively the element is taken up by the roots from the soil. This is dependent on the maturity of the root system and the variety of the tree, as well as on the concentration and the chemical form of the selenium in the soil, soil pH, and other factors (Reilly, 1999).

Brazil nuts are harvested from naturally grown forest trees over an enormous area of the Amazon basin, in Brazil, Bolivia, and neighboring countries. Not all soil types and conditions across the growing areas are the same. In some, such as the Manaus to Belem region, stretching for nearly 1,000 miles across the lower reaches of the Amazon basin, soil levels of available selenium are high. Nuts from the region contain between 1.25 and 512.0 µg/g, with an average of 36.0 ± 50.0 µg/g. In contrast, nuts from the Acre–Rondonia region, on the upper Amazon, where soil selenium levels are low, contain on average of 3.06 ± 4.01 µg/g, with a range of 0.03 to 3.17 µg (Sector and Lisk, 1989). Such differences can account for the range of 0.085 to 6.86 µg/g in Brazil nuts sold in the UK (Molnar et al., 1995).

While Brazil nuts can be considered as a good, if somewhat variable, source of dietary selenium and have been advocated as an ideal dietary supplement, it is well to recognize that there could also be a health hazard (Reilly, 1999). Brazil nut kernels average about 3 g in weight. If the selenium content of one kernel was to be 50 µg/g, a level not infrequently found in some on sale in supermarkets, consumption of just three nuts could result in ingestion of about 450 µg of the element. This is the amount of selenium that the UK Department of Health considers to be the safe maximum intake for an adult. Half a nut could well exceed the safe maximum intake of a 10 kg infant (Department of Health, 1991).

9.2 Selenium in Drinking Water

Although generally selenium levels in water used for domestic purposes, in the absence of contamination from industrial or other sources, are very low, there are occasions on which selenium intake in water is unacceptably high. Usually levels in natural surface and domestic fresh water are less than a few micrograms per litre. A maximum standard of 0.01 mg/l has been set by WHO (World Health Organization, 1971). This standard has been adopted by many countries, including the USA (US Public Health Service, 1967). Typical concentrations in domestic, piped, water supplies in many countries range between 0.05 and 5 μg/l (Oelschlager and Menke, 1969). A mean concentration of 0.06 μg/l have been recorded in Australian urban water (Tinggi et al., 1992).

Higher levels of selenium in domestic water supplies are found in a number of countries. In an area of China in which endemic human selenosis occurs, levels up to 12.27 μg/l have been recorded (Yang et al., 1989). Well water in a small municipality in northern Italy was found to have a mean concentration of 7 μg/l, leading to a ban by health authorities on its use (Vivoli et al., 1993). In areas of high soil selenium in South Dakota in the USA, a very high level of 1.6 mg/l was recorded in well water used for human consumption (Byers, 1936). An extreme case, though not used for domestic purposes, was the finding of levels of 260 mg/l in runoff from irrigated crops into the Kesterton reserve in the San Joaquin Valley, California, where environmental contamination with selenium is a serious problem (University of California Agricultural Issues Center, 1998). However, apart from such special situations, drinking water is unlikely to be a significant source of selenium in the human diet.

References

Adams, M.L., Lombi, E., Zhao, F.J., and McGrath, S.P., 2002, Evidence of low selenium concentrations in UK bread-making wheat grain, *J. Food Sci. Agric.* **82**, 116–1165.

Alejos, M.S. and Romero, C.D., 1995, Selenium concentrations in milk, *Food Chem.* **52**, 1–18.

AMAP, 1998, *Heavy Metals*, in: *Assessment Report: Arctic Pollution Issues*, Arctic Monitoring and Assessment Programme, Oslo, Norway, Chapter 7, pp. 373–524, cited in: Hansen, J.C., 2000, Dietary selenium intake among Greenlanders, *Selenium-Tellurium Development Association Bulletin*, October, STDA, Grimbergen, Belgium.

Barclay, M.N.I., MacPherson, A., and Dixon, J., 1995, Selenium content of a range of UK foods, *J. Food Comp. Anal.* **8**, 307–318.

Block, E., 1998, The organosulfur and organoselenium components of garlic and onions, in: Bidlack, W.R., Omaye, S.T., Meskin, M.S., and Jahner, D. (eds), *Phytochemicals — a New Paradigm*, Technomic, Lancaster, PA, pp. 129–141.

British Nutrition Foundation, 2001, *Briefing Papers: Selenium and Health*, British Nutrition Foundation, London, p. 5.

Byers, H.G., 1936, Selenium occurrence in certain soils in the United States, with a discussion of certain topics, *US Department of Agriculture Technical Bulletin*, No. 530, pp. 1–78, USDA, Washington, DC.

Clarkson, T.W. and Strain, J.J., 2003, Nutritional factors may modify the toxic action of methyl mercury in fish-eating populations, *J. Nutr.* **133**, 1539S–1543S.

Combs, G.F., 2001, Selenium in global food systems, *Br. J. Nutr.* **85**, 517–547.

Cumming, F.J., Fardy, J.J., and Woodward, D.R., 1992, Selenium and human lactation in Australia: milk and blood selenium levels in lactating women, and selenium intakes of their breast-fed infants, *Acta Paediatr.* **81**, 292–295.

Debski, B., Finley, D.A., Picciano, M.F., Lonnerdal, B., and Milner, J., 1989, Selenium content and glutathione peroxidase activity of milk from vegetarian and nonvegetarian women, *J. Nutr.* **119**, 215–220.

Department of Health, 1991, Dietary Reference Values for Food Energy and Nutrients for the United Kingdom. *Report on Health and Social Subjects* 41, HMSO, London.

Dorea, J.G., 2002, Selenium and breast-feeding, *Br. J. Nutr.* **88**, 443–461.

Finley, J.W., Grusak, M.A., Keck, A.S., and Gregoire, B.R., 2004, Bioavailability of selenium from meat and broccoli as determined by retention and distribution of Se-75, *Biol. Trace Elem. Res.* **99**, 191–204.

Food Standards Agency, 2002, *McCance and Widdowson's The Composition of Foods*, 6th summary edition, Royal Society of Chemistry, Cambridge, UK.

Funk, M.A., Hamlin, L., Picciano, M.F., and Milner, J.A., 1990, Milk selenium of rural African women: influence of maternal nutrition, parity, and length of lactation, *Am. J. Clin. Nutr.* **51**, 220–224.

Grandjean, P., Weihe, P., Jorgensen, P., et al., 1992, Impact of maternal seafood diet on fetal exposure to mercury, selenium and lead, *Arch. Environ. Health* **47**, 185–195.

Hansen, J.C., Kromann, N., and Wulf, H.C., 1984, Selenium and its interrelation with mercury in wholeblood and hair in an East Greenland population, *Sci. Tot. Environ.* **38**, 33–40.

Higashi, A., Nommsen, L.A., Kuroki, Y., and Matsuda, I., 1983, Longitudinal changes in selenium content of breast milk, *Acta Paediatr. Scand.* **72**, 433–436.

Hinks, L.J., Inwards, K.D., Lloyd, B., and Clayton, B.E., 1984, Body content of selenium in coeliac disease, *Br. Med. J.* **288**, 1862–1863.

Holden, J.M., Gebhardt, S., Davis, C.S., and Lurie, D.G., 1991, A nationwide study of the selenium contents and variability in white bread, *J. Food Comp. Anal.* **4**, 183–195.

Holland, B., Welch, A.A., Unwin, D., et al., 1991, *Mc Cance and Widdowson's The Composition of Foods*, 5th edn., Royal Society of Chemistry/Ministry of Agriculture, Fisheries and Food, London.

Institute of Medicine, 1991, *Nutrition During Lactation*, National Academy Press, Washington, DC.

Institute of Medicine, 2000, *Dietary Reference Intakes for Vitamin C, Vitamin E, Selenium, and Carotenoids*, National Academy Press, Washington, DC, p. 308, http://www.nap.edu/books/0309069351/html/308.html.

Iyengar, V. and Wooittiez, J, 1988, Trace elements in human clinical specimens: evaluation of literature to identify reference values, *Clin. Chem.* **34**, 474–481.

Koutnik, V. and Ingr, I., 1998, Meat as a source of selenium in human nutrition, *Fleischwirtschaft* **78**, 534–536.

Kuhnlein, H.V., Chan, H.M., Leggee, D., and Barthet, V., 2002, Macronutrient, mineral and fatty acid composition of Canadian Arctic traditional food, *J. Food Comp. Anal.* **15**, 545–566.

Labbé, M.R., Trick, K.D., and Koshy, A., 1996, The selenium content of Canadian infant formulas and breast milk, *J. Food Comp. Anal.* **9**, 119–126.

Lázló, R. and Csaba, H., 2004, Iodine and selenium intake from soil to cultivated mushrooms, *2nd International IUPAC Symposium—Trace Metals in Food, Abstracts*, Brussels, Belgium, 7–8 October 2004, p. 21.

Levander, O.A., Moser, P.B., and Morris, V.C., 1987, Dietary selenium intake and selenium concentrations of plasma and breast milk in pregnant and postpartum lactating and nonlactating women, *Am. J. Clin. Nutr.* **46**, 694–698.

Lombeck, I., Kasparek, K., Bonnermann, B., et al., 1975, Selenium content of human milk, cow's milk and cow's milk infant formulas, *Eur. J. Pedriatr.* **129**, 139–145.

Margolin, S., 1980, Mercury in marine seafood: the scientific medical margin of safety as a guide to the potential risk to public health, *World Rev. Nutr. Diet* **34**, 182–265.

Marro, N., 1996, *The 1994 Australian Market Basket Survey*, Australian Government Publishing Service, Canberra, p. 116.

McNaughton, S.A. and Marks, G.C., 2002, Selenium content of Australian food: a review of literature values, *J. Food Comp. Anal.* **15**, 169–182.

Ministry of Agriculture, Fisheries and Food, 1996, *National Food Survey 1995*, HMSO, London.

Ministry of Agriculture, Fisheries and Food, 1999, *Metals and Other Elements in Infant Foods*, Joint Food Safety and Standards Group Food Surveillance Information Sheet, No. 190, http://www.foodstandards.gov.uk/ma...ood/infsheet/1999/no190/190inf.htm.

Molnar, J., MacPherson, A., Barclay, I., and Molnar, P., 1995, Selenium content of convenience and fast foods in Ayreshire, Scotland, *Int. J. Food Sci. Nutr.* **82**, 343–352.

Morris, V.C. and Levander, O.A., 1970, Selenium content of foods, *J. Nutr.* **100**, 1383–1388.

Murphy, J. and Cashman, K.D., 2001, Selenium content of a range of Irish foods, *Food Chem.* **74**, 493–498.

Murphy, J., Hannon, E.M., Kieley, M., Flynn, A., and Cashman, K.D., 2002, Selenium intakes in 18–64-y-old Irish adults, *Eur. J. Clin. Nutr.* **56**, 402–408.

Oelschlager, W. and Menke, K.H., 1969, Concerning the selenium content of plant, animal and other materials. II. The selenium and sulfur content of foods (in German, English Abstract), *Zeitschrift für Ernahrungswissenschaft* **9**, 216–222.

Peattie, M.E., Buss, D.H., Lindsay, D.G., and Smart, G.A., 1983, Reorganization of the British Total Diet Study for monitoring food constituents from 1981, *Food Chem. Toxicol.* **21**, 503–507.

Pennington, J.A.T., 1983, Revision of total diet study food lists and diets, J. *Am. Diet Assoc.* **82**, 166–173.

Pennington, J.A.T., 1992, Revision of Food and Drug Administration's total diet study, *J. Nutr. Educ.* **24**, 173–178.

Pennington, J.A.T., 2001, Use of the core food model to estimate mineral intakes. Part 1. Selection of US core foods, *J. Food Comp. Anal.* **14**, 295–300.

Pennington, J.A.T. and Young, B., 1990, Iron, zinc, copper, manganese, selenium, and iodine in foods from the United States Total Diet Study, *J. Food Comp. Anal.* **3**, 166–184.

Piepponen, S., Liukkonen-Lilja, H., and Kuusi, T., 1983, The selenium content of edible mushrooms in Finland, *Zeitschrift für Lebensmittel Untersuchung und Forschung* [*Z.Lebensm. Unters. Forsch.*] **177**, 257–260.

Räihä, N.C., 1989, Protein quality and whey-casein ratio in infant formulas, in: Atkinson, S.A. and Lönnerdal, B. (eds), *Protein and NonProtein Nitrogen in Human Milk*, CRC Press, Boca Raton, FL, pp. 137–144.

Reilly, C., 1996, *Selenium in Food and Health*, 1st edn., Blackie Academic and Professional, London, p. 203.

Reilly, C., 1999, Brazil nuts—a selenium supplement? *BNF Nutr. Bull.* **24**, 177–184.

Rodríguez, E.M., Sanz Alaejos, M., and Díaz Romero, C., 1998, Concentrations of selenium in human milk, *Zeitschrift für Lebensmittel Untersuchung und Forschung* **207**, 174–179.

Schubert, A., Holden, J.M., and Wolfe, W.R., 1987, Selenium content of a core group of foods based on a critical evaluation of published analytical data, *J. Am. Dietet. Assoc.* **87**, 285–299.

Sector, C.L. and Lisk, D.J., 1989, Variations in the selenium content of individual Brazil nuts, *J. Food Safety* **9**, 279–281.

Shirichakwal, P.P., Puwastien, P., Polngam, J., and Kongkachuichai, R., 2005, Selenium content of Thai food, *J. Food Comp. Anal.* **18**, 47–59.

Smith, A.M., Picciano, M.F., and Milner, J.A., 1982, Selenium intakes and status of human milk and formula fed infants, *Am. J. Clin. Nutr.* **35**, 521–526.

Thomson, C.D. and Robinson, M.F., 1980, Selenium in human health and disease with emphasis on those aspects particular to New Zealand, *Am. J. Clin. Nutr.* **33**, 303–323.

Thorn, J., Robertson, J., Bass, D.H., and Bunton, N.G., 1978, Trace nutrients: selenium in British foods, *Br. J. Nutr.* **39**, 391–396.

Tinggi, U., Reilly, C., and Patterson, C.M., 1992, Determination of selenium in foodstuffs using spectrofluorimetry and hydride generation atomic absorption spectrophotometry, *J. Food Comp. Anal.* **5**, 269–280.

Tinggi, U., Patterson, C., and Reilly, C., 2001, Selenium levels in cow's milk from different regions in Australia, *Int. J. Food Sci. Nutr.* **52**, 43–51.

Turner, M.D., Marsh, D.O., Smith, J.C., et al., 1980, Methyl mercury in populations eating large quantities of marine fish, *Arch. Environ. Health* **35**, 367–378.

University of California Agricultural Issues Center, 1998, Selenium, human health and agricultural issues, in: *Resources at Risk in the San Joaquin Valley*, University of California, Davis, CA.

US Public Health Service, 1967, *Code of Regulations, Drinking Water*, Title 42, US Public Health Service, Washington, DC.

Versieck, J. and Cornelis, R., 1989, *Trace Elements in Human Plasma or Serum*, CRC Press, Boca Raton, FL, p. 76.

Vivoli, G., Vinceti, M., Rovesti, M., and Bergomi, M., 1993, Selenium in drinking water and mortality for chronic diseases. in: Anke, M., Meissner, D., and Mills, C.F. (eds), *Trace Elements in Man and Animals—TEMA 8*, Verlag Media Touristik, Gersdorf, Germany, pp. 951–954.

Vlieg, P., 1990, Selenium concentration of edible part of 74 New Zealand fish species, *J. Food Comp. Anal.* **3**, 67–72.

Wang, G., Parpia, B., and Wen, Z., 1997, *The Composition of Chinese Foods*, Institute of Nutrition and Food Hygiene, Chinese Academy of Preventive Medicine, ILSI Press, Washington, DC.

World Health Organization, 1971, *International Standards for Drinking Water*, World Health Organization, Geneva.

World Health Organization, 1987, *Selenium. A Report of the International Programme on Chemical Safety.* Environmental Health Criteria 58, World Health Organization, Geneva.

World Health Organization/International Atomic Energy Agency, 1989, *Minor and Trace Elements in Milk*, World Health Organization, Geneva, p. vii.

Yang, G., Zhou, R., Gu, L., and Li, X., 1989, Studies of safe maximal daily dietary selenium intake in the seleniferous area of China. I. Selenium intake and tissue selenium levels of the inhabitants, *Trace Elem. Health Dis.* **3**, 77–87.

Yoshida, M. and Yasumoto, K., 1987, Selenium contents of rice grown at various sites in Japan, *J. Food Comp. Anal.* **1**, 71–75.

10 Selenium in Diets

10.1 Selenium Status and Dietary Intakes

Since dietary intakes of selenium generally depend on levels of the element in the soil on which the foods consumed are produced, and since soil selenium levels can show considerable differences between different parts of the world, per capita intakes can vary widely between countries. Other factors, besides soil levels, can also be involved, such as geographical conditions, agricultural practices, type of diet, whether vegetarian or meat-eating, rich in fish or not and, not least, the economic conditions of the consumers. The worldwide range in selenium status is reflected in selenium levels in plasma or serum as recorded in different countries. Although blood levels do not necessarily provide an ideal criterion for assessing selenium status, they do give a useful overall indication of the dietary intakes on which blood levels depend. This is illustrated by data reviewed in Combs' detailed review of selenium in global food systems (Combs, 2001). This includes a table of blood selenium concentrations of healthy adults reported from 69 different countries, from Austria to Zambia. These range from a low of 15 ± 2 μg/l in Burundi, to a high of 315 ± 135 μg/l in Venezuela and nearly 500 μg/l in a selenosis region of China. Some of this data is reproduced here in Table 10.1.

These interregional differences in selenium status, as indicated by blood selenium levels, can, as Combs notes, be interpreted as manifestations of differences in food composition and intake. Combs also makes the pertinent comment that, due to differences in geography, agronomic practices, food availability, and preferences, most of which are difficult to quantify, evaluations of selenium intakes of different human population groups are seldom specific. The same can be said of evaluations of selenium status, especially when these are based on measurement of blood levels of the element. Nevertheless, such evaluations are useful in providing an overall picture of the situation in different countries and communities

TABLE 10.1 Mean selenium levels in serum or plasma of healthy adults in different countries

Country	Selenium level (μg/l)	Reference
Austria	67 ± 24	Tiran et al. (1992)
Australia	91 ± 12	McOrist and Fardy (1989)
Canada	146 ± 27	Vézina et al. (1996)
China (Eastern urban areas)	80 ± 10	Whanger et al. (1994)
(Keshan areas)	21 ± 6	Whanger et al. (1994)
(Selenosis areas)	494 ± 140	Whanger et al. (1994)
England	88 ± 21	Thuluvath and Vath (1992)
Finland (pre-1984)	66 ± 11	Westermarck (1977)
(post-1984)	110 ± 8	Korpela et al. (1989)
France	83 ± 4	Ducros et al. (1997)
Germany	86 ± 13	Meissner (1997)
Ireland	94 ± 14	Darling et al. (1992)
Italy	87 ± 17	Casaril et al. (1995)
Japan	117 ± 16	Matsuda et al. (1997)
The Netherlands	69 ± 6	Van der Torre et al. (1991)
New Zealand (South Island)	53 ± 6	Thomson and Robinson (1993)
Norway	119 ± 16	Meltzer and Huang (1995)
Spain	94 ± 3	Ferrer et al. (1999)
Turkey	71 ± 2	Ozata et al. (1999)
USA (Eastern states)	113 ± 15	Salvini et al. (1995)
(Central states)	133 ± 15	Smith et al. (2000)
Zaire	82 ± 3	Vanderpas et al. (1993)

Source: Adapted from Combs, G.F., 2001, Selenium in global food systems, *Br. J. Nutr.* **85**, 517–547.

10.2 Dietary Intakes of Selenium in Different Countries

On the basis of data available in the scientific literature, it can be estimated that the normal average per capita adult intake of selenium worldwide ranges from about 10 to 200 μg/day. When extremes of intake, as seen in such areas as the Keshan and selenosis regions of China, are included, the range is dramatically increased to about 3 to >6,500 μg/day, as is shown in Table 10.2. This represents a spread from, at the lower end, intakes capable of causing severe clinical deficiency to, at the upper, chronic and acute selenosis, with, in between, what the US Food and Nutrition Board (1980) considered to be the Estimated Safe and Adequate Daily Dietary Intake (ESADDI) for selenium of 50 to 200 μg.

TABLE 10.2 Dietary intakes of selenium in countries with extreme soil selenium levels

Country	Intake (μg/day) (range)	Reference
China:		
Enshi Province	3200–6690	Yang et al. (1983)
Keshan area	3–11	Yang et al. (1983)
Venezuela	80–500	Brätter et al. (1993)
New Zealand	5–102	Stewart et al. (1978)
Finland (pre-1984)	25–60	Mutanen et al. (1983)

There are, however, problems in compiling a table of dietary intakes of selenium in different countries based on published results. The data reported for individual countries vary considerably, depending on the methods used to assess intakes, as well as on several other causes, not least, whether the findings were based on a truly representative population sample. Even in the UK, which, geographically and demographically, is relatively homogeneous, estimates of intake reported by different investigators in the same year can differ considerably, from 234 μg/day (Cross et al., 1978) to 60 μg/day (Thorn et al., 1978), and, more recently, 30 μg/day (MacPherson et al., 1993) to 62 μg/day (Butcher et al., 1994).

A major reason for variation in selenium intakes between countries is, of course, the difference in food consumption patterns and, especially, in the types of staple foods consumed. The major sources of selenium in many diets are cereals, meat products, and seafoods. Only small amounts are usually contributed by dairy products, and still less by vegetables and fruits. A US survey found that five foods, beef, pork, chicken, eggs, and bread contributed about 50% of the total in a typical diet (Schubert et al., 1987). In the UK, the relative contributions to selenium intake made by different components of the diet are, meat and meat products 32%, bread and cereals 22%, dairy products and eggs 22%, vegetables 6%, and other foods 5%, including 1.2% of the latter from nuts (Ministry of Agriculture, Fisheries and Food, 1999).

While differences in eating practices, especially in relation to the relative amounts of cereal and meat consumed, can be assumed to account for some of the considerable differences in overall intake of selenium between certain countries, for example, 29 μg/day in Egypt (Maxia et al., 1972) compared to 224 μg/day in Canada (Thomson et al., 1975), they can also account for interindividual variations within large population groups (Combs, 2001).

Table 10.3 gives a selection of estimated daily selenium intakes by adults in a number of countries. These range from a low of 3 μg/day in parts of China where endemic selenium deficiency occurs, to a high of nearly 5 mg/day in another part of the same country where selenosis has been reported. In a country like New Zealand that has a history of selenium-deficiency diseases in farm animals, human selenium intake is approximately 2 to 10 times higher than in the selenium-deficient parts of China, nevertheless still well below adequate intake (AI) levels. Although less extreme than levels reported in China, average intakes in Venezuela approach the limits of safe intake. In between these extremes, intakes in many countries appear to be both safe and adequate.

10.3 Variations in Dietary Intakes Between Countries and Population Groups

Since meat and fish are, for some the principal sources of dietary selenium, it might be expected that people who for various reasons do not consume these foods at all, or only in limited amounts, could be at risk of having an inadequate intake of

TABLE 10.3 Estimated selenium intakes (μg/day) of adults in different countries

Country	Intake (mean and/or range)	Reference
Australia	55–87	McOrist and Fardy (1989)
Bangladesh	63–122	Bieri and Ahmed (1976)
Belgium	30	Amiard et al. (1993)
Canada	98–224	Giessel-Nielsen (1998)
China (Eastern urban areas)	53–80	Zhang et al. (2001)
(Keshan areas)	7–11	Combs and Combs (1986)
(Selenosis areas)	750–4990	Yang et al. (1989)
England	29–60	BNF (2001)
Finland (pre-1984)	25–60	Westermarck (1977)
(post-1984)	67–110	Korpela et al. (1989)
France	29–43	Ducros et al. (1997)
Germany	38–47	Oster and Prellwitz (1989)
India	28–105	Dang et al. (2001)
Ireland	44	Murphy et al. (2002)
Japan	104–127	Yoshita et al. (1998)
Mexico	61–73	Valentine et al. (1994)
New Zealand (South Island)	19–80	Thomson and Robinson (1993)
Poland	30–40	Wasowicz et al. (2003)
Russia	54–80	Aro and Alfthan (1998)
Serbia	30	Djujic et al. (1995)
Slovakia	27–43	Kadrabová et al. (1998)
Turkey	18–53	Aras et al. (2001)
USA	60–220	Longnecker et al. (2001)
Venezuela	200–350	Combs and Combs (1986)

the trace element. However, this is not necessarily so, especially if cereals are consumed in sufficient quantity.

10.3.1 Selenium Intake by Vegans and Other Vegetarians

A UK study did find that the mean dietary intake of a group of vegetarians was 28 μg/day, which is lower than that of the general population (Ministry of Agriculture, Fisheries and Food, 2000). However, another study found higher selenium intakes by vegetarians than by nonvegetarians (Gregory et al., 2000). In contrast, Lightowler and Davies (2000) who studied micronutrient intake in a group of UK vegans, some of whom were using dietary supplements, found that the selenium intake of 65% of the nonsupplement users was below the UK's Lower Reference Nutrient Intake (LRNI) of 40 μg/day (Department of Health, 1991). Even in those who were taking supplements, selenium intakes of 33% of the group were below the LRNI.

10.3.2 Selenium Intake by Young Swedish Vegans

A Swedish study (Larsson and Johansson, 2002) has confirmed these findings. The diet of a group of 30 vegans (15 of each sex, with a mean age of 17.5 ± 1.0 years) was found to contain higher intakes of vegetables, including legumes, as well as dietary supplements, and lower intakes of cakes and other confectionery and chocolates, than did that of omnivores. In spite of their consumption of nutritional supplements, the vegans had less selenium in their diet than did the omnivores.

10.3.3 Selenium Intake by Sikh Vegetarians

Selenium levels in the diet of 196 Sikh migrants, both male and female, living in Sydney, Australia, were investigated as part of a study into possible causes of their higher than average risk of cardiovascular disease than other residents of the city (Dhindsa et al., 1998). Twenty percent of the subjects were vegetarians, none were smokers, all the females were teetotal, while more than half of the males drank alcohol. The mean age was 36.5 ± 11.5 years, with a range of 18 to 73 years. The overall mean selenium level in plasma of the whole group was 91.8 ± 15.0 µg/l, which was comparable to that reported for the general population. Levels in the same gender group for vegetarians and nonvegetarians were similar. However, a significantly higher mean level was observed in vegetarian males than in females (93.7 ± 12.1 v. 81.0 ± 11.1 µg/l). It was concluded by the investigators that, even though a vegetarian diet is common in the group, as is the use of alcohol by males, selenium intake and status were adequate.

10.3.4 Selenium Intake in Fish-Eating Populations

The effect of eating marine foods on selenium intake and status is demonstrated clearly in Greenland, as has been noted by Hansen (2000). The North Atlantic island has a population of some 55,000, of which 87% are Inuit, and 13% nonInuit, mainly Danes. Although in recent years consumption of traditional foods by the Inuit has been decreasing, and has been largely replaced by imported foods from Denmark, fish and other marine products still make up a high proportion of food intake, especially in the hunting areas of the north

The traditional foods eaten by the hunting Inuit are rich in selenium. Whale liver levels can contain between approximately 2 and 24 µg selenium/g, seal liver 35 µg/g, while muscle of seabirds, such as common eider and little auk, contain up to 5 µg/g, while their liver levels can range from about 1.0 to more than 20 µg/g. A diet rich in such foods is reflected in the high selenium status of traditional Greenlanders. Mean whole blood selenium levels of 2,563 (range 880 to 4,400) µg/l have been recorded in Inuit villagers living in the Thule district, in the north. In contrast, Danish immigrants living in the same district, whose diet consisted largely of imported food, had a mean blood level of 68, with a range of 40 to 80 µg/l (Hansen and Pedersen, 1986).

A significant comment made by Hansen (2000) is that although 66% of the Inuit had blood levels and intakes well above 1,000 µg/l, well above the level of 400 µg/day considered to be the maximum safe intake in China (Yang et al., 1989), no symptoms of selenosis, apart from longitudinal striation on the nails, had been reported. The reasons for this are not clear, though they possibly include adaptations to a high selenium intake and interactions with other antagonistic trace elements, including mercury. Speciation of the ingested selenium in the marine foods, as well as seasonal variation in exposure and intake of other antioxidant micronutrients may also play a part. Hansen concluded that these findings indicate that selenium supplied through a marine diet can be tolerated at levels much higher than the normally considered safe. This is a view that had already been put forward 20 years before by Margolin (1980) as well as by Ohi et al. (1980), though from a consideration of levels of mercury, rather than of selenium in seafoods.

Although not to the levels found in the Inuit of Greenland, selenium levels in blood of another island people were also found to be high as a result of consuming large amounts of fish and other seafoods. The Faroe Islands, which lie between Scotland and Iceland, has a population of about 50,000 people whose principal occupation is fishing. The average daily adult intake of fish is 72 g, along with 12 g of whale muscle and 7 g of seal blubber (Grandjean et al., 1992). All of these foods are rich in both mercury and selenium. An investigation of levels in umbilical cord blood from more than 1,000 births found that mercury averaged 24.2 μg/l (range 13 to 40 μg/l) and selenium 110 μg/l (range 100 to 122 μg/l). The mercury and selenium levels were significantly correlated ($r_s = 0.35$; $p < 0.001$), with selenium generally in excess on a molar basis. The investigators surmised that the selenium ingested offered some protection against mercury toxicity.

10.4 Changes in Dietary Intakes of Selenium

Records of dietary intakes in some countries and regions show that, over recent decades, there have been significant changes in the levels of selenium in the diet. These changes have been attributed to a number of causes, from direct intervention by health authorities, especially provision of dietary supplements, to indirect effects of changes in economic and trade conditions. The increase in selenium intake and the corresponding fall observed in recent years in occurrence of both Keshan and Kashin-Beck disease in China, is a good example of both of these effects (Wang et al., 1987; Ge and Yang, 1993). A search of the literature shows that similar changes in selenium status, with possible effects on health, have occurred in several other regions of the world.

10.4.1 Changes in Selenium Intake in Finland

In the 1980s health authorities in Finland became concerned that selenium intakes of the general population were suboptimal and that there was a possibility of a serious public health problem. It was decided that a dramatic dietary intervention was required to prevent this happening (Ministry of Agriculture and Forestry, 1984). A law was passed which required that sodium selenate be added to all multielement agricultural fertilizers used in the country. The intention was that, by increasing levels of available selenium in the soil, levels in crops and animal feeds, and consequently in human foods, would also be increased, leading to an improvement in national selenium status.

The decision was based on the knowledge that Finnish soils were selenium-poor and that locally produced plant and animal foodstuffs had lower levels of the element than did imported products, especially those from North America (Koljonen, 1975). It had also been shown that dietary selenium intakes in Finland were about 25 to 60 μg/day, which were then believed to be among the lowest in the world (Mutanen and Koivistoinen, 1983).

The enrichment law required that, starting in Spring 1985, sodium selenate was to be added to all NPK (nitrogen–phosphorus–potassium) fertilizers at a rate of 16 mg/kg on cereals and 6 mg/kg on grassland. The effects were almost immediate and remarkable. Within the first growing season, increased levels of selenium were observed in animal feeds and in a variety of human foods. Cow's milk was the first food to show an increase, rising from a prefertilization level of 0.02 to 0.19 μg/g (both dry wt.). This was followed by meat, with, for example, pork from 0.02 to 0.70 μg/g (dry wt). Notable increases were also observed in vegetables and cereals. A particularly impressive change occurred in broccoli, with an increase from <0.01 to 1.70 μg/g (dry wt.).

These increases in selenium concentrations in foods were accompanied by significant increases in dietary levels of the element. Selenium intakes in adults increased two- and three-fold compared to presupplementation levels over the first year of intervention. By the 3rd year intakes had reached 110 to 120 μg/10 MJ, or approximately 100 μg/day (Varo et al., 1994). Indeed, so successful was the outcome that concerns were raised about possible adverse effects of high selenium intakes on animal and human health. As a result, in 1990, it was decided to decrease the required supplementation levels to 6 mg selenate/kg fertilizer for all crops and grasslands. As a result, by 1993, adult intakes had fallen back to a mean of 85 μg/10 MJ, and serum levels to a mean of 100 μg/l in both urban and rural populations.

The requirement for the addition of selenium to agricultural fertilizers remains in force in Finland. Blood selenium levels continue to be among the highest in Europe and on a par with those observed in North America. Moreover, Finland has not seen the decline in selenium intakes that has been reported in the UK and certain other European countries over the past 2 decades (Rayman, 1997).

Although nationwide supplementation with selenium has been in place in Finland for some 20 years, it is still not clear whether the practice has resulted in improvement in the health of the population. A major reason for this uncertainty is that it is not easy to isolate the effects of a single factor, such as an increased trace element intake, from others that can affect the etiology of conditions such as cancer and heart disease (Froslie, 1993). There have been reports of decreases in heart disease and certain types of cancer in Finland since 1985 (Mussalo-Rauhamaa et al., 1993). These claims have been questioned, however, by other investigators on the grounds that in the absence of adequate controls, they are inconclusive (Giessel-Nielsen, 1994). Although there is evidence that coronary heart disease mortality declined in Finland by 55% among men and 68% among women between 1972 and 1992 (Pietinen et al., 1996), this has been attributed mainly to a reduction in the total fat content of the diet, accompanied by decreased serum cholesterol levels. Other factors involved are believed to be a decrease in smoking as well as of consumption of boiled coffee, as well as a two- to threefold increase in consumption of fruits and vegetables. The question as to whether the selenium supplementation program, which has undoubtedly succeeded in elevating the selenium status of the Finnish population, has had a significant effect on health is still unresolved (Varo et al., 1994). As has been commented by one of the investigating groups (Wang et al., 1998), long-term follow-up studies are still required in order to resolve the question.

No other country has, as yet, followed the example of Finland in legislating for selenium supplementation of the diet through enrichment of fertilizers. New Zealand, where soil selenium levels are also low and selenium deficiency causes serious problems in farm animals, permits, but does not require the use of selenium fertilizers on deficient soil. Although there has been pressure from some health professionals and sections of the public concerned at the low selenium status of many New Zealanders, authorities in the country could see no reason for universal supplementation, though it might be necessary for certain vulnerable groups (Thomson and Robinson, 1980).

10.4.2 The Changing Selenium Status of the UK Population

There is evidence of a substantial fall in dietary selenium intakes in the UK over recent decades. Nearly 30 years ago Thorn et al. (1978) found that the average selenium intake of UK adults was 60 μg/day. Similar intakes continued to be reported throughout the 1980s, but by 1994 they averaged 43 μg/day (BNF, 2001). In 1995 the Laboratory of the Government Chemist (LGC) estimated that intakes by adults ranged from 29 to 39 μg/day (Ministry of Agriculture, Fisheries and Food, 1997).

The current UK Reference Nutrient Intake (RNI) is 75 μg/day for men and 60 μg/day for women. These levels are considered to be necessary to maximize activity of GPX in blood that occurs at a plasma selenium concentration of about 95 (range 89 to 114) μg/l (MacPherson et al., 1997). Recently recorded levels of intake by UK adults are considerably below RNI and are close to LRNI of 40 μg/day. The LNRI is an intake, which is estimated to meet the needs of only a few people in the population who have a low need for a nutrient (Ministry of Agriculture, Fisheries and Food, 1997).

Similar falls in selenium intakes have been observed in other countries in Europe and the decline has been reflected in a decrease in blood selenium levels. Plasma selenium levels in seven countries of the European Union (EU), as noted by Rayman (1997) fell from around 100 to 79 μg/l between 1983 and 1993. This reduction, she notes, could have implications for normal cell metabolism and disease risk, and points to a need to increase levels of selenium in the diet, as has been done in Finland.

10.4.3 Effect of Changes in Wheat Imports on Selenium Intakes

There is evidence that the decline in selenium intake in UK and certain other countries is to an extent due to a reduction in the importation of selenium-rich high protein wheat and bread-making flour from North America. In 1970 the proportion of wheat used in the UK that was imported from North America was 45%. By 1995 this had fallen to 30%, and by 1993 to 15%. The reason for the reduction was twofold: firstly, EU policy required the substitution of local and, though unintended, low-selenium wheat for imported and selenium-rich US and Canadian wheat; secondly, new baking technology allowed hard high-protein North American flour to be replaced by the lower-protein and softer European flour. As a consequence, UK and other European bread contained lower levels of selenium than formerly. There was at the same time a reduction in household consumption of cereals, especially of bread that fell from 1,080 g/person/week in 1970 to 765 g/person/week in 1995 (Ministry of Agriculture, Fisheries and Food, 1997).

Changes in trade patterns which affect importation of wheat have been found to have unexpected consequences on the selenium status of other countries, besides the UK and elsewhere in Europe. The consequences are by no means always to the detriment of nutritional status in importing countries. In Finland it was noted, even before supplementation of fertilizers had been introduced, that importation of US wheat resulted in a marked improvement in selenium intakes of the population (Wang et al., 1998). The high level of serum selenium levels observed in Norway in the late 1980s, the highest known in Europe, were attributed, not to the high consumption of fish, but to the consumption of selenium-rich imported wheat (Solvang and Rimestad, 1985). Importation of US wheat has also been responsible for an increase of selenium intakes in Transbaikalian Russia where soil selenium and locally produced food levels are naturally low (Aro et al., 1994).

10.4.4 Changing Selenium Status in New Zealand

New Zealand, in spite of low selenium levels of its soil and low dietary selenium intakes of its people, did not follow the example of Finland by imposing compulsory nationwide supplementation through the addition of selenium to fertilizers. Instead, voluntary use of selenium-enriched fertilizers and animal feeds was encouraged. This was an option readily adopted by farmers whose cattle and sheep had long, and expensively, suffered from white muscle disease and other selenium deficiency-related conditions (Thomson and Robinson, 1980). Surprisingly, though selenium intakes by farm animals were increased by these means and the incidence of selenium-deficiency disease reduced among herds, an increase in levels of the element in human foodstuffs was not observed nor was the selenium status of the population noticeably improved. Dietary intakes remained at about 28 μg/day and blood levels continued at a mean of 68 μg/l, similar to levels recorded in presupplementation Finland (Reilly, 1996). In spite of this, investigators reported that there was no convincing evidence of selenium-responsive clinical conditions in the general population, and the official policy against imposition of nationwide selenium supplementation was maintained (Thomson and Robinson, 1996).

There have been a number of observations that suggest that there may, in fact, be certain consequences of their low selenium intake at least for some groups in the New Zealand population. An increased risk of myocardial infarction was reported in New Zealanders who had a low selenium status, and were also smokers (Beaglehole et al., 1990). A further indication of a possible association between low selenium intake and cardiovascular health was the finding that selenium supplementation reduced total and LDL cholesterol in subjects with a low selenium status who were hyperlipidemic (Thomson, 1992). Though claims that cot death in New Zealand was related to low selenium intake have not received wide support from experts in the field (Dolamore et al., 1992), there are indications that the high incidence of asthma, particularly among children, may have a selenium connection (Flatt et al., 1990).

As a result of such findings, there has been continuing pressure from some members of the health professions, as well as from sections of the public, for a change in official attitudes towards selenium supplementation and for introduction of legislation similar to that in Finland requiring addition of selenate to fertilizers. However, an unexpected improvement in the selenium status in recent years may have removed the need for official intervention. In 1993 blood selenium levels of New Zealanders were found to be 94 μg/l, compared to around the 61 μg/l recorded 2 decades previously (Thomson and Robinson, 1996). The improvement is believed to have been largely due to deregulation of importation of wheat from Australia and the USA as well as the availability of a variety of imported selenium-rich breakfast cereals (Winterbourne et al., 1992). Other dietary changes, such as an increase in consumption of fish, may also have played a part in the improvement (Public Health Commission, 1993).

10.5 Use of Dietary Supplements to Change Selenium Status

Many people today consume selenium supplements on a regular basis to increase their intake and improve their nutritional status. They do this in the belief either that selenium levels in the diet are inadequate or that the additional intake will provide protection against a variety of health problems. It is widely believed also that selenium plays a protective role against oxidative damage caused by environmental pollutants, ultraviolet radiation, and other hazards of modern living. Casey (1988), in a somewhat critical review, gave the name *selenophilia* (or love of selenium) to what she described as "the current strong interest in the use of selenium, over and above normal and apparently adequate levels of dietary intake, for the prevention, alleviation or cure of a variety of disorders that have not been shown to be directly associated with selenium." However, while some of the expectations of supplement users can be attributed to uncritical reporting of medical matters in the popular media, others are not without support from well recognized and serious health professionals. Indeed much of today's interest in selenium as a supplement was triggered by the report of Clark and his highly professional team, published in 1996 in very highly regarded *Journal of the American Medical Association* (Clark et al., 1996). The group's finding that selenium supplementation, at levels above normally recommended intakes, caused a reduction in risk of certain forms of cancer caused a flurry of interest, in the scientific as well as the general media. The report led many health professionals, as well as nonmedical members of the general public, to accept that selenium has antitumorigenic properties (Combs, 2001). It also contributed to a widescale practice of self-medication, sometimes with high doses of selenium, as a preventive against cancer (Reilly, 1997). According to one recent review (Veatch et al., 2005), the increased use of these products in the USA and elsewhere is the direct result of epidemiological studies that indicate that protection is best provided by a "supranutritional" intake of selenium several times in excess of the nutritional requirement.

The use of dietary supplements in many countries is considerable and appears to be increasing. In the USA more than 62% of respondents to the National Health Survey in 2002 said that they had used a supplement in the previous year. In 1987 the figure had been 23.7% (National Center for Health Statistics, 2005). The NHANES III Survey of 1998–1994 found that 9% of all adults used supplements containing selenium (Institute of Medicine, 2000). Equivalent uses of selenium and other supplements are reported in other countries of the developed world.

Many different types of selenium supplements, with considerable variations in concentrations, are available both as "over-the-counter" (OTC) and medically prescribed products. They include inorganic forms, such as sodium selenite and selenate, defined organic forms, including selenoamino acids, principally selenomethionine and selenocysteine, and more complex organic forms found in selenium-enriched yeast and other foods. The inorganic forms and the selenoamino acids are well-defined chemical entities with known physicochemical characteristics. The selenoamino acids are available as racemates or as either D- or L-isomeric forms (Nève, 1995).

These products are available, normally in tablet form, in quantities up to 200 μg, and sometimes more, per tablet. Though these amounts exceed the recommended daily intakes in the USA and many other countries, a dosage of 200 μg is generally considered safe and adequate for an adult of average weight subsisting on the typical American diet according to Schrauzer (2001).

10.5.1 Selenium-Enriched Yeast

There is some uncertainty about the composition of selenium-enriched yeast. This is usually prepared by growing brewers' or baker's yeast (*Saccharomyces cerevisiae*) in a selenium-rich nutrient medium under conditions of sulfur limitation. This encourages the uptake of selenium to form seleno-analogs of organic compounds of sulfur. The yeast is usually prepared for pharmacological use by isolation and washing, followed by lyophilization, and is then made into tablets (Power, 1995).

Many different commercial preparations of selenium yeast are available. Their chemical composition varies, depending on the different culture conditions used. The preparations can contain different amounts of different selenium compounds, including selenoamino acids, selenoproteins, selenosulfides, and inorganic forms of the element (Korhola et al., 1986). Levels of organically bound selenium have been reported to range, in some commercial preparations of selenium yeast, from 0 to 97% of the total selenium content (Uden et al., 2003). Rayman (2004) found that selenomethione accounted for between 60 and 84% of selenium species in ten different kinds of commercial selenium yeasts. Other species in these yeasts included Se-cystine, Se-cysteine, Se-methyl-Se-cysteine, and Se-cystathione, all at less than 1%. Though a few selenium yeasts contain predominantly selenite or selenate (Schrauzer and McGinness, 1979), the majority of commercial preparations contain mainly selenomethionine (Rayman, 2004).

In 2002 the European Parliament and Council of the EU issued a directive on permitted food supplements. This specified a “positive list” of approved supplements that included inorganic forms of selenium, but not selenium yeast. This means that once the directive is put into effect, the sale of selenium yeast will no longer be permitted in the EU (Rayman 2004). The decision was based on the opinion of the Scientific Committee on Food of the European Commission (EC) that selenium yeast supplements were poorly characterized and that there was danger that selenium from the selenomethionine in the yeast could build up to toxic levels in body tissues.

10.5.2 Selenomethionine in Selenium Yeast

The reasoning behind the directive has been challenged by Rayman in a well-reasoned review. She points to the wide use of selenium yeast, both in carefully monitored clinical trials and as a dietary supplement. She produces evidence to show that, when manufactured by reputable manufacturers, selenium yeast is of reproducible quality and defined selenomethionine content. Moreover there is no evidence of toxicity from selenomethionine even at levels far above the EC tolerable upper limit (UL) of 300 μg/day. This is also the view of Schrauzer (2000) who believes that concern at the possibility that incorporation of selenomethionine into body proteins could increase selenium to toxic levels, is not warranted because a steady state is established, which prevents uncontrolled accumulation of the element. Moreover the release of selenomethionine from body proteins could not result in selenium toxicity since no mechanism for the selective release of selenomethionine during catabolism exists. Indeed, he argues that selenomethionine, or enriched food sources of it, are appropriate forms of selenium for human nutritional supplementation. He believes that, since higher animals cannot synthesize the amino acid, yet from it all needed forms of selenium are produced, selenomethionine meets the criteria for an essential amino acid (Schrauzer, 2003).

10.5.3 Variations in Levels of Selenium in Supplements

The concern expressed by the EC Scientific Committee at the absence of information about the composition of selenium yeast and its poor characterization, has been echoed by others. Combs (2001) noted that published composition data, especially relating to different selenium species in yeast, were very limited. At the time he wrote he could only find information on a single commercial selenium yeast product. He commented that in the absence of compositional information, and with no published standards of product identity for selenium-enriched yeast, it was not clear whether the data he had found described general characteristics of selenium-enriched yeasts or merely specific traits of that particular product. Consumer acceptance, he noted, called for inclusion on labels of information about the selenium content of the product, as well as for the establishment of quality control procedures. These were necessary to minimize risk of selenium overexposure and to ensure delivery of known forms of the element.

The absence of regulations on the purity and potency of supplements, and, in the case of selenium supplements, the hazard associated with the absence of good manufacturing practices has been noted by Veatch et al. (2005). They believe that their neglect accounts for the unacceptable wide variations in levels of selenium sometimes observed even in the same batch of some commercial products. Among the examples they cite is a value of 27.3 mg selenium per tablet in a single manufacturing lot, a value 182 times higher than stated on the label. They believe that this is not an isolated case, and could account for the 13 cases of selenium toxicity from consumption of OTC selenium supplements reported in the USA in 1 year. Their own investigation, which examined levels in 15 commercial products, found differences between their analytical data and that stated on the labels ranging from −13.4 to + 19.5%, with individual tablets ranging from 0.78 to 1.6 times the stated dose. While these figures, according to the authors, do indicate that, compared to earlier reports, the accuracy of selenium supplements has improved over recent years, they still give cause for concern. They point out that one popular multivitamin, labeled at 200 μg/tablet, contained selenium in excess of 300 μg and that many of its users could well exceed the 400 μg/day tolerable UL of intake.

10.6 Enhancing Selenium Content of Foods

As the growing use of selenium supplements shows, many people believe that an increase in intake of the element will have beneficial effects on their health. However, not everyone is willing to use dietary supplements, whether OTC or prescribed by a physician, to bring about an improvement in selenium status, not least because of possible toxic effects of "chemical" ingestion. They would prefer to do so in a more "natural" way by consuming foods that are enriched in selenium. Food producers are making considerable efforts to meet this consumer demand.

A relatively simple way to achieve an increase in selenium levels in food crops is, as has been seen, by adding selenium to fertilizers. This has been advocated by Rayman (1997) as a practical way of addressing the problem of falling selenium intakes in the UK. As has been commented by Arthur (2003), experience in Finland suggests that it is indeed a convenient and economical way of increasing dietary intake and can be implemented without introducing toxic levels of selenium in crops, animals fed on them, or in the human population. However, as Arthur has also noted, it is difficult to associate changes in selenium intake in Finland with any improvement in chronic disease or health. The UK Department of Health, through its Committee on Medical Aspects of Food Policy (COMA), made it clear in 1998 that legislation requiring the addition of selenium to fertilizers was unlikely to be introduced in the country. This was on the grounds that there was insufficient evidence that fortification of fertilizers with selenium would be of any practical benefit, either with respect to cancer prevention or in the promotion of a more general improvement in health (COMA, 1998). No other country has, as yet, followed Finland's legislative lead, though, as we have seen, the use of selenium-enriched fertilizers is permitted in New Zealand and selenium is legally added to animal rations and licks in the UK and other countries.

There is no doubt that selenium-enriched fertilizers can be used effectively to increase the selenium content of a variety of food crops, as has been demonstrated in numerous laboratory and field trials. The fertilizer can be applied in a number of different ways. Foliate application has been shown to increase the selenium content of rice by more than 30% compared to untreated grain (Chen et al., 2002). Selenium-containing fertilizers, applied either to roots or leaves, can increase levels in *Brassicae* vegetables, including Brussels sprouts (Stoewsand et al., 1989) and broccoli (Finley, 1999). High-selenium onions and garlic and a variety of other vegetables and other plants foods, such as mint and chamomile (Sekulovic et al., 1996) have also been produced by similar means. There is currently considerable interest in the possibility of developing selenium-accumulating cultivars of different food plants by the use of selective plants breeding techniques, as well as by genetic engineering (Reilly, 1998).

Even without the use of selenium-enriched fertilizers, crops with a higher than usual selenium content can be produced if they are grown on naturally seleniferous soils. We have already seen this in the case of wheat grown on seleniferous soils of North America (Rayman, 2000) and Australia (Lyons et al., 2003). In seleniferous regions of China a selenium-enriched tea is grown which is used to produce an elixir promoted as a natural dietary supplement (Anon, 1989). A variety of vegetables, such as broccoli and other *Brassicae*, onions and garlic, which are able to accumulate selenium to a higher than average level, especially from selenium-rich soils, are promoted as a safe means of increasing intake of the element (BNF, 2001).

Animal foodstuffs are also enriched with selenium. This is achieved by adding selenium supplements, both inorganic and organic, to their rations. These value-added products, according to a recent report, include selenium-enriched milk developed in Korea, the "Mega egg" which has added vitamin E as well as selenium (developed in Ireland), as well as selenium-enriched chicken and pork (Foley, 2005).

10.6.1 Selenium in Functional Foods

Selenium-enriched manufactured foods of several types have been developed and are promoted to consumers as a convenient way of increasing their selenium intake. These products are sometimes described as *nutraceuticals* or *functional foods*. They include foods that are normal items in the diet, but have been fortified with selenium, either in inorganic forms, such as sodium selenite, or organic forms, mainly selenium-enriched yeast. Several different types of selenium-fortified breakfast cereal have been produced, as well as table salt, margarine, sports drink, and other such products and are available for sale in some countries (Reilly, 1994). In the UK selenium-enriched bread is sold in supermarkets and is promoted with the claim that two slices will meet more than half the daily requirement for the element (Waitrose, 2005).

10.6.2 Chemical Forms of Selenium Used to Fortify Foods

There has been controversy with regard to the forms of selenium used to fortify bread and other foods. Those normally used by manufacturers range from inorganic compounds, such as sodium selenite, sodium hydrogenselenite, and sodium selenate, to organic forms which include selenoamino acids (selenomethionine and selenocysteine) as well as selenium-enriched yeast. These have all been in use in various countries for many years. However, a 2002 directive issued by the EU has excluded the use of organic forms, including selenium-enriched yeast, and allows only inorganic forms to be used as a supplement (Rayman, 2004). This decision is at least partly based on a fear that an increased intake of selenomethionine, could lead to its accumulation in body tissues to toxic levels.

10.6.2.1 Use of Selenomethione as a Food Fortificant

Selenomethionine has long been suspected of contributing to the toxic properties of seleniferous plants (Franke and Painter, 1938). It has been shown to be present in seleniferous wheat protein extracts. Selenomethionine can cause both acute and chronic toxicity when injected into or fed to animals. Unlike selenite or selenate, the amino acid is not used directly in the body for selenoprotein synthesis but is incorporated into body proteins. Thus it is stored in the organism and is reversibly released by normal metabolic processes (Schrauzer, 2003). It has been suggested by some investigators that this could pose a danger of toxicity if the stored amino acids were to be released during times of catabolism (Waschulewski and Sunde, 1968). Schrauzer (2000) and Rayman (2004) believe that there is no danger of this occurring and that, on the contrary, selenomethionine and selenium-enriched yeast are safe and suitable for use in food. Moreover, Schrauzer (2003) argues that selenomethionine not only represents the major nutritional source of selenium for humans but also has specific physiological functions not shared by other naturally occurring selenoamino acids, and hence it meets the criteria of an essential amino acid and could be considered to be the 23rd amino acid in protein synthesis (Schrauzer, 2004).

10.7 Dietary Reference Values for Selenium

Dietary recommendations for selenium have been the subject of considerable debate since they were first published in a number of countries in the 1980s and 1990s. There have been several reasons for this, particularly the difficulty encountered by expert committees in attempting to arrive at a definition of requirements based on the interpretation of biochemical markers of selenium status (Nève, 2000). Plasma GPX activity has generally been taken as the key measure of selenium status and it has been assumed that maximal activity of the enzyme is necessary for optimal health. The validity of this approach has been questioned by a number of nutritionists, including Combs (1994) who has pointed out that other measures, such as activities of different selenoproteins, might be more appropriately used for this purpose. Another complication has been the changing attitudes among experts in recent years, particularly towards the development of new concepts of "optimal" nutrition, complementary to "adequate" nutrition (Johnson, 1996). As a consequence there are uncertainties and a lack of uniformity between recommendations in different countries. In several of them, expert committees have already completed, or are currently undertaking reviews of dietary guidelines for selenium, among other nutrients. Recommendations that have been made have, in some cases, been controversial. In the USA, for instance, in spite of strong pressure from several leading nutritionists for an increase, the recommended dietary intake (RDA) was lowered in the year 2000 (Food and Nutrition Board, 2000).

The first country to publish an official recommended intake for selenium was Australia. In 1987 the Australian National Health and Medical Research Council (NHMRC) proposed an RDI of 80 μg for men and 70 μg for women (NHMRC, 1987). Two years later the US National Research Council proposed an RDA of 70 and 55 μg for men and women, respectively (National Research Council, 1989). In 1991 the UK's COMA published an RNI of 75 μg/day for men and 60 μg/day for women, with an LRNI of 40 μg/day for both male and female adults (Department of Health, 1991).

Several other national and international bodies have also made dietary recommendations for selenium. In 1996 the World Health Organization proposed a "normative" requirement (designed to provide an intake sufficient to maintain twothirds of maximal GPX activity and provide a desirable body store) of 40 and 30 μg/day to meet the needs of adult men and women, respectively (WHO, 1996). In the Nordic countries a population reference intake (PRI—equivalent to the RDA) of 60 and 30 μg/day for adult men and women, respectively, was published in 1992 (EEC Scientific Committee for Food, 1992). Some of these recommendations have been modified in subsequent reviews.

Differences between intake recommendations for different countries reflect, to a considerable extent, differences between expert committees in approaches and in interpretations of data. Nève (2000) has discussed the problems caused by such differences in a review that provides some insightful comments, especially with regard to the reasoning behind the decision of the US experts to reduce the adult RDA to 55 μg/day. In spite of criticism of the decision and the continuing pressure from many nutrition experts worldwide to increase rather than decrease recommendations for selenium intake, some other countries seem likely to follow the example of the USA. The proposed joint Australian and New Zealand nutrient reference values, for example, are for an RNI of 60 and 55 μg/day for adult males and females, respectively, which is lower than the current Australian values of 85 and 70 μg/day (Thomson, 2003).

The current UK and USA recommendations for dietary selenium intakes are summarized in Tables 10.4 and 10.5. These recommendations differ from those issued in some other countries in having a greater number of life-stage groups and also by including more than one category of DRI. Thus, the UK table includes a LRNI, which is the amount of selenium sufficient only for those with lower needs, while the US table gives a tolerable UL as the maximum level of daily intake unlikely to pose risks of adverse health effects to almost all individuals. Also in the US table recommendations for infants are given as AIs, which are based on observed or experimentally determined approximations, in the absence of sufficient scientific evidence with which to determine an RDA. The RNI in the UK table, and the RDA in the US table, are equivalent to each other and are the amounts of selenium that will meet the requirements of almost all (97 to 98%) healthy individuals in each group.

TABLE 10.4 UK dietary reference values (μg/day) for selenium

Age	Lower reference nutrient intake (LRNI)	Reference nutrient intake (RNI)
0–3 months	4	10
4–6 months	5	13
7–9 months	5	10
10–12 months	6	10
1–3 years	7	15
4–6 years	10	20
7–10 years	16	30
Men		
11–14 years	25	45
15–18 years	40	70
19–50 years	40	75
50 + years	40	75
Women		
11–14 years	25	45
15–18 years	40	60
19–50 years	40	60
50+ years	40	60
Lactation	+15	+15

Adapted from Department of Health, 1991, *Dietary Reference Values for Food Energy and Nutrients for the UK*, COMA, HMSO, London.

TABLE 10.5 US dietary reference intakes (μg/day) for selenium

Life-stage group	RDA/AI[a]	UL
Infants		
0–6 months	15[a]	45
7–12 months	20[a]	60
Children		
1–3 years	**20**	90
4–8 years	**30**	150
Males		
9–13 years	**40**	280
14–18 years	**55**	400
19–30 years	**55**	400
31–50 years	**55**	400
50–70 years	**55**	400
>70 years	**55**	400
Females		
9–13 years	**40**	280
14–18 years	**55**	400
19–30 years	**55**	400
31–50 years	**55**	400
50–70 years	**55**	400
>70 years	**55**	400
Pregnancy		
≤18 years	**60**	400
19–30 years	**60**	400
31–50 years	**60**	400
Lactation		
≤18 years	**70**	400
19–30 years	**70**	400
31–50 years	**70**	400

RDA: Recommended Dietary Allowances are shown in bold.
[a]Adequate Intakes (AIs) are shown in ordinary type.
Source: Adapted from: Food and Nutrition Board National Academy of Sciences (2002) *US Dietary Reference Intakes: Elements. http://www4.nationalacademies.org/10M/10Mhome.nst/pages/Food+and+Nutrition+Board.*

10.8 The Future—Is Supplementation the Way Forward?

Selenium continues to be a subject of very wide-ranging and intensive research, in many fields of investigation related to food and nutrition. To judge from the number of papers appearing in the scientific and medical literature, that interest seems likely to continue for many years. In spite of this concentration of interest by so many investigators, there remain many unanswered questions, not least about the potential implications of selenium supplementation of the diet.

In several countries, such as the UK, dietary intakes fall far short of official recommendations. Even in the USA and Canada, where intakes normally exceed the RDAs, it is argued by several leading experts in the nutrition field, that the health of many people would be improved by increasing selenium intakes well above recommended levels. If this advice is to be followed, how should this supplementation be carried out, improving health, while at the same time making sure not to expose consumers to risk of toxicity?

The authorities in Finland, as we have seen, did agree that that the health of the general community would benefit by increasing their intake of selenium. The method they adopted to achieve this increase was by the addition of the element to fertilizers. This has been shown to be an effective and economical way of increasing the selenium status of the general population. Whether it has had a direct beneficial effect on health has not yet been clearly established (Varo et al., 1994).

The UK authorities have been urged to follow the Finnish example because of evidence that selenium intakes in Britain do not meet recommended levels (Rayman, 1997). However, COMA experts concluded that such measures should not be encouraged in the absence of evidence of adverse effects of the UK's relative low selenium intake (COMA, 1998). Arthur (2003), in a discussion of whether or not selenium supplementation of the soil, as practiced in Finland, has the potential to be beneficial for the UK population, emphasizes the importance in general of maintaining AIs of the micronutrient. He notes that supplementation trials have shown that some people could indeed benefit from an increased intake. This increase would potentially improve the efficiency of biochemical pathways dependent on selenoproteins, with several possible effects, such as prevention of cancer, improvement in thyroid metabolism, and stimulation of immune function. However, he cautions, these potential beneficial effects need to be confirmed by further studies. The actual health benefits can only be predicted after extensive supplementation trials in which the effect of selenium can be separated from any other dietary and medical interventions taking place.

It is significant, in the light of the above comments, that, as has been noted by Combs (2001), the antitumorigenic effects of selenium observed in experimental carcinogenesis models have been associated with selenium intakes that are, in many trials 200 to 300 μg/day, up to tenfold levels required to prevent signs of selenium deficiency. They are also much greater than the dietary intake of most people worldwide and greater also than recommended intakes in the USA and other countries. It is true that such intakes are below the upper limit of 400 μg/day set by WHO and also the UK's recommended maximum safe intake of 450 μg/day. However, concern has been expressed about possible adverse outcomes of long-term use of such high selenium doses (Vinceti et al., 1998). A review by the US EPA has concluded that the NOAEL for an adult is 853 μg selenium/day (Poirier, 1994). The Agency's Reference Dose (RfD) of selenium for a 70 kg human is 350 μg/day, which is what an American adult, consuming as a normal diet, with an additional supplementary intake of 200 μg, might be expected to consume in a day (Schrauzer, 2000). A similar intake in the UK would require, on an average, consumption of a supplement of at least 300 μg/day.

A second point that should be taken into account when the use of selenium supplements is being considered is that there is evidence of individual variations in the way in which people respond to selenium intake (Hesketh and Villette, 2002). These differences appear to be due, at least in part, to single nucleotide polymorphisms (SNPs) in genes for selenium-containing proteins (Arthur, 2003). Their discovery has been made possible by the availability of human genome sequence data and the use of genomic technologies that allow the investigation of gene regulatory mechanisms that underlie phenotypic variations in individual responses to components of the diet. These studies are still at relatively early stages of development, but undoubtedly will, in combination with both molecular biology and human nutrition studies, help to clarify many of the still unanswered questions relating to selenium supplementation. It can be expected that, within probably the next decade, the use of such molecular approaches with gene-expression studies to address nutritional problems will transform our understanding of the role of selenium in human metabolism and health.

References

Alfthan, G. and Neve, J., 1996, Reference values for serum selenium in various areas—evaluated according to TRACY protocol, *J. Trace Elem. Med. Biol.* **10**, 77–87.

Amiard, J.-C., Berthet, H., and Boutaghou, S., 1993, Seasonal selenium variations in mussels and oysters from a French marine farm, *J. Food Comp. Anal.* **6**, 370–380.

Anon, 1989, Oral selenium solution for ageing-retardation and heart protection, *The People's Daily, Overseas Edition*, August 17, Beijing, Peoples' Republic of China.

Aras, N.K., Nazli, A., Zhang, W., and Chatt, A., 2001, Dietary intake of zinc and selenium in Turkey, *J. Radioanal. Nuc. Chem.* **249**, 33–37.

Aro, A. and Alfthan, G., 1998, Effects of selenium supplementation of fertilizers on human nutrition and selenium status, in: Frankenberger, W.G. and Engberg, R.A. (eds), *Environmental Chemistry of Selenium*, Dekker, New York, pp. 81–97.

Aro, A., Kumpulainen, A., Alfthan, G. et al., 1994, Factors affecting the selenium intake of people in Transbaikalian Russia, *Biol. Trace Elem. Res.* **40**, 277–285.

Arthur, J.R., 2003, Selenium supplementation: does soil supplementation help and why? *Proc. Nutr. Soc.* **62**, 1–5.

Beaglehole, R., Jackson, R., Watkinson, J. et al., 1990, Decreased blood selenium and the risk of myocardial infarction, *Int. J. Epidemiol.* **19**, 918–922.

Bieri, J.G. and Ahmed, K., 1976, Selenium in the Bangladesh diet, *J. Agric. Food Chem.* **34**, 1073–1079.

BNF, 2001, *Selenium and Health*, British Nutrition Foundation, London, p. 10.

Butcher, M.A., Judd, P.A., Caygill, C., et al., 1994, Current selenium content of foods and an estimate of average intakes in the United Kingdom, *Proc. Nutr. Soc.* **54**, 131A.

Casaril, M., Stanzial, A.M., Menini, C., et al., 1995, Serum selenium in a healthy population in the Venetian region: relation to age, sex, weight and population intake, *Eur. J. Med.* **3**, 35–39.

Casey, C.E., 1988, Selenophilia, *Proc. Nutr. Soc.* **47**, 55–62.

Chen, L.C., Yang, F.M., Xu, J., et al., 2002, Determination of selenium concentration of rice in China and the effect of fertilization of selenite and selenate on selenium content of rice, *J. Agric. Food Chem.* **50**, 5128–5130.

Clark, L.C., Combs, G.F., Jr., Turnbill, B.W., et al., 1996, Effects of selenium supplementation for cancer prevention in patients with carcinoma of the skin: a randomized controlled trial, *J. Am. Med. Assoc.* **276**, 1957–1963.

COMA, 1998, Statement from the Committee on Medical Aspects of Food and Nutrition Policy on Selenium. Food Safety Information Bulletin No. 93, Ministry of Agriculture, Fisheries and Food/Department of Health, London.

Combs, G.F., 2001, Selenium in global food systems, *Br. J. Nutr.* **85**, 517–547.

Combs, G.F., Jr., 1994, Essentiality and toxicity of selenium: a critique of the recommended dietary allowances and the reference dose, in: Mertz, W., Abernathy, C.O., and Olin, S.S. (eds), *Risk Assessment of Essential Elements*, ILSI, Washington, DC, pp. 167–183.

Combs, G.F., Jr. and Combs, S.B., 1986, The biological availability of selenium in foods and feeds, in: *The Role of Selenium in Nutrition*, Academic Press, New York, pp. 127–177.

Cross, J.D., Raie, R.M., Smith, H., and Smith, L.B., 1978, Dietary selenium in the Glasgow area, *Radioanalyt. Letts* **35**, 281–290.

Dang, H.S., Jaiswal, D.D., and Nair, S., 2001, Daily intake of trace elements of radiological and nutritional importance by the adult Indian population, *J. Radioanal. Nucl. Chem.* **249**, 95–101.

Darling, G., Mathias, P., O'Regan, M., and Naughten, E., 1992, Serum selenium levels in individuals on PKU diets, *J. Inher. Metabol. Dis.* **15**, 769–773.

Department of Health, 1991, Dietary Reference Values for Food Energy and Nutrients for the United Kingdom. Report on Health and Social Subjects, No. 41, London, HMSO.

Dhindsa, H.S., Bermingham, M.A., Mierzwa, J., and Sullivan, D., 1998, Plasma selenium concentrations in a Sikh population in Sydney, Australia, *Analyst* **123**, 885–887.

Dolamore, B.A., Brown, J., Barlow, B.A., et al., 1992, Selenium status of Christchurch infants and the effect of diet, *NZ Med. J.* **105**, 139–142.

Ducros, V., Faure, P., Ferry, M., et al., 1997, The sizes of the exchangeable pools of selenium in elderly women and their relation to institutionalization, *Br. J. Nutr.* **78**, 379–396.

Djujic, I.S., Jozanov-Stankov, O.N., Milovac, M., et al., 2000, Bioavailability and possible benefits of wheat intake enriched with selenium and its products, *Biol. Trace Elem. Res.* **77**, 273–285.

EEC Scientific Committee for Food, 1992, *Reference Nutrient Intakes for the European Community*. European Community, Brussels.

Ferrer, E., Alegria, A., Barbera, R., et al., 1999, Whole blood selenium content in pregnant women, *Sci. Tot. Environ.* **227**, 139–143.

Finley, J.W., 1999, The retention and distribution by healthy young men of stable isotopes of selenium consumed as selenite, selenate or hyrdoponically grown broccoli are dependent on the isotopic form, *J. Nutr.* **129**, 865–871.

Flatt, A., Pearce, N., Thomson, C.D., et al., 1990, Reduced selenium status in asthma subjects in New Zealand, *Thorax* **45**, 95–99.

Foley, A.M., 2005, Research news, *Technology Ireland*, 24 Sep. pp. 1–2, http://www.technologyireland.ie.

Food and Nutrition Board National Academy of Sciences, 2002, *US Dietary Reference Intakes: Elements*, http://www4.nationalacademies.org/10M/10Mhome.nst/pages/Food±and±Nutrition±Board.

Food and Nutrition Board, Institute of Medicine, 2000, *Dietary Reference Intakes for Vitamin C, Vitamin E, Selenium, and Carotenoids*, National Academy Press, Washington, DC, pp. 284–324.

Food and Nutrition Board, 1980, *Recommended Dietary Allowances*, 9th edn., National Academy of Sciences, Washington, DC, pp. 162–164.

Franke, K.W. and Painter, E.P., 1938, A study of the toxicity and selenium content of seleniferous diets: with statistical consideration, *Cereal Chem.* **15**, 1–24.

Froslie, A., 1993, Problems of selenium in animal nutrition, *Norwegian J. Agric. Sci.* **11**, 221.

Ge, K. and Yang, G., 1993, The epidemiology of selenium deficiency in the etiology of endemic diseases in China, *Am. J. Clin. Nutr.* **57**, 259S–263S.

Giessel-Nielsen, G., 1998, Effects of selenium supplementation on field crops, in: Frankenberger, W.T., Jr. and Engberg, R.A. (eds), *Environmental Chemistry of Selenium*, Dekker, New York, pp. 99–112.

Giessel-Nielsen, G., 1994, Effects of selenium supplementation of field crops, in: *Proceedings of STDA's 5th International Symposium*, Selenium–Tellurium Development Association, Grimbergen, Belgium, pp. 103–105.

Grandjean, P., Weihe, P., Jorgensen, P.J., et al., 1992, Impact of maternal seafood diet on fetal exposure to mercury, selenium and lead, *Arch. Environ. Health* **47**, 185–195.

Gregory, J., Lowe, S., Bates, C., et al., 2000, National Diet and Nutrition Survey: young people aged 4 to 18 years, Vol. 1: Findings, The Stationery Office, London.

Hansen, J.C., 2000, Dietary selenium intake among Greenlanders, *Bulletin of the Selenium-Tellurium Development Association*, October 2000, Selenium–Tellurium Development Association, Grimbergen, Belgium, pp. 1–4.

Hansen, J.C. and Pedersen, H.S., 1986, Environmental exposure to heavy metals in North Greenland, *Arctic Med. Res.* **41**, 21–34.

Hesketh, J.E. and Villette, S., 2002, Intracellular trafficking of micronutrients: from gene regulation to nutrient requirements, *Proc. Nutr. Soc.* **61**, 405–414.

Institute of Medicine, 2000, *Dietary Reference Intakes for Vitamin C, Vitamin E, Selenium, and Carotenoids*, National Academy Press, Washington, DC, pp. 310–311. http://www.nap.edu/books/0309069351/html/310.html.

Johnson, P.E., 1996, New approaches to establish mineral element requirements and recommendations: an introduction, *J. Nutr.* **126**, 2309S–2311S.

Kadrabova, J., Madaric, A., and Ginter, E., 1997, The selenium content of selected food from the Slovak Republic, *Food Chem.* **58**, 29–32.

Koljonen, T., 1975, The behavior of selenium in Finnish soils, *Ann. Agric. Fenn.* **41**, 240–247.

Korhola, M., Vainio, A., and Edelmann, K., 1986, Selenium yeast, *Ann. Clin. Res.* **18**, 65–68.

Korpela, H., Nuutinen, L.S., and Kumpulainen, J., 1989, Low serum selenium and glutathione peroxidase activity in patients receiving short-term total parenteral nutrition, *Int. J. Vit. Min. Res.* **59**, 80–84.

Larsson, C.L. and Johansson, G.K., 2002, Dietary intake and nutritional status of young vegans and omnivores in Sweden, *Am. J. Clin. Nutr.* **76**, 100–106.

Lightowler, H.J. and Davies, G.J., 2000, Micronutrient intakes in a group of UK vegans and the contribution of self-selected dietary supplements, *J. Roy. Soc. Protect. Health* **120**, 117–124.

Longnecker, M.P., Taylor, P.R., Levander, O.A., et al., 1991, Selenium in diet, blood, and toenails in relation to human health in a seleniferous area, *Am. J. Clin. Nutr.* **53**, 1288–1294.

Lyons, G., Stangoulis, J., and Graham, R., 2003, Nutriprevention of disease with high selenium wheat, *J. Aust. Coll. Nutr. Env. Med.* **22**, 3–9.

MacPherson, A., Barclay, M.N.I., Dixon, J., et al., 1993, Decline in dietary intake and effect on plasma concentrations, in: Anke, M., Meissner, D., and Mills, C.F. (eds), *Trace Elements in Man and Animals—TEMA8*, Verlag Media Touristik, Gersdorf, Germany, pp. 269–270.

MacPherson, A., Barclay, M.N.I., Scott, R., and Yates, R.W.S., 1997, Loss of Canadian wheat lowers selenium intake and status of the Scottish population, in: Fischer, P.W.F.,

L'Abbé, M.P., Cockrell, K.A., and Gibson, R.S. (eds), *Trace Elements in Man and Animals 9—TEMA 9*, NRC, Ottawa, pp. 203–205.
Margolin, S., 1980, Mercury in marine seafood: the scientific medical margin of safety as a guide to the potential risk to public health, *World Rev. Nutr. Diet.* **34**, 182–265.
McOrist, G.D. and Fardy, J.J., 1989, Selenium status in the blood of Australians using neutron activation analysis, *J. Radioanal. Nucl. Chem.* **134**, 65–72.
Matsuda, A., Kimura, M., and Itokawa, Y., 1997, Selenium level and glutathione peroxidase activity in plasma, erythrocytes and platelets of healthy Japanese volunteers, *J. Nutr. Sci. Vitaminol.* **43**, 497–504.
Maxia, V., Meloni, R., Rollier, M.A., et al., 1972, *I.A.E.A. Report SM-157/67*, International Atomic Energy Agency, Vienna.
Meissner, D., 1997, Reference values for blood and serum selenium in the Dresden area, *Medicine Klinische* **92**, Suppl. 3, 41–42.
Meltzer, H.M. and Huang, E., 1995, Oral intake of selenium and its effect on the serum concentrations of growth hormone-like growth factor-1, insulin-like growth factor-binding 1 and 3 in healthy women, *Eur. J. Biochem.* **33**, 411–415.
Ministry of Agriculture and Forestry, 1984, *Proposal for Addition of Selenium to Fertilizers. Working Group Report No. 7*, Helsinki (in Finnish), cited in Eurola, M., Ekholm, P., Koivistoinen, P., et al., 1989, Effects of selenium fertilization on the selenium content of selected Finnish fruits and vegetables, *Acta Agric. Scand.* **39**, 345–350.
Ministry of Agriculture, Fisheries and Food, 1997, Dietary intake of selenium, *Food Surveillance Information Sheet, No. 126*, Ministry of Agriculture, Fisheries and Food, London.
Ministry of Agriculture, Fisheries and Food, 1999, 1997 Total Diet Study—aluminum, arsenic, cadmium, chromium, copper, lead, mercury, nickel, selenium, tin, and zinc, *Food Surveillance Sheet, No. 191*, Ministry of Agriculture, Fisheries and Food, London.
Ministry of Agriculture, Fisheries and Food, 2000, Duplicate diet study of vegetarians—dietary exposure to 12 metals and other elements, *Food Surveillance Information Sheet* No. 193, Ministry of Agriculture, Fisheries and Food, London.
Murphy, J., Hannon, E.M., Kiely, M., et al., Selenium intakes in 18–64-year-old Irish adults, *Eur. J. Clin. Nutr.* **56**, 402–408.
Mussalo-Rauhamaa, H., Vuori, E., Lento, J.J., et al., 1993, Increase in serum selenium levels in Finnish children and young adults during 1980–1986: a correlation between the serum levels and the estimated uptake, *Eur. J. Clin. Nutr.* **47**, 711–717.
Mutanen, M. and Koivistoinen, P., 1983, The role of imported grain in the selenium intake of the Finnish population in 1941–1948, *Int. J. Vit. Min. Res.* **53**, 102–108.
National Center for Health Statistics, 2005, *Use of Dietary Supplements in the United States*, http://www.cdc.gov/nchs/products/pubs/pubd/sr11/pre-241/sr11–244.htm.
National Research Council, 1989, *Recommended Dietary Allowances*, 10th edn., National Academy Press, Washington, DC.
Nève, J., 1995, Assessing the biological activity of selenium supplements: interest of blood selenium and glutathione peroxidase, in: *Proceeding of the Selenium-Tellurium Development Association 5th International Symposium, Brussels, 8–10 May*, Selenium-Tellurium Development Association, Grimbergen, Belgium, pp. 123–130.
Nève, J., 2000, New approaches to assess selenium status and requirement, *Nutr. Revs* **58**, 363–369.
NHMRC, 1987, *Recommended Dietary Intakes for Use in Australia*, Australian Government Publishing Services, Canberra.

Ohi, G., Seki, N.H., Tamura, Y., et al., 1980, The protective potency of marine animal meat against the neurotoxicity of methylmercury: its relationship with the organ distribution of mercury and selenium in the rat, *Food Cosmet. Toxicol.* **18**, 139–145.

Oster, O. and Prellwitz, W., 1989, The daily dietary selenium intake of West German adults, *Biol. Trace Elem. Res.* **20**, 1–7.

Ozata, M., Salik, M., Aydin, A., et al., 1999, Iodine and zinc, but not selenium and copper, deficiency exists in a male Turkish population with endemic goitre, *Biol. Trace Elem. Res.* **69**, 211–216.

Pietinen, P., Vartiainen, E., Seppänen, R., et al., 1996, Changes in diet in Finland from 1972 to 1992: impact on coronary heart disease risk, *Prev. Med.* **25**, 243–250.

Poirier, K.A., 1994, Summary of the derivation of the reference dose for selenium, in: Mertz, W., Abernathathy, C.O., and Olin, S.S. (eds), *Risk Assessment for Essential Elements*, International Life Sciences Institute, Washington, DC, pp. 157–166.

Power, R., 1995, Selenium-enriched yeast: form and applications, in: *Proceedings of the Selenium-Tellurium Development Association 5th International Symposium*, Brussels, 8–10 May, Selenium–Tellurium Development Association, Grimbergen, Belgium, pp. 89–94.

Public Health Commission, 1993, *Our Health our Future: Honora Pakari, Koiora Roa.* The State of the Public Health in New Zealand, Public Health Commission, Wellington, New Zealand.

Rayman, M.P., 2004, The use of high-selenium yeast to raise selenium status: how does it measure up? *Br. J. Nutr.* **92**, 557–573.

Rayman, M., 1997, Dietary selenium: time to act, *Br. Med. J.* **314**, 387–388.

Reilly, C., 1994, Functional foods—a challenge for consumers, *Trends Food Sci. Technol.* **5**, 121–123.

Reilly, C., 1996, Selenium supplementation—the Finnish experiment, *BNF Nutr. Bull.* **21**, 167–173.

Reilly, C., 1997, Dietary selenium: a call for action, *BNF Nutr. Bull.* **22**, 85–87.

Reilly, C., 1998, Selenium: a new entrant into the functional food arena, *Trends Food Sci. Technol.* **9**, 114–118.

Salvini, S., Hennekens, C.H., Morris, J.S., et al., 1995, Plasma levels of the antioxidant selenium and risk of myocardial infarction among US physicians, *Am. J. Cardiol.* **76**, 1218–1221.

Schrauzer, G.N., 2000, Selenomethionine: a review of its nutritional significance, metabolism and toxicity, *J. Nutr.* **130**, 1653–1656.

Schrauzer, G.N., 2001, Nutritional selenium supplements: product types, quality, and safety, *J. Am. Coll. Nutr.* **20**, 1–4.

Schrauzer, G.N., 2003, The nutritional significance, metabolism and toxicology of selenomethionine, *Adv. Food Nutr. Res.* **47**, 73–112.

Schrauzer, G.N., 2004, Nutritional selenium supplements, in: *Book of Abstracts, 2nd International IUPAC symposium—Trace Elements in Food, Brussels, 7–8 October*, European Commission, Directorate General Joint Research Center, Brussels, p. 5.

Schrauzer, G.N. and McGinness, J.E., 1979, Observations on human selenium supplementation, *Trace Subst. Environ. Health* **13**, 64–67.

Schubert, A., Holden, J.M., and Wolf, W.R., 1987, Selenium content of a core group of foods based on a critical evaluation of published analytical data, *J. Am. Diet. Assoc.* **87**, 285–292.

Sekulovic, D., Maksimovic, S., Jakovljevic, M., et al., 1996, Application of Se-fertilizers in cultivated mint and chamomile production in order to improve their pharmacological properties, *J. Sci. Agric. Res.* **57**, 93–99.

Smith, A.M., Chang, M.P.H., and Medeiros, L.C., 2000, Generational differences in selenium status of women, *Biol. Trace Elem. Res.* **75**, 157–165.

Solvang, A. and Rimestad, A., 1985, Beregning av noen sporelementer i norsk kosthold, *Näringsforskning* **29**, 139–143.

Stoewsand, G.S., Andrews, J.L., Munson. L., and Lisk, D.J., 1989, Effect of dietary Brussels sprouts with increased selenium content on mammary carcinogenesis in the rat, *Cancer Lett.* **45**, 43–48.

Thomson, C.D., 1992, Is there a case for selenium supplementation in New Zealand, in: *Trace Elements: Roles, Risks and Remedies. Proceedings of the New Zealand Trace Elements Group Conference*, University of Otago, Dunedin, NZ.

Thomson, C.D., 2003, Proposed Australian and New Zealand nutrient reference values for selenium and iodine, *J. Nutr. Suppl.* **133**, 278E (Abstract).

Thomson, C.D. and Robinson, M., 1980, Selenium in human health and disease with emphasis on those aspects peculiar to New Zealand, *Am. J. Clin. Nutr.* **33**, 303–323.

Thomson, C.D. and Robinson, M.F., 1993, Long-term supplementation with selenate and selenomethionine: selenium and glutathione peroxidase (*EC* 1.11.1.9) in blood components of New Zealand women, *Br. J. Nutr.* **69**, 577–588.

Thomson, C.D. and Robinson, M.F., 1996, The changing status of New Zealand residents, *Eur. J. Clin. Nutr.* **50**, 107–114.

Thomson, J.N., Erdody, P., and Smith, D.C., 1975, Selenium in Canadian foods and diets, *J. Nutr.* **105**, 274–279.

Thorn, J., Robertson, J., Buss, D.H., and Bunton, N.G., 1978, Trace nutrients: selenium in British food, *Br. J. Nutr.* **39**, 391–396.

Thuluvath, P.J. and Triger, D.R., 1992, Selenium and chronic disease, *J. Haematol.* **14**, 176–182.

Tiran, B., Tiran, A., Petck, W., et al., 1992, Selenium status of healthy children and adults in Styria (Austria). Investigation of a possible undersupply in the Styrian population, *Trace Elem. Med.* **9**, 75–79.

Uden, P.C., Totoe Boakye, H., Kahakachchi, C., et al., 2003, Element selective characterization of stability and reactivity of selenium species in selenized yeast, *J. Anal. At. Spectrom.* **18**, 1–10.

Valentine J.L., Cebrian, M.E., Garcia-Vargas, G.G., et al., 1994, Daily selenium intake estimates for residents of arsenic endemic areas, *Environ. Res.* **64**, 1–9.

Vanderpas, J.B., Contrempre, B., Duale, N., 1993, Selenium deficiency mitigates hypothyroxinemia in iodine-deficient subjects, *Am. J. Clin. Nutr.* **57**, 271S–275S.

Van der Torre, H., van Dokkum, W., Schaafsma, G., Wendel, M., and Ockhuizen, T., 1991, Effects of various levels of selenium in wheat and meat on blood selenium status indices and on selenium balance in Dutch men, *Br. J. Nutr.* **65**, 69–80.

Varo, P., Alfthan, G., Huttunen, J.K., and Aro, A., 1994, Nationwide selenium supplementation in Finland—effects on diet, blood and tissue levels, and health, in: Burk, R.F. (ed.), *Selenium in Biology and Medicine*, Springer, New York, pp. 198–218.

Veatch, A.E., Brockman, J.D., Spate, V.L., 2005, Selenium and nutrition: the accuracy and variability of the selenium content in commercial supplements, *J. Radioanal. Nucl. Chem.* **264**, 33–38.

Vénzina, D., Mauffette, F., Roberets, K.D., and Bleau, B., 1996, Selenium-vitamin E, supplementation in infertile men. Effects on semen parameters and micronutrient levels and distribution, *Biol. Trace Elem. Res.* **53**, 65–83.

Vinceti, M., Rothman, K.J., Bergomi, M., et al., 1998, Commentary re: Vinceti et al., Excess melanoma incidence in a cohort exposed to high levels of environmental selenium, *Cancer Epidemiol. Biomark. Prevent.* **7**, 851–852.

Waitrose, K., 2005, *Knead to enrich a slice of your life*, http://www.waitrose.com/about/press-resources/pr-merchandise/201.asp.

Wang, W.C., Mäkelä, Nänto, V., et al., 1998, The serum concentrations in children and young adults: a long-term study during the Finnish fertilization programme, *Eur. J. Clin. Nutr.* **52**, 529–535.

Wang, Z.W., Li, I.Q., Liu, J.X., et al., 1987, The analysis of the development of Kashin-Beck disease in Hulin County, Heilongjiang Province, *Chin. J. Epidemiol.* **6**, 299–231 (in Chinese) cited in Ge and Yang (1993).

Waschulewski, I.H. and Sunde, R.A., 1968, Effect of dietary methionine of tissue selenium and glutathione peroxidase on tissue selenium and glutathione peroxidase (EC 1.11.1.9) activity given selenomethionine, *Br. J. Nutr.* **60**, 57–68.

Wasowicz, W., Gromadinska, J., Rydzynski, K., and Tomczak, J., 2003, Selenium status of low-selenium area residents: Polish experience, *Toxicol Lett.* **137**, 95–101.

Westermarck, T., 1977, Selenium content of tissues in Finnish infants and adults with various diseases, and studies on the effects of selenium supplementation in neuronal ceroid lipofuscinosis patients, *Acta Pharmacol. Toxicol.* **41**, 121–128.

Whanger, P.D., Xia, Y., and Thomson, C.D., 1994, Protein technics for selenium speciation in human body fluids, *J. Trace Elem. Electrolytes Health Dis.* **8**, 1–7.

Winterbourne, C.C., Saville, D.J., George, P.M., et al., 1992, Increase in selenium status of Christchurch adults associated with deregulation of the wheat market, *New Zealand Med. J.* **105**, 466–468.

WHO, 1996, Trace Elements in Human Nutrition and Health, Prepared in collaboration with the Food and Agricultural Organization of the United Nations and the Atomic Energy Agency, World Health Organization, Geneva.

Yang, G., Wang, S., Zhou, R., et al., 1989, Studies of safe maximal daily dietary Se intake in a seleniferous area of China. Part II: Relation between Se intake and the manifestation of clinical signs and certain biochemical alterations in blood and urine, *J. Trace Elem. Electrolytes Health Dis.* **3**, 123–130.

Yoshita, K., Tabata, M., Kimura, R., et al., 1998, Relationship between selenium intake and foods intake and nutrients intake in middle aged men, *Eiyogaku Zasshi* **56**, 19–148.

Zhang, Z.W., Shimbo, S., Qu, J.B., et al., 2001, Dietary selenium intake of Chinese adult women in the 1990s, *Biol. Trace Elem. Res.* **80**, 125–138.

Index

A
Acquired immunity, of body, *see* Adaptive immunity
Acquired immunodeficiency syndrome (AIDS), and selenium, 140–141
Acute phase proteins, 133
Adaptive immunity, of body, 133
Aflatoxin B1 (AFB1), 116
Ageing and selenium, 147–148
Age-related degenerative disorders of eye, and selenium
  AMD, 148–149
  cataract, 149
Age-related macular degeneration (AMD), selenium and, 148–149
Agriculture, selenium and, 65
AIDS, *see* Acquired immunodeficiency syndrome
Alkali disease and "blind staggers," 66–68
Allium family, selenium levels in, 165
Allotropic forms of selenium, 3–4
ALS, *see* Amyotrophic lateral sclerosis
AMD, *see* Age-related macular degeneration
American yeast
  Factor 2 in, 70
  Factor 3 in, 70
Aminoacrylyl-tRNA^{Sec}, 52
Amyotrophic lateral sclerosis (ALS), and high selenium intake, 87–88
Antidandruff shampoo, 9
Antitumorigenic metabolites, 120
Astragalus, 22, 67
Asymmetrical conductivity, of selenium, 4
Atomic absorption spectrophotometry, 12–13

B
Bacterial Sec insertion sequence (bSECIS), 52
Basophils, in immune system, 135
B cells, in immune system, 134
Bertholletia excelsa, 84, 166
Berzelius, predecessors of, 2–3
"Blind staggers," 3
Brain function and selenium, 150–151
Brazil nuts, 84–85
  selenium levels in other and, 166
Bread and flour, selenium levels in, 161–162
Breast milk, selenium levels in, 159–160
Broccoli *(Brassica oleracea),* selenium levels in, 165
Bursa of Fabricius, 134

C
Cadmium sulfide-selenide, 9
Cancer and selenium, 112; *see also* Cancer prevention
  case-control studies of, 113–114
  epidemiological studies of the relation between, 113
  intervention trials for
    Linxian intervention trials, 115–116
    NPC trial, 116–118
    PRECISE intervention trial, 118
    Qidong intervention trial, 116
    SELECT intervention trial, 118–119
    SU.VI.MAX trial, 119
  "nested" case-control studies in, 114–115
Cancer prevention
  evidence for association between selenium and, 119
    baseline selenium levels and dose size in trials of, 120
  selenium compounds role in, 120–123
Cardiomyopathy, selenium deficiency-related, 96
  other causes of, 110–111

Cardiovascular disease (CVD), and selenium, 123
epidemiological studies of CVD incidence, 124
prospective epidemiological studies of, 124–125
Case-control studies of selenium and cancer associations, 113–114
nested, 114–115
Cataract, age-related, selenium and, 149
Cell-mediated immunity, 134
Change hoof disease, 3
CHF, *see* Congestive heart failure
China
regional studies of KD in, 90–91
selenium intoxication in, 85–86
Chronic hypoxemia, 150
"Classical" GPX1, 44
Clausthalite (PbSe), 8
Clostridium barkeri, 50
Clostridium sticklandii, 20–21
Cocksackievirus, 139–140
Commonwealth Scientific and Industrial Research Organization (CSIRO), 77
Congestive heart failure (CHF), 152
Cot death, *see* Sudden infant death syndrome
Cow's milk, selenium levels in, 159
infant formulae based on, 160–161
C-reactive proteins, 133
Crib death, *see* Sudden infant death syndrome
Crops grown
on adequate-selenium soils, 26
on high-selenium soils, 26–27
on low-selenium soils, 25–26
CSIRO, *see* Commonwealth Scientific and Industrial Research Organization
CVD, *see* Cardiovascular disease
Cytosolic TR, 47

D

DAN, *see* 2,3-Diaminonaphthalene
Degenerative eye disorders, *see* Age-related degenerative disorders of eye, and selenium
Degnala disease, 67
Dental caries, and high selenium intake, 87
"Derbyshire neck ," 99
2,3-Diaminonaphthalene (DAN), 5, 12
Diet
PKU, 111–112
role of inadequate, in cardiomyopathy, 110–111
Dietary intakes of selenium, 171
changes in
effect of changes in wheat imports on selenium intakes, 179
in Finland, 176–178
in New Zealand, 179–180
in UK, 178
between countries and population groups, variation in, 173
in fish-eating populations, 175–176
by Sikh vegetarians, 175
by vegans and other vegetarians, 174
by young Swedish vegans, 174–175
in different countries, 172–173
Dietary reference values for selenium, 186–187
in UK, 187t
in US, 188t
Dietary selenium, for cancer prevention, 121–123
Dietary selenium supplements, to change selenium status, 180
selenium-enriched yeast, 181–182
selenomethionine in selenium yeast, 182
variations in levels of selenium in, 183
Dimethylselenide (DMSe), 24
Dipeptide γ-glutamyl-seleno-methyl-selenocysteine, 24
Drinking water, selenium levels in, 166–167
Dry ashing, 10–11
Dry photocopying, 9

E

ED, *see* Exudative diathesis
EF-Tu, elongation factor, 52
Endemic diseases related to selenium deficiency in humans, 88
Kashin-Bek disease (KBD), 96–97
etiology of, 97–98
Keshan disease (KD), 89
etiology of, 91–93
features of, 91
interventions in the management of, 94–96
regional studies of, in China, 90–91
in Russia, 96
Endemic selenium and iodine deficiencies, combined
role of selenium deficiency in endemic goiter, 99–102
selenium, KBD, goiter, 98–99
thyroid biochemistry and selenium, 102–103
Enshi County, selenium intoxication in, 85–86
Enteral nutrition (EN), 109
Enteroviruses, and KD, 92

Enzootic myopathies in cattle and sheep, role of selenium in treatment of, 71
Eosinophils, in immune system, 135
Esophageal cancer prevention, 115
Eukaryotes, selenoprotein synthesis in, 53
Extracellular GPX, 45
Exudative diathesis (ED), 73–74

F

Factor 2, in American yeast, 70
Farm animals, selenium-responsive conditions in
  exudative diathesis, 73–74
  hepatosis dietetica, 74
  ill thrift, 74–75
  impaired immune response, 75–77
  impaired reproduction, 75
  pancreatic degeneration, 74
  white muscle disease, 72–73
Farm animals, selenium toxicity in
  alkali disease and "blind staggers," 66–68
  selenosis in farm animals outside USA
    selenosis in Irish farms, 68–70
Fertilizers, selenium-enriched, 184
Finland, changes in selenium dietary intakes in, 176–178
Fish and other sea foods, selenium levels in, 163–164
Flame atomic emission spectrophotometry (FAES), 13
Flavine adenine dinucleotide (FAD), 47
Food composition databases, selenium in, 157–158
Fulminant syndrome, 73
Fulvic acid (FA), 97–98
Functional foods, selenium in, 185
Fusarium, 67
Fusarium tricinatum, 98

G

Glutathione peroxidase (GPX), 43, 58–59, 75–76, 101
Goiter
  role of selenium deficiency in endemic, 99–102
  selenium, KBD, and, 98–99
GPX, *see* Glutathione peroxidase
GPX4, 45–46, 56
  role in CVD, 123–124
GPX6, 46
GPX2 and GPX3, 45
GPX-like selenoproteins, 141

Graphite furnace or electrothermal AAS (GFAAS/ ETAAS), 13

H

HCC, *see* Hepatocellular carcinoma
HD, *see* Hepatosis dietetica
Hepatocellular carcinoma (HCC), 114, 116
Hepatosis dietetica (HD), 74
HGAAS, *see* Hydride generation atomic absorption spectrophotometry
High-resolution mass analyzer (HRMA), 14
Human fertility and selenium, 141–142
Human immunodeficiency virus (HIV), and selenium, 140–141
Human selenoprotein genes, 45
Humoral immunity, of body, 134
Hydride generation atomic absorption spectrophotometry (HGAAS), 12
Hyperaccumulators, 21
Hypothyroidism, 138, 151

I

Iatrogenic selenium deficiencies, 111–112
IDI enzyme, 102
Immune response
  impaired, 75–77
  role of selenium in, 135–136
    selenium and immune response to infection, 137–138
    selenium and inflammatory diseases, 138–139
Immune system
  components of, 132–135
  enhancement by selenium, 122
Immunoglobulins, 134, 135
Inductively coupled plasma atomic emission spectrophotometry, 13
Inductively coupled plasma mass spectrometry, 13–14
Infant formula, selenium levels in, 160–161
Infertility, due to selenium intoxication, 88
Inflammatory diseases and selenium, 138–139
Innate immunity, *see* Natural immunity
Inorganic compounds of selenium, 4–5
Inorganic forms of selenium supplements, 181
Instrumental neutron activation analysis (INAA), 14
Intervention trials for protective effects of selenium against cancer
  Linxian intervention trials, 115–116
  NPC trial, 116–118
  PRECISE intervention trial, 118

Intervention trials for protective effects of selenium against cancer (*Contd.*)
Qidong intervention trial, 116
SELECT intervention trial, 118–119
SU.VI.MAX trial, 119
Intracellular (or cytosolic) GPX (cGPX), 44
Iodine deficiency in humans
a caution: selenium supplementation and, 102–103
combination of selenium and, 98–103
Iodine supplementation, 103
Irish farms, selenosis in, 68
symptoms of extreme concentrations of selenium, 69–70
Isotopes of selenium, 6–7

K
Kashin-Beck disease (KBD), 96–97
etiology of, 97–98
selenium, goiter, and, 98–99
KBD, *see* Kashin-Beck disease
KD, *see* Keshan disease
Keshan and Kashin-Beck diseases, 26
Keshan disease (KD), 89
etiology of, 91–93
features of, 91
interventions in the management of, 94–96
regional studies of, in China, 90–91
in Russia, 96
Keshan disease areas, selenium status of residents in, 93–95
Kwashiorkor, 152

L
Lecythis elliptica, 84
Lecythis ollaria, 85
Linxian intervention trials, 115–116
Lipoprotein, low-density, (LDL), oxidation of, 123
Liver necrosis, 74
Locoweeds, 22
Lupinosis-associated myopathy (LAM), 73
Lymphocytes, 133–134

M
Major histocompatibility complex (MCH) molecules, 134
Marasmus, 151–152
Mast cells, in immune system, 135
Meat and meat products, selenium levels in, 163
Memory cells, in immune system, 134
Mercury, relation between selenium and, in sea foods, 164–165
Metallic selenides, 4
Metallic selenium, 4
Methylselenol, 122–123
Microwave-heated sealed polytetrafluoroethylene (PTFE) tubes, 11
Mitochondrion, 123
"Monkey coconut," 85
Motor neuron disease, *see* Amyotrophic lateral sclerosis
Multifocal myocardial necrosis (MMN), 91
Muscular problems and low selenium intake in New Zealand, 111
Mushrooms (*Agaricus spp.*) selenium levels in, 165
Myxedematous endemic cretinism, 100

N
Natural immunity, of immune system, 133
Neurological cretinism, 100
New Zealand, changes in selenium dietary intake in, 179–180
Nonendemic selenium deficiency in humans, 109–111
Nonmelanoma carcinoma, 116, 117
NPC trial, *see* Nutritional Prevention of Cancer trial
Nutraceuticals, *see* Functional foods, selenium in
Nutritional Prevention of Cancer (NPC) trial, for selenium against cancer, 116–118

O
Opsonization, 133
Organo-selenium compounds, 5–6
"Orphan selenoproteins," 49
Osteoarthropathy, 97
Oxygen bomb, 11

P
Pancreatic degeneration, 74
PEM, *see* Protein-energy malnutrition
Peridinium gatuense, 21
Peroxynitrite, 142
Phagocytes, 133
Phenylalanine, 111
Phenylketonuria (PKU), 111–112
Phomopsis leptostromiformis, 73
Phospholipid hydroperoxide GPX (PHGPx), 45
Physical properties, of selenium, 4
Phytolectin mitogens, 136–137

Phytoremedation, 25
Piazoselenol, 12
PKU, *see* Phenylketonuria
Placebo, for muscular problems, 111
Placebo-controlled intervention trial, 116–117
Polymorphonuclear neutrophil leucocytes (PMN), 133
Potassium ammonium sulfoselenide, 9
PRECISE trial, *see* Prevention of Cancer with Selenium in Europe and America trial
Preeclampsia and selenium, 142–143
Prevention of Cancer with Selenium in Europe and America (PRECISE) trial, 118
Primary indicator plants, 21
Prokaryotes
  biological role of selenium in, 20–21
  selenoprotein synthesis in, 51–52
Protein-energy malnutrition (PEM), 151
Pyrrolysine, 50–51

Q
Qidong intervention trial, 116
Quadripole mass analyser (PQ), 14

R
Reactive oxygen species (ROS)
  in ageing, 147
  by neutrophils, 137
Reproduction, defective, due to selenium intoxication, 88
Reticulo-endothelial system, 133
Rice, selenium levels in, 162–163
Rutin and silymarin, effect on ED, 74

S
Salicornia bigelovii (pickleweed), 25
Salt , fortification of domestic, with selenium, 116
SBP2, 55
Sea foods, relation between selenium and mercury in, 164–165
Seborrheic dermatitis, 9
Sec, 50–51
SelB, 52
SelC, 52
SelD, 52
SELECT, *see* Selenium and Vitamin E Cancer Prevention Trail
Selenates, 7, 23
Seleniferous soils, 69
Selenites, 122
Selenium; *see also specific* Selenium
  ageing and, 147–148
  age-related degenerative disorders of eye and
    age-related macular degeneration, 148–149
    cataract, 149
  agricultural and horticultural applications, 9
  agriculture and, 65
  allotropic forms of, 3–4
  brain function and, 150–151
  dietary reference values for, 186–188
  direct application of to agricultural land, 78
  discovery of, 2
    Predecessors of Berzelius, 3–4
  as essential nutritional factor, 70–71
  in functional foods, 185
  HIV, AIDS, and, 140–141
  human fertility and, 141–142
  and immune response to infection, 137–138
  industrial and other applications of, 8–9
  inflammatory diseases and, 138–139
  other health conditions and, 153
  in pharmaceutical industry, 9
  preeclampsia and, 142–143
  in prokaryotes, biological role of, 20–21
  in rice from KD-affected and non-affected countries, 94t
  role in treatment of enzootic myopathies in cattle and sheep, 71
  SIDS and, 149–150
  sources and production of, 8
  viral infections and, 139–141
  vitamin E and, 76–77
Selenium, metabolic roles of
  selenoproteins, 43
    glutathione peroxidases, 44–46
    iodothyronine deiodinases, 46–47
Selenium accumulators, 3
  and nonaccumulators in higher plants, 21–22
Selenium analysis
  end-determination methods for selenium analysis, 12
    atomic absorption spectrophotometry, 12–13
    inductively coupled plasma
      atomic emission spectrophotometry, 13
    inductively coupled plasma mass spectrometry, 13–14
    spectrofluorimetry, 12
  sample preparation
    dry ashing, 10–11
    wet ashing, 11
  speciation analysis, 14
    analytical quality control, 15–16

Selenium and cancer, 112; *see also* Cancer prevention
case-control studies of, 113–114
epidemiological studies of the relation between, 113
intervention trials for
Linxian intervention trials, 115–116
NPC trial, 116–118
PRECISE intervention trial, 118
Qidong intervention trial, 116
SELECT intervention trial, 118–119
SU.VI.MAX trial, 119
"nested" case-control studies in, 114–115
Selenium and cancer-prevention, evidence for association between, 119
baseline selenium levels and dose size in cancer prevention trials, 120
Selenium and cardiovascular disease (CVD), 123
epidemiological studies of CVD incidence, 124
prospective epidemiological studies of, 124–125
Selenium and Vitamin E Cancer Prevention Trail (SELECT), 118–119
Selenium assimilation and modification within plant tissues, 23–24
Selenium chemistry
allotropic forms of selenium, 3–4
inorganic compounds of selenium, 4–5
isotopes of selenium, 6–7
organo-selenium compounds, 5–6
physical properties of selenium, 4
Selenium compounds
carcinostatic properties of, 120–121
role in cancer prevention, 120–123
Selenium content of foods, enhancement of, 183–184
chemical forms of selenium used to fortify foods
use of selenomethione as a food fortificant, 185–186
selenium in functional foods, 185
Selenium deficiency-associated cardiomyopathies
other causes of, 110–111
Selenium deficiency(ies)
combination of iodine deficiency and, 98–103
in endemic goiter, role of, 99–102
and KBD, 97–98
subclinical, 77
TPN- induced, 109
and viral infection in KD, 91–92
Selenium deficiency-related cardiomyopathy, 96
Selenium dioxide, 5
Selenium-enriched fertilizers, 184
Selenium in animal tissues
absorption, transport, and excretion of selenium, 28–29
enteric absorption of selenium, 29
selenium distribution and retention in the human body, 30–31
selenium levels in blood
in other blood fractions, 33–34
in serum and plasma, 31–33
in whole blood, 31
selenium pools and stores in the body, 36
selenium retention and excretion from the body
fecal excretion of selenium, 35–36
losses of selenium in hair and nails, 36
pulmonary excretion of selenium, 36
urinary excretion of selenium, 34–35
transport of selenium in the body, 29–30
Selenium in diets
changes in dietary intakes of
effect of changes in wheat imports on selenium intakes, 179
in Finland, 176–178
in New Zealand, 179–180
in UK, 178
dietary intakes of, 171
in different countries, 172–173
dietary intakes of, between countries and population groups, variation in, 173
in fish-eating populations, 175–176
by Sikh vegetarians, 175
by vegans and other vegetarians, 174
by young Swedish vegans, 174–175
status of, 171
Selenium in food plants
crops grown on adequate-selenium soils, 26
crops grown on high-selenium soils, 26–27
crops grown on low-selenium soils, 25–26
risk of selenosis in humans from eating selenium-rich crops, 27–28
Selenium in lithosphere, distribution of
in soil, 7
in water, 7
Selenium in plants
selenium in food plants
crops grown on adequate-selenium soils, 26
crops grown on high-selenium soils, 26–27
crops grown on low-selenium soils, 25–26
risk of selenosis in humans from eating selenium-rich crops, 27–28
selenium in higher plants, 21

selenium accumulators and nonaccumulators, 22
selenium metabolism in plants, 22
selenium assimilation and modification within plant tissues, 23–24
selenium toxicity and tolerance in plants, 24–25
selenium uptake and transport in plants, 23
volatilization of selenium by plants, 25
Selenium intake, low, and muscular problems in New Zealand, 111
Selenium intakes, consequences of high levels of, 86
amyotrophic lateral sclerosis, 87–88
defective reproduction, 88
dental caries, 87
Selenium levels in blood
in other blood fractions, 33–34
in serum and plasma, 31–33
in whole blood, 31
Selenium levels in body organs, 31t
Selenium levels in food, 156
from different countries, 157t
food composition databases, 157
selenium in total diet studies, 158
in individual foodstuffs
in brazil and other nuts, 166
in bread and flour, 161–162
in cow's milk, 159
in drinking water, 166–167
in fish and other sea foods, 163–164
in human breast milk, 159–160
in infant formula, 160–161
in meat and meat products, 163
in other cereals, 162–163
selenium and mercury in sea foods, relation between, 164–165
in vegetables and fruits, 165
national and international databases of, 156–157
variations in levels of, 158
Selenium levels in serum or plasma of healthy adults in different countries, 172t
Selenium metabolism in plants, 22
selenium assimilation and modification within plant tissues, 23–24
selenium toxicity and tolerance in plants, 24–25
selenium uptake and transport in plants, 23
volatilization of selenium by plants, 25
Selenium oxychloride, 5
Selenium poisoning, *see* Selenosis
Selenium-responsive conditions in farm animals
ED, 73–74
WMD, 72–73
Selenium retention and excretion from body
fecal excretion of selenium, 35–36
losses of selenium in hair and nails, 36
pulmonary excretion of selenium, 36
urinary excretion of selenium, 34–35
Selenium-rich crops, risk of selenosis in humans from eating, 27–28
Selenium ruby glass, 9
Selenium status
assessment of, 57
hair, nail, and urinary selenium, 58–59
other potential markers of selenium functional status, 60–61
use of blood selenium levels for, 58
use of functional indicators of selenium status, 59–60
Selenium supplementation
a caution: iodine deficiency and, 102–103
future aspects of, 188–190
of livestock, 77–78
for pancreatitis, 139
for patients with mood and behavior problems, 151
for rheumatoid arthritis, 138–139
Selenium supplements, variations in levels of selenium in, 183
Selenium toxicity and tolerance in plants, 24–25
Selenium toxicity in farm animals
alkali disease and "blind staggers," 66–68
selenosis in farm animals outside USA
selenosis in Irish farms, 68–70
Selenium toxicity in humans, 83
in China, 85–86
consequences of, 86
amyotrophic lateral sclerosis, 87–88
defective reproduction, 88
dental caries, 87
in Latin America, 84–85
in seleniferous regions of North America, 83–84
Selenium trioxide, 5
Selenium uptake and transport in plants, 23
Selenium yeast, 181
selenomethionine in, 182
Selenocystathionine, 24
Selenocysteine, 23, 28, 50
dual function of UGA codon, 51
Selenoenzymes, 21, 47, 102
in CVD, 123
Selenols, 5–6
Selenomethione, as a food fortificant, 185–186

Selenomethionine, 24, 28
in selenium yeast, 182
Selenophobia, 84
Selenoproteins, 43, 44
glutathione peroxidases, 44–46
iodothyronine deiodinases, 46–47
other selenoproteins, 49–50
selenophosphate synthetase, 48
selenoprotein P, 48–49
thioredoxin reductases, 47–48
Selenoprotein expression, regulation of, 53–54
complexities of regulation of selenoprotein synthesis, 55
regulatory role for tRNA$^{[SER] SEC}$ in selenoprotein synthesis, 56
single nucleotide polymorphisms and regulation of selenoprotein synthesis, 57
Selenoprotein P (Se-P), 48–49
15 kDa Selenoprotein (Sel15), 49
Selenoprotein synthesis
in eukaryotes, 53, 54f
in prokaryotes, 51–52
selenocysteine: the 21st amino acid, 50
dual function of UGA codon, 51
Selenoprotein W (Se-W), 49–50
Selenosis; *see also* Selenium toxicity in humans
endemic, in China, 85–86
human, in Latin America, 84–85
Selenosis in farm animals outside USA
in Irish farms, 68
symptoms of extreme concentrations of selenium, 69–70
Selenosugars, 35
Se-P, *see* Selenoprotein P
Se-W, *see* Selenoprotein W
Sheep red blood cells (SRBC), 136
SIDS, *see* Sudden infant death syndrome
Sodium selenate, 9
Sodium selenite tablets, 95–96
Soil, selenium in, 7
Spectrofluorimetry, 12
"Stiff lamb disease," 72
Sudden infant death syndrome (SIDS), 89
and selenium, 149–150
Supplementation en Vitamines et Mineraux AntioXydants (SU.VI.MAX) trial, 119
SU.VI.MAX trial, *see* Supplementation en Vitamines et Mineraux AntioXydants trial

T
T cell receptors (TCR), 134
T cells, in immune system, 135
Thiobarbituric reactive substances (TBARS), 147
Thioredoxin reductase 1 (TR1), 47
Thyroid biochemistry and selenium, 102–103
Thyroid hormone metabolism, 102
Thyroid stimulating hormone (TSH), 101–103
Thyrotrophin, 101
Tinea versicolor, 9
α-Tocopherol (vitamin E), 70–71
Toenail selenium, and coronary heart disease, 125
Total diet study (TDS), of selenium, 158
Total parenteral nutrition (TPN)- induced selenium deficiency, 109
Toxic liver dystrophy, 74
TPN-related KD-like cardiomyopathies, 110
TR, *see* Thioredoxin reductase 1
Trace elements, analytical techniques for, 12
Transcriptomics, 60
Trimethylselenonium (TMSe), 35
TR/Trx system, 47–48

U
UGA codon, 51
Urov disease, *see* Kashin-Bek disease

V
Vegetables and fruits, selenium levels in, 165
Viral infections
and selenium, 139–141
and selenium deficiency, in KD, 91–92
Vitamin and mineral supplements on chronic disease risk, effect of, 119
Volatilization of selenium by plants, 25

W
Water, selenium in, 7
Wells rating scale, 26
Wet ashing, 11
Whale skin, selenium levels in, 164
Wheat imports, effect of changes in, on selenium intakes, 179
White muscle disease (WMD), 72–73
WMD, *see* White muscle disease

X
Xerography, 9

Y
Yeast, selenium-enriched, 181
selenomethionine in, 182